A
Clinical
REPERTORY

to the

Dictionary of Materia Medica

TOGETHER WITH REPERTORIE OF

- *Causation* • *Temperaments*
- *Clinical Relationships* • *Natural Relationships*

John Henry Clarke, M.D.

B. Jain Publishers (P) Ltd.

An ISO 9001 : 2000 Certified Company
USA — EUROPE — INDIA

A Clinical **REPERTORY**
to the **Dictionary of Materia Medica**

Edition: 2007

Published in India by
Kuldeep Jain
for

B. Jain Publishers (P) Ltd.
An ISO 9001 : 2000 Certified Company
1921, Street No. 10, Chuna Mandi,
Paharganj, New Delhi 110 055 (INDIA)
Phones: 91-11-2358 0800, 2358 1100, 2358 1300
Fax: 91-11-2358 0471; *Email:* bjain@vsnl.com
Website: www.bjainbooks.com

Printed in India by
J.J. Offset Printers
522, FIE, Patpar Ganj, Delhi - 110 092
Phones: 91-11-2216 9633, 2215 6128

ISBN: 81-7021-066-6
BOOK CODE: BC-2161

To The Memory of

ROBERT THOMAS COOPER,
M.A., M.D. (T.C.D.)

This volume is inscribed in undying
affection and admiration by his friend

THE AUTHOR

Publisher's Note

This new edition has been upgraded in the following ways:
- Improved and more readable font has been introduced with increased font size.
- Modern book designing has been used which markes the book user-friendly.
- The printing, paper and binding are of best quality.

We hope all the above changes will make this new edition a pleasure to read.

Kuldeep Jain
CEO, B. Jain Publishers

Preface

I must ask my readers to do me the favour to give particular attention to the prefaces to this work—not only to this, the general preface, but also to the introductory notes to each separate division; for, though the uses of each division are fairly obvious, and the arrangements simple, the REPERTORY is capable of subserving other uses besides the obvious ones, and these I shall endeavour to point out. That prince of Repertory-makers, Von Boenninghausen, described his well-known *"Pocket Book"* as being intended for use at the beside *"and in the study of the materia medica."* I may in the same way describe my REPERTORY as being designed "for use in the study of the materia medica" no less than as an instrument for finding out the indicated remedies. Homoeopathic practice consists in knowledge of materia medica and knowledge how to use it. This demands unlimited patience and application in the study of drug comparisons. My REPERTORY will enable the practitioner to compare any remedy with any similar remedy in five different points, all of great importance in practice.

In my *Dictionary of Practical Materia Medica* every remedy is described from a number of different points of view. The clinical point of view is one of these, and under the heading "CLINICAL" I have prefixed to each remedy a list of the affections in which it has been found most frequently indicated in practice. In compiling these clinical lists I had in view the project of preparing, later on, an Index of these headings to enable the reader to find at a glance all the remedies which have been accredited with the cure or alleviation of any given state. The CLINICAL REPERTORY herewith presented constitutes this Index.

Whilst the preparation of this work was in progress it occurred to me that it would greatly extend the usefulness of the CLINICAL REPERTORY if I were to add one or two other indices at the same time.

One of the sections under which I have described remedies in the *Dictionary* is headed "CAUSATION." This tells how remedies are related to conditions due to definite *Causes*. I have therefore added an alphabetical list of CAUSES, under any one of which will be found named all the drugs which have been observed to be curative in conditions produced by it.

Another index deals with TEMPERAMENTS. Acute observers, from the time of Hahnemann onwards, have noticed that some remedies act well on some types of persons and not at all so well on others. The respective types of *Nux vomica* and *Pulsatilla* are well known; but many other remedies have preferences more or less well marked for particular temperaments. These are mentioned in the *Dictionary* under the heading "CHARACTERISTICS" as the types of constitutions the particular remedy is specially "suited to." In the second and third volumes I have put the words "suited to" in italics so that they may be more easily found. In the *Repertory of Temperaments* they will all be found completely indexed. This, I think, is of no little importance, since type of constitution is very often a determining factor in the choice of a remedy. There are some patients whose constitutions correspond so accurately to a particular medicinal type, that the corresponding remedy will cure almost any indisposition they may happen to have. But under "SUITED TO" are included not temperaments, persons, and constitutions only, but also *complaints* occurring in persons of particular age and type; so that this section becomes in a way a complement of the *Clinical Repertory*—the first and most important division of this work. The user of the *Repertory*, therefore, who may not find the remedy he is in search of in the *Clinical Repertory*, may possibly find it in the Repertory of Temperaments under the heading of the complaint the patient is suffering from.

The last of the repertories included in this volume is a REPERTORY OF RELATIONSHIPS. This is twofold, and includes Clinical Relationships and Natural Relationships. The *Repertory of Natural Relationships* shows at a glance the place in nature of any remedy in question—mineral, vegetable, or animal—and how it stands in regard to its closest congeners. For instance, if a reader wishes to find the nearest botanical relations of any plant remedy he will be able to find them without difficulty. In the *Dictionary* is given the natural order of each plant. In the Repertory will be found an alphabetical list of all the natural orders represented, and under each is given in alphabetical order a list of all the plants of that order included in the materia medica.

But there is also given a list of the natural orders in their systematic or evolutionary order; so that every order is here given in juxtaposition with its allied orders. In this list I have prefixed a number to each order; and in the alphabetical list I have given each order the same number. Thus on consulting the alphabetical list, not only will all the individual members of that order be found there, but the number attached to the order will enable the reader to refer to the numerical list and find in that the orders most nearly allied to it. On reference to these orders in the alphabetical list, all the members of each will be found.

This is often to importance, since there is a strong therapeutic likeness between members of the same botanical group. The chief function of homoeopathy, it is true, is to individualise. This must be effected with the greatest possible completeness. But when once this has been done—and to effect this was one of the main objects I kept before me in compiling my *Dictionary*—grouping can be of the utmost value in the study and use of the materia medica. The mistake some first, and thinking that this might prove a short-cut to learning the materia medica. It is nothing of the kind: it merely results in muddling the materia medica unless each individual remedy has been first of all depicted in full detail.

When this indidualising of remedies has been mastered, the grouping becomes of great importance in practice. Of this both Dr. Burnett and Dr. Cooper made the most brilliant use. I need only instance the working out of the Lobelias by Dr. Burnett.

Those who wish to follow up the successes of these great therapeutists will have a light to guide them in my *Repertory of Natural Relationships.*

But, quite independently of all known natural relationships—I say "known relationships" because there is nothing in nature really unreleated to anything else—medicines are inter-related in various ways in point of therapeutic action. A knowledge of these relations is all-important to thse who aim at accurate prescribing. Take the antidotal relation, for example. It is often as important to be able to arrest a medicinal action as it is to start it. A prescriber who cannot antidote a drug effect is like a driver of a motor who cannot put on the brake. Hahnemann was always careful to observe and record the antidotes to the remedies he proved, and later observers have largely added to his observations. Some remedies have been observed to prepare the way for other remedies; some to follow others well. Such remedies are termed compatibles. Some spoil the effects of others, and such are called incompatibles. When a remedy has done good and has ceased to be indicated, the choice of the remedy to follow will be greatly assisted by a knowledge of CLNICAL RELATIONSHIPS. I have therefore given a tabulated list of all the remedies in the materia medica with their antidotes and other related remedies. In compiling this table I have made use of the excellent table published by Dr. Gibson Miller in the *Homoeopathic World* of September, 1902. It will be noticed that many of the remedies have no related remedies placed to their credit. This does not mean that such do not exist, but only that they have not been observed and recorded. I have not on that account omitted them from the list, and the vacant spaces will serve the purpose of providing a place of their entry whenever they may be found.

It will therefore be seen the CLINICAL REPERTORY is a clinical repertory and much more besides. The practitioner who consults it will not be tied down to a mere list of names of diseaes : he will be able to test his choice of a remedy from other points of view, and if further information should be required, the *Dictionary of Materia Medica,* which this REPERTORY is designed to make more accessible, will supply it.

A necessary preliminary to the compilation of work of this nature was to fix the abbreviation which should always represent each remedy named. In making choice of these abbreviations I have followed largely those selected by the compilers of the *Cypher Repertory.* The chief object aimed at in the selection has been to choose a combination of letters which shall at once suggest the remedy and not suggest any other remedy. This, as a matter of course, is an ideal which cannot always be attained, but to make identification as easy as possible I have given two lists— first a list of remedies in alphabetical order with the abbreviations appended to each, and next a list of abbreviations in alphabetical order with the remedy it stands for appended. It will be observed that I have followd the *Cypher Repertory* in using the letter "x." to signify "acid" ; "Nt. x." is "nitric acid"; "Fl. x." "fluoric acid," &c. Every time a medicine is mentioned it begins with a capital letter. When a name has two parts the second part always begins with a small letter. Thus, in the text, it will be impossible to mistake where the name of one remedy ends and the other begins.

It will be gathered from the above that the CLINICAL REPERTORY is intended to serve a purpose of its own. It is given to the world as complete in itself within the range of its aims. A *Symptom-Repertory* to the *Dictionary* is a very different matter and a much larger undertaking. But I do not despair of seeing that work accomplished one day. Some little progress has, in fact, already been made towards the carrying out of this project.

John Henery Clarke
8, Bolton Street, Piccadilly,
London, W.
September 14, 1904.

Contents

List of Remedies with

ABBREVIATIONS

Abies canadensis	Ab. c.	Agaricus phalloides	Ag. p.
Abies nigra	Ab. n.	Agave americana	Agv.
Abrotanum	Abt.	Agnus castus	Agn.
Absinthium	Abs.	Agraphis nutans	Agr. n.
Acalypha indica	Acal.	Agrostemma githago	Ags.
Acetanilidum	Antf.	Ailanthus glandulosa	Ail.
(*see* Anti-fibrinum)		Aletris farinose	Alet.
Aceticum acidum	Ac. x.	Allium cepa	Cep.
Aconitinum	Acn.	Allium sativum	All.
Aconitum cammarum	Ac. c.	Alnus	Alns.
Aconitum ferox	Ac. f.	Aloe socotrina	Alo.
Aconitum lycoctonum	Ac. l.	Alstonia constricta	Als.
Aconitum napellus	Aco.	Alumen	Aln.
Actaea racemosa	Act. r.	Alumina	Alm.
Actaea spicata	Act. s.	Ambra grisea	Amb.
Adonis vernalis	Ado.	Ambrosia artemisiaefolia	Abrs.
Adrenalin	Adr.	Ammoniacum	Amc.
Aesculus glabra	Aes. g.	Ammonium aceticum	Am.ac.
Aesculus hippocastanum	Aesc.	Ammonium benzoicum	Am.bz.
Aethiops antimonialis	Aeps.	Ammonium bromatum	Am. br.
Aethusa cynapium	Aeth.	Ammonium carbonicum	Am. c.
Agaricus emeticus	Ag. e.	Ammonium causticum	Amm.
Agaricus muscarius	Aga.	Ammonium muriaticum	Am. m.

Ammonium phosphoricum	Am. p.	Apis	Aps.
Ammonium picricum	Am. pi.	Apium graveolens	Api. g.
Ampelopsis	Ampl.	Apocynum	Ap. a.
Amphisbaena	Amph.	androsaemifolium	
Amygdalae amarae aqua	Amg.	Apocynum cannabinum	Apo.
Amylenum nitrosum	Aml.	Apomorphinum	Apm.
Anacardium occidentale	An. oc.	Aqua marina	Aq. m.
Anacardium orientale	Ana.	Aquilegia vulgaris	Aqui.
Anagallis arvensis	Anag.	Aralia racemosa	Aral.
Anantherum muriaticum	Anan.	Aranea diadema	Aran.
Ancistrodon contortrix	Cen.	Aranea scinencia	Ar. sc.
(see Cenchris contortrix)		Aranearum tela	Ara. t.
Angophora	Ago.	Arbutus andrachne	Arb.
Angustura spuria	Bru.	Arctium lappa	Ar. lp.
(see Brucea antidysenterica)		Areca	Arec.
Angustura Vera	Ang.	Argentum cyanatum	Ag. cy.
Anhalonium lewinii	Anh.	Argentum iodatum	Ag. i.
Anilinum	Anil.	Argentum metallicum	Arg.
Anisum stellatum	Ill.	Argentum nitricum	Ag. n.
(see Illicium)		Aristolochia milhomens	Ari.
Anthemis nobilis	Anth. n.	Aristolochia serpentaria	Ari. s.
Anthoxanthum	Antho.	Armoracia sativa	Arm.
Anthracinum	Athra.	Arnica	Arn.
Anthrokokali	Ank.	Arsenicum album	Ars.
Antifebrinum	Antf.	Arsenicum bromatum	As. br.
Antimonium arsenicicum	Ant. a.	Arsenicum hydrogenisatum	As. h.
Antimonium crudum	Ant. c.	Arsenicum iodatum	As. i.
Antimonium iodatum	Ant. i.	Arsenicum metallicum	As. mt.
Antimonium muriaticum	Ant. m.	Arsenicum stibiatum	Ant. a.
Antimonium	Ant. s. a.	(see Antimonium ars.)	
sulphuratum aureum		Arsenicum	As. f.
Antimonium tartaricum	Ant. t.	sulphuratum flavum	
Antipyrinum	Atp.	Arsenicum	As. r.
Aphis chenopodii glauci	Aph.	sulphuratum rubrum	

Artemisia abrotanum	Abr.	Aurum sulphuratum	Au. s.
(see Abrotanum)		Avena sativa	Avn.
Artemisia absinthium	Abs.	Aviaire	Avi.
(see Absinthium)		Azadirachta indica	Az.
Artemisia contra and Judaica	Cin.		
(see Cina)		Bacillinum	Bac.
Artemisia vulgaris	Art. v.	Bacillinum testium	Bac. t.
Arum dracontium	Ar. dm.	Badiaga	Bad.
Arum dracunculus	Ar. ds.	Balsamum peruvianum	Bal.
Arum italicum	Ar. it.	Baptisia confusea acetica	Bap. c.
Arum maculatum	Ar. m.	Baptisia tinctoria	Bap.
Arum triphyllum	Ar. t.	Barosma	Baro.
Arundo mauritanica	Ard.	Baryta acetica	Ba. ac.
Asafoetida	Asa.	(see Baryta carbonica)	
Asarum europaeum	Asr.	Baryta carbonica	Ba. c.
Asclepias syriaca	Asc. s.	Baryta iodata	Ba. i.
Asclepias tuberose	Asc. t.	Baryta muriatica	Ba. m.
Asimina triloba	Asi.	Belladonna	Bel.
Asparagus	Asp.	Bellis perennis	Bls.
Astacus fluviatilis	Ast. f.	Benzinum	Bnz.
Asterias rubens	Ast. r.	Benzinum dinitricum	Bz. d.
Astragalus menziesii	Astg.	Benzinum nitricum	Bz. n.
Athamanta	Ath.	Benzoicum acidum	Bz. x.
Atropinum	Atr.	Benzoin	Bzn.
Aurantium	Arnt.	Berberis aquifolium	Ber. a.
Aurum arsenicicum	Au. ar.	Berberis vulgaris	Ber.
Aurum bromatum	Au. br.	Bismuthum	Bis.
Aurum iodatum	Au.i.	Blatta americana	Bl. a.
Aurum metallicum	Aur.	Blatta orientalis	Bl. o.
Aurum muriaticum	Au. m.	Boletus laricis	Bo. la.
Aurum muriaticum kalinatum	Au. m. k.	Boletus luridus	Bo. lu.
		Boletus satanas	Bo. s.
Aurum muriaticum natronatum	Au. m. n.	Bombyx processionea	Bom.
		Boracicum acidum	Brc. x.

Borax	Bor.	Calcarea phosphorica	Ca. p.
Bothrops lanceolatus	Bth.	Calcarea picrica	Ca. pi.
Bovista	Bov.	Calcarea renalis	Ca. ren.
Brachyglottis repens	Brac.	Calcarea silicica	Ca. si.
Brassica napus	Brs.	Calcarea silico-fluorica	Lp.a.
Bromium	Bro.	(see Lapis albus)	
Brucea antidysenterica	Bru.	Calcarea sulphurica	Ca. s.
Brucinum	Brcn.	Calendula	Caln.
Bryonia	Bry.	Calotropis	Cltr.
Buchu (see Barosma)	Baro.	Caltha palustris	Clt.
Bufo	Buf.	Camphora	Cam.
Bursa pastoris	Thl.	Camphora bromata	Cm. br.
(see Thlaspi bursa pastoris)		Cancer fluviatilis	Ast. f.
		(see Astacus fluviatilis)	
Cactus grandiflorus	Cac.	Canchalagua	Cnu.
Cadmium bromatum	Cd. br.	Cannabis indica	Cn. i.
Cadmium sulphuratum	Cd. s.	Cannabis sativa	Can. s.
Cainca	Cai.	Cantharis	Cth.
Cajuputum	Caj.	Capsicum	Cap.
Calabar	Phst.	Carbo animalis	Cb. a.
(see Physostigma)		Carbo vegetabilis	Cb. v.
Caladium	Cld.	Carbolicum acidum	Cbl. x.
Calcarea acetica	Ca. ac.	Carboneum	Cbn.
Calcarea arsenicosa	Ca. ar.	Carboneum hydrogenisatum	Crb. h.
Calcarea bromata	Ca. br.	Carboneum oxygenisatum	Crb. o.
Calcarea carbonica	Calc.	Carboneum sulphuratum	Crb. s.
Calcarea caustica	Ca. cs.	Carduus benedictus	Crd. b.
Calcarea chlorinata	Ca. chl.	Carduus marianus	Crd. m.
Calcarea fluorata	Ca. fl.	Carlsbad	Carl.
Calcarea hypophosphorosa	Ca. hp.	Carya alba	Cry. a.
Calcarea iodata	Ca. i.	Cascara sagrada	Cas. s.
Calcarea muriatica	Ca. m.	Cascarilla	Csc.
Calcarea ovi testae	Ca. o. t.	Castanea vesca	Cst. v.
Calcarea oxalica	Ca. ox.	Castor equi	Ct. eq.

Castoreum	Cast.	Chromicum acidum	Chr. x.
Caulophyllum	Caul.	Chromium oxydatum	Chr. o.
Causticum	Caus.	Chrysophanicum acidum	Chs. x.
Ceanothus americanus	Cean.	Cichorium	Cich.
Cedron	Ced.	Cicuta maculata	Cic. m.
Cenchris contortrix	Cen.	Cicuta virosa	Cic. v.
Centraurea tagana	Cnt.	Cimex	Cim.
Cepa (Allium cepa)	Cep.	Cina	Cin.
Cereus bonplandii	Ce. b.	Cinchoninum sulphuricum	Chn. s.
Cereus serpentinus	Ce. s.	Cineraria maritima	Cin. m.
Cerium oxalicum	Cer. o.	Cinnabaris	Cnb.
Cervus	Crv.	Cinnamomum	Cinm.
Cetraria islandica	Cet.	Cistus canadensis	Cis.
Chamomilla	Cham.	Citrus limonum	Cit.
Chaparro amargoso	Chp.	Citrus vulgaris	Arnt.
Cheiranthus cheiri	Chei.	(see Aurantium)	
Chelidonium	Chel.	Clematis erecta	Clem.
Chelone	Chne.	Cobaltum	Cob.
Chenopodium anthelminticum	Chn. a.	Coca	Coca
		Coccinella septempunctata	Ccn. s.
Chenopodium vulvaria	Chn. v.	Cocculus indicus	Coc. i.
Chimaphila maculata	Chm. m.	Coccus cacti	Ccs. c.
Chimaphila umbellata	Chm. u	Cochlearia armoracia	Arm.
China boliviana	Chi. b.	(see Armoracia sativa)	
China officinalis	Chi.	Codeinum	Cod.
Chininum arsenicosum	Ch. ar.	Coffea cruda	Cof.
Chininum muriaticum	Ch. m.	Coffea tosta	Cf. t.
Chininum salicylicum	Ch. sal.	Coffeinum	Cfn.
Chininum sulphuricum	Ch. s.	Colchicinum	Cchn.
Chionanthus virginica	Chio.	Colchicum	Clch.
Chloralum	Chl. h.	Collinsonia canadensis	Coll.
Chloroformum	Chlf.	Colocynthinum	Clcn.
Chlorum	Chlm.	Colocynthis	Col.
Cholesterinum	Chlst.	Colostrum	Clost.

Coniinum	Cnn.
Coniinum bromatum	Cn. br.
Conium maculatum	Con.
Convallaria majalis	Cvl.
Convolvulus duartinus	Clv. d.
Copaiva	Cop.
Corallium rubrum	Crl.
Coriaria ruscifolia	Cri. r.
Cornus alternifolia	Co. a.
Cornus circinata	Co. c.
Cornus florida	Co. fl.
Corydalis	Cry.
Coto bark	Cto.
Cotyledon	Cty.
Crataegus oxyacantha	Crat.
Crocus sativus	Cro.
Crotalus caseavella	Crt. c.
Crotalus horridus	Crt. h.
Croton chloral	Ctn. ch.
Croton tiglium	Ctn.
Cubeba	Cub.
Cucurbita pepo	Cuc. p.
Culex musea	Cul.
Cundurango	Cnd.
Cuphea viscosissima	Cph.
Cupressus australis	Cp. a.
Cupressus lawsoniana	Cp. l.
Cuprum aceticum	Cp. a.
Cuprum arsenicosum	Cu. as.
Cuprum metallicum	Cup.
Cuprum sulphuricum	Cu. s.
Curare	Cur.
Cyclamen	Cyc.
Cypripedium	Cyp.

Damiana	Tur.
(see Turnera aphrodisiaca)	
Daphne indica	Dph.
Datura arborea	Dt. a.
Datura ferox	Dt. f.
Datura metel	Dt. m.
Derris pinnata	Der.
Diadema	Aran.
(see Aranea)	
Dictamnus	Dct.
Digitalinum	Dgn.
Digitalis	Dig.
Digitoxinum	Dxn.
Dioscorea	Dio.
Diphtherinum	Dphn.
Direa palustris	Dir.
Dolichos	Dol.
Doryphora	Dor.
Drosera	Drs.
Duboisinum	Dbn.
Dulcamara	Dul.
Echinacea angustifolia	Ech. a.
Echinacea purpurea	Ech. p.
Elaeis guineensis	Elae.
Elaps corallinus	Elp.
Elaterium	Elt.
Electricitas	Elc.
Ephedra vulgaris	Eph.
Epigea repens	Epg.
Epilobium palustre	Epl.
Epiphegus	Eps.
Equisetum	Equ.
Erechthites	Ere.

Ergotinum	Erg.	Fagus sylvatica	Fgs.
Erigeron	Erig.	Fel tauri	Fel.
Eriodictyon glutinosum	Erio.	Ferrum metallicum,	Fer.
Erodium	Erod.	*including* :—	
Eryngium aquaticum	Ery. a.	Ferrum aceticum	Fe. ac.
Eryngium maritimum	Ery. m.	*and*	
Erythrinus	Eryth.	Ferrum carbonicum	Fe. c.
Erythroxylon	Coca	Ferrum arsenicicum	Fe. as.
(*see* Coca)		Ferrum bromatum	Fe. br.
Eserinum	Eser.	Ferrum iodatum	Fe. i.
Etherum	Eth.	Ferrum magneticum	Fe. mg.
Ethylum nitricum	Eth. n.	Ferrum muriaticum	Fe. m.
Eucalyptus	Euc.	Ferrum pernitricum	Fe. pn.
Eugenia jambos	Eug.	Ferrum phosphoricum	Fe. p.
Euonyminum	Evm.	Ferrum phosphoricum	Fe. p. h.
Euonymus atropurpurea	Ev. a.	hydricum	
Eunymus europaea	Evo.	Ferrum picricum	Fe. pi.
Eupatorium aromaticum	E. ar.	Ferrum pyrophosphoricum	Fe. py.
Eupatorium perfoliatum	E. pf.	Ferrum sulphuricum	Fe. s.
Eupatorium purpureum	E. pu.	Ferrum tartaricum	Fe. t.
Euphorbia amygdaloides	Eu. a.	Ferula glauca	Frl.
Euphorbia corallata	Eu. co.	Ficus religiosa	Fic. r.
Euphorbia cyparissias	Eu. cy.	Filix mas	Fil.
Euphorbia heterodoxa	Eu. ht.	Fluoricum acidum	Fl. x.
Euphorbia hypericifolia	Eu. hp.	Formica	For.
Euphorbia ipecacuanha	Eu. i.	Fragaria vesca	Frg.
Euphorbia lathyris	Eu. l.	Franciscea uniflora	Fnc.
Euphorbia peplus	Eu. pp.	Franzensbad	Frz.
Euphorbia pilulifera	Eu. pi.	Fraxinus americana	Frx.
Euphorbium	Eub.	Fucus vesiculosus	Fuc.
Euphrasia	Ephr.		
Eupionum	Epn.	Gadus morrhua	Gad.
		Galega officinalis	Glg.
Fagopyrum	Fag.	Galium aparine	Gli.

Gallicum acidum	Ga. x.	Hecla	Hec.
Galvanisumus	Glv.	Hedeoma	Hdm.
Gambogia	Gam.	Hedera helix	Hd. h.
Gastein	Gas.	Hedysarum ildefonsianum	Hdy.
Gultheria	Gau.	Helianthus	Hli.
Gelsemium	Gel.	Heliotropium	Hlt.
Genista	Gen.	Helix tosta	Hlx.
Gentiana cruciata	Gn. c.	Helleborus foetidus	Hl. f.
Gentiana lutea	Gn. l.	Helleborus niger	Hel.
Gentiana quinqueflora	Gn. q.	Helleborus orientalis	Hl. o.
Geranium meculatum	Ger.	Helleborus viridis	Hl. v.
Gettysburg	Get.	Heloderma	Hlod.
Geum rivale	Geu.	Helonias	Hlon.
Ginseng	Gin.	Hepar	Hep.
Glonoinum	Glo.	Hepatica	Hpt.
Gnaphalium	Gna.	Heracleum	Her.
Gossypium herbaceum	Gos.	Hippomanes	Hpm.
Granatum	Grn.	Hippozaeninum	Hpz.
Graphites	Gph.	Hoang-nan	Hoa.
Gratiola	Grt.	Homarus	Homa.
Grindelia	Gnd.	Homeria	Hmer.
Guaco	Guac.	Hura brasiliensis	Hur.
Guaiacum	Gui.	Hura crepitans	Hur. c.
Guarana	Grna.	Hydrangea arborescens	Hdrn. a.
Guarea	Gre.	Hydrastinium muriaticum	Hnn. m.
Gummi gutti	Gam.	Hydrastinum muriaticum	Hn. m.
(see Gambogia)		Hydrastis candadensis	Hdr.
Gymnema sylvestre	Gne.	Hydrocotyle asiatica	Hyd.
Gymnocladus canadensis	Gno.	Hydrocyanicum acidum	Hy. x.
		Hydrophobinum	Hfb.
		Hydrophyllum virginianum	Hph. v.
Haematoxylon	Haem.	Hyoscyaminum	Hyn.
Hall	Hal.	Hyoscyamus	Hyo.
Hamamelis	Ham.	Hypericum	Hyp.

Iberis	Ibe.	Juniperus virginianus	Jn. v.
Ichthyolum	Icth.		
Ictodes feotida	Ict.	Kali aceticum	K.ac.
Ignatia	Ign.	Kali arsenicosum	K. as.
Ilex aquifolium	Ilx.	Kali bichromicum	K. bi.
Illicium anisatum	Ill.	Kali bromatum	K. br.
Imperatoria	Imp.	Kali carbonicum	K. ca.
Indigo	Ind.	Kali chloricum	K.chl.
Indium	Idm.	Kali chlorosum	K.chs.
Inula	Inu.	Kali citricum	K. cit.
Iodium	Iod.	Kali cyanatum	K. ey.
Iodoformum	Iof.	Kali Ferrocyanatum	K. fe.
Ipecacuanha	Ipc.	Kali iodatum	K. i.
Ipomoea	Clv. d.	Kali manganicum	
(*see* Convolvulus duratinus)		(Kali permanganicum)	K. Pm.
Iridium	Ird.	Kali muriaticum	K. m.
Iris florentina	Ir. fl.	Kali nitricum	K. n.
Iris foetidissima	Ir. foe.	Kali oxalicum	K. ox.
Iris germanica	Ir. g.	Kali permanganicum	K. pm.
Iris tenax	Ir. t.	Kali phosphoricum	K. ph.
Iris versicolor	Iris	Kali picricum	K. pi.
Itu	Itu	Kali sulphuratum	K. s.
		Kali sulphuricum	K. s. c.
Jaborandi	Jab.	Kali tartaricum	K. trt.
Jacaranda caroba	Ja. c.	Kali telluricum	K. tel.
Jacaranda gualandai	Ja. g.	Kalmia latifolia	Klm.
Jalapa	Jal.	Kamala	Kam.
Jasminum	Jas.	Kaolin	Kao.
Jatropha	Jat.	Karaka	Kar.
Jatropha urens	Jt. u.	Katipo	Lt. k.
Jequirity	Jeq.	(*see* Latrodectus katipo)	
Juglans cinerea	Jg. c.	Kava	Pip. m.
Juglans regia	Jg. r.	(*see* Piper methysticum)	
Juncus	Jnc.	Kerosolenum	Ker.

Kino	Ago.	Leptandra	Lpt.
(*see* Angophora)		Levico	Lev.
Kissingen	Kis.	Liatris spicata	Lia.
Kousso	Kou.	Lilium tigrinum	Lil.
Krameria	Rat.	Limulus	Lim.
(*see* Ratanhia)		Linaria	Lina.
Kreosotum	Kre.	Linum catharticum	Ln. c.
		Linum usitatissinum	Ln. u.
Laburnum	Lab.	Lippia mexicana	Lip. u.
Lac caninum	Lc. c.	Lippspringe	Lips.
Lac felinum	Lc. f.	Lithium benzoicum	Li. bz.
Lac vaccinum	Lc. v.	Lithium bromatum	Li. br.
Lac vaccinum coagulatum	Lc. v. c.	Lithium carbonicum	Li. c
Lac vaccinum defloratum	Lc. v. d.	Lithium lacticum	Li. l.
Lacerta	Lcrt.	Lithium muriatcum	Li. m.
Lachesis	Lach.	Lobelia cardinalis	Lo. c.
Lachnanthes	Lchn.	Lobelia dortmanna	Lo. d.
Lactis acidum	Lc.x.	Lobelia erinus	Lo.e.
Lactis vaccini flos	Lc. v. f.	Lobelia inflata	Lo. i.
Lactuca virosa	Let. v.	Lobelia purpurascens	Lo. p.
Lamium	Lam.	Lobelia syphilitica	Lo. s.
Lapathum	L. a. p.	Loco-weed	Oxt.
Lappa	Ar. lp.	(*see* Oxytropis Lamberti)	
(*see* Acretium lappa)		Lolium temulentum	Lol.
Lapsana communis	Lpsa.	Lonicera Periclymenum	Ln. p.
Lathyrus	Lth.	Lonicera xylosteum	Lon.
Latrodectus katipo	Lt. k.	Luesinum or Lueticum	Syph.
Latrodectus mactans	Lt.m.	(*see* Syphilinum)	
Laurocerasus	Vb. t.	Luna	Lun.
(*see* Viburnum tinus)		Lupulus	Lup.
Ledum	Led.	Lycopersicum	Lrs.
Lemna minor	Lmn.	Lycopodium	Lyc.
Leonurus cardiaca	Leo.	Lycopus	Lcs.
Lepidium bonariense	Lpi.	Lysidinum	Lys.

Lyssinum	Hfb.
(see Hydrophobinum)	
Macrotinum	Mac.
Mangnesia carbonica	Mag. c.
Magnesia muriatica	Mag. m.
Magnesia phosphorica	Mag. p.
Magnesia sulphurica	Mag. s.
Magnetis poli ambo	Mgt.
Magnetis polus australis	Mgt. s.
Magnolia glauca	Mgn. gl
Magnolia grandiflora	Mgn. gr.
Mais and Stigmata maidis	Zea.
(see Zea mays)	
Malandrinum	Mld.
Malaria offieinalis	Mlr.
Mancinella	Mnc.
Mandragora	Mnd.
Manganum	Man.
Including :—	
(1) Manganum aceticum	Mn. a.
(2) Manganum carbonicum	Mn. c.
Manganum muriaticum	Mn.m.
Manganum oxydatumnativum	Mn. o.
Manganums sulphuricum	Mn. s.
Matthiola graeca	Mat.
Medorrhinum	Med.
Medusa	Mds.
Melastoma	Mla.
Melilotus	Mli.
Melitagrinum	Mlt.
Menispermum	Mns.
Mentha piperita	Mth. pi.
Mentha pulegium	Mth. pu.

Menyanthes	Men.
Mephitis	Mep.
Mercurialis perennis	Mrl.
Mercurius	Merc.
Including :-	
(1) Mercuris	Mr. sol.
oxydulatus niger	
(M. solubilis Hahn.)	
(2) Mecuris vivius	Mr. v.
Mercurius aceticus	Mr. ac.
Mercurius binodatus	Mr. bin.
Mercurius binodatus	Mr. K. i.
cum Kali iodatum	
Mercurius corrosivus	Mr. c.
Mercurius cyanatus	Mr. cy.
Mercurius dulcis	Mr. d.
Mercurius nitricus	Mr. n.
Mercurius praecipitatus albus	Mr.p.a.
Mercurius praecipitatus ruber	Mr. p. r.
Mercurius protoiodatus	Mr. i. f.
Mercurius sulphocy anatus	Mr. scy.
Mercurius sulphuratus ruber	Cnb.
(see Cinnabaris)	
Mercurius sulphuricus	Mr. s.
Methylene-blue	Mth. b.
Mezereum	Mez.
Millefolium	Mil.
Mimosa	Mim.
Mitchella	Mit.
Momordica	Mom.
Morphinum	Mor.
Morphinum aceticum	Mo. a.
Morphinum muriaticum	Mo. m.
Morphinum sulphuricum	Mo. s.

Moschus	Mos.	Niccolum	Nic.
Mucuna pruriens	Dol.	*Including :—*	
(*see* Dolichos)		(1) Niccolum metallicum	Nic.
Mucuna urens	Mu. u.	(2) Niccolum carbonicum	Ni. c.
Murex	Mur.	Niccolum sulphuricum	Ni. s.
Muriaticum acidum	Mu. x.	Nicotinum	Nct.
Musa	Mus.	Nitri spiritus dulcis	Nt. s. d.
Mygale	Myg.	Nitricum acidum	Nt. x.
Myosotis	Myo.	Nitrogenum oxygenatum	Nt.o.
Myrica cerifera	My. c.	Nitroso muriaticum acidum	Nm. x.
Myristica sebifera	Mst. s.	Nitrun	K. n.
Myrtus communis	Mrt.	(*see* Kali nitricum)	
		Nuphar luteum	Nup.
Nabalus	Nab.	Nux juglans	Jg. r.
Naja	Naj.	(*see* Juglans regia)	
Naphthalinum	Nph.	Nux moschata	Nx. m.
Narcissus	Nrs.	Nux vomica	Nux
Narcotinum	Nrn.	Nyctanthes	Nyc.
Natrum arsenicicum	Na. as.	Nymphaea odorata	Nym.
Natrum cacodylicum	Na. cc.		
Natrum carbonicum	Na. c.	Ocimum canum	Ocm.
Natrum hypochlorosum	Na. hch.	Oenanthe crocata	OEna.
Natrum iodatum	Na. i.	Oenothera	OEno.
Natrum lacticum	Na. l.	Oleander	Oln.
Natrum muriaticum	Na. m.	Oleum animale	Ol. a.
Natrum nitricum	Na. n.	Oleum jecoris aselli	Ol. j.
Natrum nitrosum	Na. ns.	Oleum ricini	
Natrum phosphoricum	Na. p.	(*see* Ricinus)	Ric.
Natrum salicylicum	Na. sa.	Oniscus	Onis.
Natrum selenicum	Na. se.	Ononis	Onon.
Natrum silicofluoricum	Na. sf.	Onosmodium	Onos.
Natrum sulphuricum	Na. s.	Oophorinum	Oop.
Natrum sulphurosum	Na. ss.	Opium	Opi.
Nectrianinum	Nec.	Opuntia	Opu.

Orchitinum	Orc.	Pepsinum	Pep.
Oreodaphne	Ore.	Persica	Per.
Origanum	Ori.	Persicaria urens	Plg.
Ornithogalum umbellatum	Orn.	(see Polygonum)	
Osmium	Osm.	Pestinum	Pest.
Ostrya	Ost.	Petiveria	Ptv.
Ovi gallinae pellicula	Ov. g. p.	Petroleum	Pet.
Ovi gallinae testa	Ca. o. t.	Petroselinum	Pts.
(see Calcarea ovi testae)		Phallus impudicus	Phal.
Oxalicum acidum	Ox. x.	Pheaseolus	Phas.
Oxydendron	Oxd.	Phellandrium	Phel.
Oxygenium	Oxg.	Phenacetinum	Phen.
Oxytropis lamberti	Oxt.	Phlorizinum	Phlo.
Ozonum	Ozo.	Phosphoricum acidum	Ph. x.
(see Oxygenium)		Phosphorus	Pho.
		Phosphorus hydrogenatus	Ph. h.
Paeonia	Paeo.	Phosphorus muriaticus	Ph. m.
Palladium	Pal.	Physalia	Phy.
Pancreatinum	Pan.	Physostigma	Phst.
Papaya (see Asimina)	Asi.	Phytolacca	Phyt.
Paraffinum	Prf.	Pichi	Pch.
Pareira	Prei.	Picricum acidum	Pi. x.
Parietaria	Priet.	Picrotoxinum	Pcx.
Paris	Par.	Pilocarpinum	Plo.
Parthenium	Prt.	Pilocarpinum muriaticum	Plo. m.
Passiflora	Pas.	Pilocarpinum nitricum	Plo. n.
Pastinaca	Pst.	Pimenta	Pmt.
Paullinia pinnata	Pau.	Pimpernel	Anag.
Paullinia sorbilis	Grna.	(see Anagallis	
(see Guarana)		Pimpinella	Pim.
Pecten	Pec.	Pinus lambertiana	Pin. l.
Pediculus	Ped.	Pinus sylvestris	Pin. s.
Pelargonium reniforme	Pel.	Piper methysticum	Pip. m.
Penthorum sedoides	Pnt.	Piper nigrum	Pip. n.

Piperazinum	Ppz.	Prunus virginiana	Pr. v.
Piscidia	Psc.	Psorinum	Pso.
Pix liquida	Pix.	Ptelea	Ptl.
Plantago	Plnt.	Pulmo vulpis	Pmo.
Platanus	Plts.	Pulsatilla	Pul.
Platinum	Plat.	Pulsatilla nuttaliana	Pl. n.
Platinum muriaticum	Pt. m.	Pyrethrum parthenium	Pyre.
Platinum muriaticum natronatum	Pt. m. n.	Pyrogenium	Pyro.
		Pyrus americana	Pyr. a
Plectranthus	Ple.		
Plumbago	Pbo.	Quassia	Qua.
Plumbum	Pb.	Quebracho	Qeb.
(including P. metallicum, P. aceticum, and P. carbonicum)		Quercus	Qer.
		Quininum	Ch. s.
		(see Chininum sulphuricum)	
Plumbum chromicum	Pb. chr.		
Plumbum iodatum	Pb. i.	Ranunculus acris	Rn. a.
Podophyllum	Pod.	Ranunculus bulbosus	Rn. b.
Polygonum	Plg.	Ranunculus ficaria	Rn. fi.
Polyporus officinalis	Bo. la.	Ranunculus flammula	Rn. fl.
(see Boletus laricis)		Ranunculus glacialis	Rn. g.
Polyporus pinicola	Plp.	Ranunculus repens	Rn. r.
Populus candicans	Pop. c.	Ranunculus sceleratus	Rn. s.
Populus tremuloides	Pop. t.	Raphanus	Rap.
Pothos foetidus	Ict.	Ratanhia	Rat.
(see Ictodes)		Rhamnus catharticus	Rm. c.
Primula obconica	Prm.o.	Rhamnus frangula	Rm.f.
Primula veris	Prm. ve.	Rheum	Rhe.
Primula vulgaris	Prm. vg.	Rhodium oxydatum nitricum	Rdm.
Prinos verticillatus	Prin.	Rhododendron	Rho.
Propylaminum	Trm.	Rhus aromatica	Rs. a.
(see Trimethylaminum)		Rhus diversiloba	Rs. d.
Prunus padus	Pr. p.	Rhus glabra	Rs. g.
Prunus spinosa	Pr. s.	Rhus radicans	Rs. r.

Rhus toxico dendron Rs. t.	Rhs.	Sanguinarinum nitricum	Sg. n.
("Rhs." implies both or either)		Sanguinarinum tartaricum	Sg. t.
Rhus venenata	Rs. v.	Sanguisuga	Sgs.
Ricinus	Ric.	Sanicula	Snc.
Robinia	Rob.	Santalum	Snt.
Rosa canina	Ro. c.	Santoninum	Sntn.
Rosa damascena	Ro. d.	Saponinum	Sap.
Rosmarinus	Rsm.	Sarracenia	Src.
Rubia tinctorum	Rub.	Sarsaparilla	Sars.
Rumex acetosa	Rx. ac.	Scammonium	Sca.
Rumex crispus	Rum.	Schinus	Sch.
Rumex obtusifolia	Lap.	Scilla maritima	Scil.
(see Lapathum)		Scirrhinum	Scir.
Russula	Rus.	Scolopendra	Scol.
Ruta	Rut.	Scorpio	Scor.
		Scrophularia	Scro.
Sabadilla	Sbd.	Scutellaria	Scu.
Sabal serrulata	Sbl.	Secale cornutum	Sec.
Sabina	Sbi.	Selenium	Sel.
Saccharum lactis	Sac. l.	Sempervivum tectorum	Smp.
Saccharum officinale	Sac. o.	Senecio aureus	Se. a.
Salicinum	Sln.	Senecio jacobaea	Se. j.
Salicylicum acidum	Sl. x.	Senega	Sga.
Salix mollissima	Sx. m.	Senna	Sna.
Salix nigra	Sx. n.	Sepia	Sep.
Salix purpurea	sx. p.	Sepsinum	Pyro.
Salol	Sll.	*(see* Pyrogenium)	
Salufer	Na. sf.	Septicaeminum	Sptn.
(see Natrum Silicofluoricum)		Shucks	Zea Sh.
Salvia	Slv.	*(see* Zea)	
Sambucus canadensis	Smb. c.	Silica	Sil.
Sambucus nigra	Smb. n.	Silica marina	Sil. m.
Sanguinaria Canadensis	Sang.	Silphium	Slp.
Sanguinarinum	Sgn.	Sinapis alba	Sin. a.

Sinapis nigra	Sin.n.	Stramonium	Stm.
Sium	Siu.	Strontium bromatum	Sto. b.
Skookum chuck	Sko.	Strontium carbonicum	Sto. c.
Slag	Sla.	Strontium nitricum	Sto. n.
Sol	Sol.	Strophanthus	Strp.
Solaninum	Son.	Strychninum	Sty.
Solaninum aceticum	Son. ac.	Strychninum nitricum	Sty.n
Solanum arrebenta	So. a.	Strychninum phosphoricum	Sty. p.
Solanum carolinense	So. c.	Strychninum sulphuricum	Sty. s.
Solanum mammosum	So. m.	Strychninum valerianicum	Sty. v.
Solanum nigrum	So. n.	Succinum	Suc.
Solanum oleraceum	So. o.	Sulfonal	Sfn.
Solanum pseudo-capsicum	So. pc.	Sulphur	Sul
Solanum tuberosum	So. t.	Sulphur hydrogenisatum	Sul. h.
Solanum	So. t. ae.	Sulphur iodatum	Sul. i.
tuberosum aegrotans		Sulphur terebinthinatum	Sul. t.
Solidago	Sld.	Sulphuricum acidum	Su. x.
Sperminum	Orc.	Sulphurosum acidum	Ss. x.
(see Orchitinum)		Sumbul	Sum.
Sphingurus	Sgu.	Symphoricarpus	Sym. r.
Spigelia	Spi.	racemosus	
Spigelia marilandica	Sp.m.	Symphytum	Symt.
Spiraea ulmaria	Spa. u.	Syphilinum	Syph.
Spiranthes	Sprn.	Syzygium	Syz.
Spongia tosta	Spo.		
Stachys betonica	Sta.	Tabacum	Tab.
Stannum	Stn.	Tamus	Tam.
Stannum iodatum	Stn. i.	Tanacetum	Tnc.
Staphisagria	Stp.	Tanghinia	Tng.
Stellaria media	Ste.	Tannin	Tnn.
Sticta pulmonaria	Sti.	Taraxacum	Trx.
Stigmata maidis	Zea. st.	Tarentula cubensis	Trn. c.
(see Zea)		Tarentula hispanica	Trn.
Stillingia sylvatica	Stil.	Tartaricum acidum	Tt. x.

Taxus baccata	Tax.	Tussilago petasites	Ts.p.
Tellurium	Tel.		
Teplitz	Tep.	Ulmus fulva	Ul. f.
Terebinthina	Ter.	Upas	Up.
Tetradymite	Ttr.	Uraninum nitricum	Ur. n.
Teucrium marum verum	Teu.	Urea	Ure.
Teucrium scorodonia	Teu. s.	Uricum acidum	Ur. x.
Thallium	Tha.	Urinum	Uri.
Thea	Tea.	Urtica urens	Urt.
Theridion	Ther.	Usnea barbata	Usn.
Thevetia	Thev.	Ustilago	Ust.
Thiosinaminum	Thio.	Uva-ursi	Uva.
Thlaspi bursa pastoris	Thl.		
Thuja	Thu.	Vaccininum	Vac.
Thyroidinum	Thyr.	Valeriana	Val.
Thyroiodinum	Thri.	Vanadium	Van.
Tilia	Til.	Variolinum	Var.
Titanium	Tit.	Veratrinum	Vrn.
Tongo	Ton.	Veratrum album	Ver.
Toxicophis	Tox.	Veratrum nigrum	Ve. n.
Trachinus	Trac.	Veratrum viride	Ve. v.
Tradescantia	Trad.	Verbascum	Vbs.
Trifolium pratense	Trf. p.	Verbens hastata	Vbn.
Trifolium repens	Trf. r.	Vesicaria	Ves.
Trillium	Trl.	Vespa	Vsp.
Trimethylaminum	Trm.	Viburnum opulus	Vb. o.
Triosteum	Tri.	Viburnum prunifolium	Vb.p.
Triticum repens	Trt.	Viburnum tinus	Vb. t.
Trombidium	Trb.	Vichy	Vic.
Tropaeolum	Trp.	Vinca minor	Vin.
Tuberculinum	Tub.	Viola odorata	Vi. o.
Turnera aphrodisiaca	Tur.	Viola tricolor	Vi. t.
Tussilago farfara	Ts. ff.	Vipera	Vip.
Tussilago fragrans	Ts. fg.	Vipera redi	Vp. r.

Vipera torva	Vp. t.	Zincum	Zin.
Viscum album	Vis.	Zincum aceticum	Zn. a.
Voeslau	Voe.	Zincum bromatum	Zn. br.
		Zincum cyantum	Zn. cy.
Wiesbaden	Wis.	Zincum iodatum	Zn. i.
Wildbad	Wil.	Zincum muriaticum	Zn. m.
Wyethia	Wye.	Zincum oxydatum	Zn. o.
		Zincum phosphoricum	Zn. p.
Xanthoxylum	Xan.	Zincum picricum	Zn. pi.
		Zincum sulphuricum	Zn. s.
Yohimbinum	Yoh.	Zincum valerianicum	Zn. v.
Yucca filamentosa	Yuc.	Zingiber	Zng.
		Zizia	Ziz.
Zea mays	Zea		

□□

Alphabetical list of Abbreviations with

REMEDIES

Ab. c.	Abies canadensis	Ag. e.	Agaricus emeticus
Ab. n.	Abies nigra	Ag. i.	Argentum iodatum
Abr.	Ambrosia artemisiaefolia	Ag. n.	Argentum nitricum
Abs.	Absinthium (Artemisia absinthium)	Ag. p.	Agaricus phalloides
		Aga.	Agaricus muscarius
Abt.	Abrotanum (Artemisia abrotanum	Agn.	Agnus castus
		Ago.	Angophora (Kino)
Ac. c.	Aconitum cammarum	Agr. n.	Agraphis nutans
Ac. f.	Aconitum ferox	Ags.	Agrostemma githago
Ac. l.	Aconitum lycoctonum	Agv.	Agave americana
Ac. x.	Aceticum acidum	Ail.	Ailanthus glandulosa
Acal.	Acalypha indica	Alet.	Aletris farinosa
Acn.	Aconitinum	All.	Allium Sativum
Aco.	Aconitum napellus	Alm.	Alumina
Act. r.	Actaea racemosa	Aln.	Alumen
Act. s.	Actaea spicata	Alns.	Alnus
Ado.	Adonis vernalis	Alo.	Aloe socotrina
Adr.	Adrenalin	Als.	Alstonia constricta
Aes. g.	Aesculus glabra	Am. ac.	Ammonium aceticum
Aesc.	Aesculus hippocastanum	Am. br.	Ammonium bromatum
Aeps.	Aethiops antimonialis	Am. bz.	Ammonium benzoicum
Aeth.	Aethusa cynapium	Am. c.	Ammonium carbonicum
Ag. cy.	Argentum cyanatum	Am. m.	Ammonium muriaticum

Am. p.	Ammonium phosphoricum
Am. pi.	Ammonium picricum
Amb.	Ambra grisea
Amc.	Ammoniacum
Amg.	Amygdalae amarae aqua
Aml.	Amylenum nitrosum
Amm.	Ammonium causticum
Amph.	Amphisbaena
Ampl.	Ampelopsis
An. oc.	Anacardium occidentale
Ana.	Anacardium orientale
Anag.	Anagallis arvensis (Pimpernel)
Anan.	Anantherum muriaticum
Ang.	Angustura uera
Anh.	Anhalonium lewinii
Anil.	Anilinum
Ank.	Anthrokokali
Ant. a.	Antimonium arsenicicum (Arsenicum stibiatum)
Ant. c.	Antimonium crudum
Ant. i.	Antimonium iodatum
Ant. m.	Antimonium muriaticum
Ant. s. a.	Antimonium sulphuratum aureum
Ant. t.	Antimonium tartaricum
Antf.	Antifebrinum (Acetanilidum)
Anth. n.	Anthemis nobilis
Antho.	Anthoxanthum
Ap. a.	Apocynum androsaemifolium
Aph.	Aphis chenopodii glauci
Api. g.	Apium graveolens
Apm.	Apomorphinum
Apo.	Apocynum cannabinum
Aps.	Apis
Aq. m.	Aqua marina
Aqui.	Aquilegia vulgaris
Ar. dm.	Arum dracontium
Ar. ds.	Arum dracunculus
Ar. it.	Arum italicum
Ar. lp.	Arctium lappa (Lappa)
Ar. m.	Arum maculatum
Ars. c.	Aranea scinencia
Ar. t.	Arum triphyllum
Ara. t.	Aranearum tela
Aral.	Aralia racemosa
Aran.	Aranea diadema (Diadema)
Arb.	Arbutus andrachne
Ard.	Arundo mauritanica
Arec.	Areca
Arg.	Argentum metallicum
Ari.	Aristolochia milhomens
Ari. s	Aristolochia serpentaria
Arm.	Armoracia sativa (cochlearia armoracia)
Arn.	Arnica
Arnt.	Aurantium (Citrus vulgaris)
Ars.	Arsenicum album
Art. v.	Artemisia vulgaris
As. br.	Arsenicum bromatum
As. f.	Arsenicum sulphuratum flavum
As. h.	Arsenicum

	hydrogenisatum		carbonica)
As. i.	Arsenicum iodatum	Ba. c.	Baryta carbonica
As. mt.	Arsenicum metallicum	Ba. i.	Baryta iodata
As. r.	Arsenicum sulphuratum rubrum	Ba. m.	Baryta muriatica
		Bac.	Bacillinum
Asa.	Asafoetida	Bac. t.	Bacillinum testium
Asc. s.	Asclepias syriaca	Bad.	Badiaga
Asc. t.	Asclepias tuberosa	Bal.	Balsamum peruvianum
Asi.	Asimina triloba (Papaya)	Bap.	Baptisia tinctoria
Asp.	Asparagus	Bap. c.	Baptisia confusa acetica
Asr.	Asarum europaeum	Baro.	Barosma (Buchu)
Ast. f.	Astacus fluviatilis (Cancer f.)	Bel.	Belladonna
		Ber.	Berberis vulgaris
Ast. r.	Asterias rubens	Ber. a.	Berberis aquifolium
Astg.	Astragalus menziesii	Bis.	Bismuthum
Ath.	Athamanta	Bl. a.	Blatta americana
Athra.	Anthracinum	Bl. o.	Blatta orientalis
Atp.	Antipyrinum	Bls.	Bellis perennis
Atr.	Atropinum	Bnz.	Benzinum
Au. ar.	Aurum arsenicicum	Bo. la.	Boletus laricis (Polyporus officinalis)
Au. br.	Aurum bromatum		
Au. i.	Aurum iodatum	Bo. lu.	Boletus luridus
Au. m.	Aurum muriaticum	Bo. s.	Boletus satanas
Au. m. k.	Aurum muriaticum kalinatum	Bom.	Bombyx processionea
		Bor.	Borax
Au. m. n.	Aurum muriaticum natronatum	Bov.	Bovista
		Brac.	Brachyglottis repens
Au. s.	Aurum sulphuratum	Brc. x.	Boracicum acidum
Aur.	Aurum metallicum	Brcn.	Brucinum
Avi.	Aviaire	Bro.	Bromium
Avn.	Avena sativa	Brs.	Brassica napus
Az.	Azadirachta indica	Bru.	Brucea antidysenterica (Angustura spuria)
Ba. ac.	Baryta acetica (*see* Baryta	Bry.	Bryonia

Bth.	Bothrops lanceolatus	Cast.	Castoreum
Buf.	Bufo	Caul.	Caulophyllum
Bz. d.	Benzinum dinitricum	Caus.	Causticum
Bz. n.	Benzinum nitricum	Cb. a.	Carbo animalis
Bz. x.	Benzoicum acidum	Cb. v.	Carbo vegetabilis
Bzn.	Benzion	Cbl. x.	Carbolicum acidum
		Cbn.	Carboneum
Ca. ac.	Calcarea acetica	Cchn.	Colchicinum
Ca. ar.	Calcarea arsenicosa	Ccn. s.	Coccinella septempunctata
Ca. br.	Calcarea bromata		
Ca. chl.	Calcarea chlorinata	Ccs. c.	Coccus cacti
Ca. cs.	Calcarea caustica	Cd. br.	Cadmium bromatum
Ca. fl.	Calcarea fluorata	Cd. s.	Cadmium sulphuratum
Ca. hp.	Calcarea hypophosphorosa	Ce. b.	Cereus bonplandii
Ca. i.	Calcarea iodata	Ce. s.	Cereus serpentinus
Ca. m.	Calcarea muriatica	Cean.	Ceanothus americanus
Ca. o. t.	Calcarea ovi testae (Ovi gallinae testa)	Ced.	Cedron
		Cen.	Cenchris contortrix (Ancitrodon c.)
Ca. ox.	Calcarea oxalica		
Ca. p.	Calcarea phosphorica	Cep.	Cepa (Allium cepa)
Ca. pi.	Calcarea picrica	Cer. o.	Cerium oxalicum
Ca. ren.	Calcarea renalis	Cet.	Cetraria islandica
Ca. s.	Calcarea Sulphurica	Cf.t.	Coffea tosta
Ca. si.	Calcarea silicica	Cfn.	Coffeinum
Cac.	Cactus grandiflorus	Ch. ar.	Chininum arsenicosum
Cai.	Cainca	Ch. m.	Chininum muriaticum
Caj.	Cajuputum	Ch. s.	Chininum sulphuricum (Quininum)
Calc.	Calcarea carbonica		
Caln.	Calendula	Ch. sal.	Chininum salicylicum
Cam.	Camphora	Cham.	Chamomilla
Can. s.	Cannabis sativa	Chei.	Cheiranthus cheiri
Cap.	Capsicum	Chel.	Chelidonium
Carl.	Carlsbad	Chi.	China officinalis
Cas. s.	Cascara sagrada	Chi. b.	China boliviana

Chio.	Chionanthus virginica	Clv. a.	Convolvulus arvensis
Chl. h.	Chloralum	Clv. d	Convolvulus duartinus
Chlf.	Chloroformum		(Ipomoea)
Chlm.	Chlorum	Cm. br.	Camphora bromata
Chlst.	Cholesterinum	Cn. br.	Coniinum bromatum
Chm. m.	Chimaphila maculata	Cn. i.	Cannabis indica
Chm. u.	Chimaphila umbellata	Cnb.	Cinnabaris (Mercurius
Chn. a.	Chenopodium		sulphuratus ruber)
	anthelminticum	Cnd.	Cundurango
Chn. s.	Cinchoninum	Cnn.	Coniinum
	sulphuricum	Cnt.	Centaurea tagana
Chn. v.	Chenopodium vulvaria	Cnu.	Canchalagua
Chne.	Chelone	Co.a.	Cornus alternifolia
Chp.	Chaparro amargoso	Co.c.	Cornus circinata
Chr. o.	Chromium oxydatum	Co. fl.	Cornus florida
Chr. x.	Chromium acidum	Cob.	Cobaltum
Chs. x.	Chrysophanicum acidum	Coc. i.	Cocculus indicus
Cic. m.	Cicuta maculata	Coca.	Coca (Erythroxylon)
Cic. v.	Cicuta virosa	Cod.	Codeinum
Cich.	Cichorium	Cof.	Coffea cruda
Cim.	Cimex	Col.	Colocynthis
Cin.	Cina (Artemisia contra	Coll.	Collinsonia canadensis
	and judaica)	Com.	Comocladia
Cin. m.	Cineraria maritima	Con.	Conium maculatum
Cinm.	Cinnamomum	Conc.	Conchiolinum
Cis.	Cistus canadensis	Cop.	Copaiva
Cit.	Citrus limonum	Cp. a.	Cupressus australis
Clch.	Colchicum	Cp. l.	Cupressus lawsoniana
Clcn.	Colocynthinum	Cph.	Cuphea vicosissima
Cld.	Caladium	Crat.	Crataegus oxyacantha
Clem.	Clematis erecta	Carb. h.	Carboneum
Clost.	Colostrum		hydrogenisatum
Clt.	Caltha palustris	Carb. s.	Carboneum sulphuratum
Cltr.	Calotropis	Crd. b.	Carduus benedictus

Crd. m.	Carduus marianus	Dio.	Dioscorea
Cri. r.	Coriaria ruscifolia	Dir.	Dirca palustris
Crl.	Corallium rubrum	Dol.	Dolichos (Mucuna
Cro.	Crocus sativus		pruriens)
Crt. c.	Crotalus cascavella	Dor.	Doryphora
Crt. h.	Crotalus horridus	Dph.	Daphne indica
Crv.	Cervus	Dphn.	Diphtherinum
Cry.	Corydalis	Drs.	Drosera
Cry. a.	Carya alba	Dt. a.	Datura arborea
Csc.	Cascarilla	Dt. f.	Datura ferox
Cst. v.	Castanea vesca	Dt. m.	Datura metel
Ct. eq.	Castor equi	Dul.	Dulcamara
Cth.	Cantharis	Dxn.	Digitoxinum
Ctn.	Croton tiglium		
Ctn. ch.	Croton chloral	E. ar.	Eupatorium aromaticum
Cto.	Coto bark	E. pf.	Eupatorium perfoliatum
Cty.	Cotyledon	E. pu.	Eupatorium purpureum
Cu. a.	Cuprum aceticum	Ech. a.	Echinacea angustifolia
Cu. as.	Cuprum arsenicosum	Ech. p.	Echinacea purpurea
Cu. s.	Cuprum sulphuricum	Elae.	Elaeis guineensis
Cub.	Cubeba	Elc.	Electricitas
Cuc. p.	Cucurbita pepo	Elp.	Elaps corallinus
Cul.	Culex musca	Elt.	Elaterium
Cup.	Cuprum metallicum	Epg.	Epigea ripens
Cur.	Curare	Eph.	Ephedra vulgaris
Cvl.	Convallaria majalis	Ephr.	Euphrasia
Cyc.	Cyclamen	Epl.	Epilobium palustre
Cyp.	Cypripedium	Epn.	Eupionum
		Eps.	Epiphegus
Dbn.	Duboisinum	Equ.	Equisetum
Dct.	Dictamnus	Ere.	Erechthites
Der.	Derris pinnata	Erg.	Ergotinum
Dgn.	Digitalinum	Erig.	Erigeron
Dig.	Digitalis	Erio.	Eriodictyon glutinosum

Erod.	Erodium		Fe. pi.	Ferrum picricum
Ery. a.	Eryngium aquaticum		Fe. pn.	Ferrum pernitricum
Ery. m.	Eryngium maritimum		Fe. py.	Ferrum pyrophosphoricum
Eryth.	Erythrinus		Fe. s.	Ferrum sulphuricum
Eser.	Eserinum		Fe. t.	Ferrum tartaricum
Eth.	Etherum		Fel.	Fel tauri
Eth. n.	Ethylum nitricum		Fer.	Ferrum (metallicum),
Eu. a.	Euphorbia amygdaloides			*including* F. aceticum
Eu. co.	Euphorbia corallata			*and* F. carbonicum
Eu. cy.	Euphorbia cyparissias			
Eu. hp.	Euphorbia hypericifolia		Fgs.	Fagus sylvatica
Eu. ht.	Euphorbia heterodoxa		Fic. r.	Ficus religiosa
Eu. i.	Euphorbia ipecacuanha		Fil.	Filix mas
Eu. l.	Euphorbia lathyris		Fl. x.	Fluoricum acidum
Eu. pi.	Euphorbia pilulifera		Fnc.	Franciscea uniflora
Eu. pp.	Euphorbia peplus		For.	Formica
Eub.	Euphorbium		Frg.	Fragaria vesca
Euc.	Eucalyptus		Frl.	Ferula glauca
Eug.	Eugenia jambos		Frx.	Fraxinus americana
Evm.	Euonyminum		Frz.	Franzensbad
Evo.	Euonymus europaea		Fuc.	Fucus vesiculosus
Ev. a.	Euonymus atropurpurea			
			Ga. x.	Gallicum acidum
			Gad.	Gadus morrhua
Fag.	Fagopyrum		Gam.	Gambogia (Gummi gutti)
Fe. ac.	Ferrum acteicum		Gas.	Gastein
Fe. as.	Ferrum arsenicicum		Gau.	Gaultheria
Fe. br.	Ferrum bromatum		Gel.	Gelsemium
Fe. c.	Ferrum carbonicum		Gen.	Genista
Fe. i.	Ferrum iodatum		Ger.	Geranium maculatum
Fe. m.	Ferrum muriaticum		Get.	Gettysburg
Fe. mg.	Ferrum magnecticum		Geu.	Geum rivale
Fe. p.	Ferrum phosphoricum		Gin.	Ginseng
Fe. p. h.	Ferrum phosphoricum hydricum		Glg.	Galega officinalis
			Gli.	Galium aparine

Glo.	Glonoinum
Glv.	Galvanismus
Gn. c.	Gentiana cruciata
Gn. l.	Gentiana lutea
Gn. q.	Gentiana quinqueflora
Gna.	Gnaphalium
Gnd.	Grindelia
Gne.	Gymnema sylverstre
Gno.	Gymnocladus canadensis
Gos.	Gossypium herbaceum
Gph.	Graphites.
Gre.	Guarea
Grn.	Granatum
Grna.	Guarana (Paullinia sorbilis)
Grt.	Gratiola
Guac.	Guaco
Gui.	Guaiacum
Haem.	Haematoxylon
Hal.	Hall
Ham.	Hamamelis
Hd. h.	Hedera helix
Hdm.	Hedeoma
Hdr.	Hydrastis canadensis
Hdrn. a	Hydrangea arborescens
Hdy.	Hedysarum ildefonsianum
Hec.	Hecla
Hel.	Helleborus niger
Hep.	Hepar
Her.	Heracleum
Hfb.	Hydrophobinum (Lyssinum)
Hl. f.	Helleborus foetidus

Hl. o.	Helleborus orientalis
Hl. v.	Helleborus viridis
Hli.	Helianthus
Hlod.	Heloderma
Hlon.	Helonias
Hlt.	Heliotropium
Hlx.	Helix tosta
Hmer.	Homeria
Hn. m.	Hydrastinum muriaticum
Hnn. m.	Hydrastininum muriaticum
Hoa.	Hoang-nan
Homa.	Homarus
Hph. v.	Hydrophyllum virginianum
Hpm.	Hippomanes
Hpt.	Hepatica
Hpz.	Hippozaeninum
Hur.	Hura brasiliensis
Hur. c.	Hura crepitans
Hy.x.	Hydrocyanicum acidum
Hyd.	Hydrocotyle asiatica
Hyn.	Hyoscyaminum
Hys.	Hyoscyamus
Hyp.	Hypericum
Ibe.	Iberis
Ict.	Ictodes foetida (Pothos foetidus)
Icth.	Ichthyolum
Idm.	Indium
Ign.	Ignatia
Ill.	Illicium anisatum (Anisum stellatum)

Ilx.	Ilex aquifolium	K. ca.	Kali carbonicum
Imp.	Imperatoria	K. chl.	Kali chloricum
Ind.	Indigo	K. chs.	Kali chlorosum
Inu.	Inula	K. cit.	Kali citricum
Iod.	Iodium	K. cy.	Kali cyantum
Iof.	Iodoformum	K. fe.	Kali ferrocyanatum
Ipc.	Ipecacuanha	K. i.	Kali iodatum
Ir. fl.	Iris florentina	K. m.	Kali muriaticum
Ir. foe.	Iris foetidissima	K. n.	Kali nitricum (Nitrum)
Ir. g.	Iris germanica	K. ox.	Kali oxalicum
Ir. t.	Iris tenax		(Kali manganicum)
Ird.	Iridium	K. ph.	Kali phosphoricum
Iris.	Iris versicolor	K. pi.	Kali picricum
Itu	Itu	K. pm.	Kali permanganicum
		K. s.	Kali sulphuratum
Ja. c.	Jacaranda caroba	K. sc.	Kali sulphuricum
Ja. g.	Jacaranda gualandai	K. tel.	Kali telluricum
Jab.	Jaborandi	K. trt.	Kali tartaricum
Jal.	Jalapa	Kam.	Kamla
Jas.	Jasminum	Kao.	Kaolin
Jat.	Jatropha	Kar.	Karaka
Jeq.	Jequirity	Ker.	Keroselenum
Jg. c.	Juglans cinerea	Kis.	Kissingen
Jg. r.	Juglans regia (Nux juglans)	Klm.	Kalmia latifolia
		Kou.	Kousso
Jn. c.	Juniperus communis	Kre.	Kreosotum
Jn. v.	Juniperus virginianus		
Jnc.	Juncus	Lab.	Laburnum
Jt. u.	Jatropha urens	Lach.	Lachesis
		Lam.	Lamium
Ka. ac.	Kali aceticum	Lap.	Lapathum (Rumex obtusifolia)
K. as.	Kali arsenicosum		
K. bi.	Kali bichromicum	Lau.	Laurocerasus
K. br.	Kali bromatum	Lc. c.	Lac caninum

Lc. f.	Lac felinum
Lc. v.	Lac vaccinum
Lc. v. c.	Lac vaccinum coagulatum
Lc. v. d.	Lac vaccinum defloratum
Lc. v. f.	Lactis vaccini flos
Lc. x.	Lacticum acidum
Lchn.	Lachnanthes
Lcrt.	Lacerta
Lcs.	Lycopus
Lct. v.	Lactuca virosa
Led.	Ledum
Leo.	Leonurus cardiaca
Lev.	Levico
Li. br.	Lithium bromatum
Li. bz.	Lithium benzoicum
Li. c.	Lithium carbonicum
Li. l.	Lithium lacticum
Li. l.	Lithium muriaticum
Lia.	Liatris spicata
Lil.	Lilium tigrnum
Lim.	Limulus
Lina.	Linaria
Lip. m.	Lippia mexicana
Lips.	Lippspringe
Lmn.	Lemna minor
Ln. c.	Linum catharticum
Ln.p.	Lonicera periclymenum
Ln.u.	Linum usitatissimum
Lo. c.	Lobelia cardinalis
Lo. d.	Lobelia dortmanna
Lo. e.	Lobelia erinus
Lo. i.	Lobelia inflata
Lo. p.	Lobelia purpurascens

Lo. s.	Lobelia syphilitica
Lol.	Lolium temulentum
Lon.	Lonicera xylosteum
Lp. a.	Lapis albus (calcarea silicofluorica)
Lpi.	Lepidium bonariense
Lpsa.	Lapsana communis
Lpt.	Leptandra
Lrs.	Lycopersicum
Lt. k.	Latrodectus katipo (Katipo)
Lt. m.	Latrodectus mactans
Lth.	Lathyrus
Lun.	Luna
Lup.	Lupulus
Lyc.	Lycopodium
Lys.	Lysidinum
Mac.	Macrotinum
Mag. c.	Mangnesia carbonica
Mag. m.	Magnesia muriatica
Mag. p.	Magnesia phosphorica
Mag. s	Magnesia sulphurica
Man.	Manganum, *including* M. aceticum *and* M. carbonicum
Mat.	Matthiola graeca
Mds.	Medusa
Med.	Medorrohinum
Men.	Menyanthes
Mep.	Mephitis
Merc.	Mercurius, *including* M. oxydulatus niger (M.sol. Hahn.) *and* M.vivus

Mez.	Mezereum
Mgn. gl.	Magnolia glauca
Mgn. gr.	Magnolia grandiflora
Mgt.	Magnetis poli ambo
Mgt. n.	Magnetis polus arcticus
Mgt. s.	Magnetis polus australis
Mil.	Millefolium
Mim.	Mimosa
Mit.	Mitchella
Mla.	Melastoma
Mld.	Malandrinum
Mli.	Melilotus
Mlr.	Malarica officinalis
Mlt.	Melitagrinum
Mn. a	Manganum aceticum
Mn. c.	Manganum carbonicum
Mn. m.	Manganum muriaticum
Mn. o.	Manganum oxydatum nativum
Mn. s.	Manganum sulphuricum
Mnc.	Mancinella
Mnd.	Mandragora
Mns.	Menispermum
Mo. a.	Morphinum aceticum
Mo. m.	Morphinum muriaticum
Mo. s.	Morphinum sulphuricum
Mom.	Momordica
Mor.	Morphinum
Mos.	Moschus
Mr. ac.	Mercurius aceticus
Mr. bin.	Mercurius biniodatus
Mr. c.	Mercurius corrosivus
Mr. cy.	Mercurius cyanatus
Mr. d.	Mercurius dulcis

Mr. i. f.	Mercurius protoiodatus
Mr. k. i.	Mercurius biniodatus *cum* Kali iodatum
Mr. n.	Mercurius nitricus
Mr. p. a.	Mercurius praecipitatus albus
Mr. p. a.	Mercurius praecipitatus ruber
Mr. s.	Mercurius sulphuricus
Mr. scy.	Mercurius sulphocyanatus
Mr. sol.	Mercurius oxydulatus niger (M. solubilis Hahn.)
Mr. v.	Mercurius vivus
Mrl.	Mercurialis perennis
Mrt.	Myrtus communis
Mst. s.	Myristica sebifera
Mth. b.	Methylene-blue
Mth. pi.	Mentha piperita
Mth. pu.	Mentha pulegium
Mu. u.	Mucuna urens
Mu. x.	Muriaticum acidum
Mur.	Murex
Mus.	Musa
My. c.	Myrica cerifera
Myg.	Mygale
Myo.	Myosotis
Na. as.	Natrum arsenicicum
Na. c.	Natrum carbonicum
Na. cc.	Natrum cacodylicum
Na. hch.	Natrum hypochlorosum
Na. i.	Natrum iodatum
Na. l.	Natrum lacticum

Na. m.	Natrum muriaticum	Oena.	Oenanthe crocata
Na. n.	Natrum nitricum	Oeno.	Oenothera
Na. ns.	Natrum nitrosum	Ol. a.	Oleum animale
Na. p.	Natrum phosphoricum	Ol. j.	Oleum jecoris aselli
Na. s.	Natrum sulphuricum	Oln.	Oleander
Na. sa.	Natrum salicylium	Onis.	Oniscus
Na. se.	Natrum selenicum	Onon.	Ononis
Na. sf.	Natrum silicofluoricum (Salufer)	Onos.	Onosomodium
		Oop.	Oophorinum
Na. ss.	Natrum sulphurosum	Opi.	Opium
Nab.	Nabalus	Opu.	Opuntia
Naj.	Naja	Orc.	Orchitinum (Sperminum)
Nct.	Nicotinum	Ori.	Origanum
Nec.	Nectrianinum	Ore.	Oreodaphne
Ni. c.	Niccolum carbonicum	Orn.	Ornithogalum umbellatum
Ni. s.	Niccolum sulphuricum	Osm.	Osmium
Nic.	Niccolum, *including* N. metallicum *and* N. carbonicum	Ost.	Ostrya
		Ov. g. p.	Ovi gallinae pellicula
		Ox. x.	Oxalicum acidum
Nm. x.	Nitroso- muriaticum acidum	Oxd.	Oxydendron
		Oxg.	Oxygenium *including* Ozonum
Nph.	Naphthalinum		
Nrn.	Narcotinum	Oxt.	Oxytropis lamberti (Locoweed)
Nrs.	Narcissus		
Nt.o.	Nitrogenum oxygenatum		
Nt. s. d.	Nitri spiritus dulcis	Paeo.	Paeonia
Nt. x.	Nitricum acidum	Pal.	Palladium
Nup.	Nuphar luteum	Pan.	Pancreatinum
Nux.	Nux vomica	Par.	Paris
Nx. m.	Nux moschata	Pas.	Passiflora
Nyc.	Nyctanthes	Pau.	Paullinia pinnata
Nym.	Nymphaea odorata	Pb.	Plumbum
		Pb. chr.	Plumbum chromicum
Ocm.	Ocimum canum	Pb. i.	Plumbum iodatum

Pbo.	Plumbago	Plnt.	Plantago
Pch.	Pichi	Plo.	Pilocarpinum
Pex.	Picrotoxinum	Plo. m.	Pilocarpinum muriacticum
Pec.	Pecten		
Ped.	Pediculus	Plo. n.	Pilocarpinum nitricum
Pel.	Pelargonium reniforme	Plp.	Polyporus pinicola
Pep.	Pepsinum	Plts.	Platanus
Per.	Persica	Pmo.	Pulmo vulpis
Pest.	Pestinum	Pmt.	Pimenta
Pet.	Petroleum	Pnt.	Penthorum sedoides
Ph. h.	Phosphorus hydrogenatus	Pod.	Podophyllum
Ph. m.	Phosphorus muriaticus	Pop. c.	Populus candicans
Ph. x.	Phosphoricum acidum	Pop. t.	Populus tremuloides
Phal.	Phallus impudicus	Ppz.	Piperazinum
Phas.	Phaseolus	Pr. p.	Prunus padus
Phel.	Phellandrium	Pr. s.	Prunus spinosa
Phen.	Phenacetinum	Pr. v.	Prunus virginiana
Phlo.	Phlorizinum	Prei.	Pareira
Pho.	Phosphorus	Prf.	Paraffinum
Phst.	Physostigma (Calabar)	Priet.	Parietaria
Phy.	Physalia	Prin.	Prinos verticillatus
Phyt.	Phytolacca	Prm. o.	Primula obconica
Pi.x.	Picricum acidum	Prm. ve.	Primula veris
Pim.	Pimpinella	Prm. vg.	Primula vulgaris
Pin. l.	Pinus lambertiana	Prt.	Parthenium
Pin. s.	Pinus sylvestris	Psc.	Piscidia
Pip. m.	Piper methysticum (Kava)	Pso.	Psorinum
Pip. n.	Piper nigrum	Pst.	Pastinaca
Pix.	Pix liquida	Pt. m.	Platinum muriaticum
Pl. n.	Pulsatilla nuttalinana	Pt. m. n.	Platinum muriaticum natronatum
Plat.	Platinum		
Ple.	Plectranthus	Ptl.	Ptelea
Plg.	Polygonum (persicaria urens)	Pts.	Petroselinum
		Ptv.	Petiveria

Pul.	Pulsatilla
Pyr. a.	Pyrus americana
Pyre.	Pyrethrum parthenium
Pyro.	Pyrogenium (Spesinum)
Qeb.	Quebracho
Qer.	Quercus
Qua.	Quassia
Rap.	Raphanus
Rat.	Ratanhia (Krameria)
Rdm.	Rhodium oxydatum nitricum
Rhe.	Rheum
Rho.	Rhododendron
Rhs.	Rhus radicans and R. toxicodendron (*both or either*)
Ric.	Ricinus (Oleum ricini)
Rm. c.	Rhamnus cathorticus
Rm. f.	Rhamnus frangula
Rn. a.	Ranunculus acris
Rn. b.	Ranunculus bulbosus
Rn. fi.	Ranunculus ficaria
Rn. fl.	Ranunculus flammula
Rn. g.	Ranunculus glacialis
Rn. r.	Ranunculus repens
Rn. s.	Ranunculus sceleratus
Ro. c.	Rosa canina
Ro. d.	Rosa damascena
Rob.	Robinia
Rs. a.	Rhus aromatica
Rs. d.	Rhus diversiloba
Rs. g.	Rhus glabra

Rs. r.	Rhus radicans
Rs. t.	Rhus toxicodendron
Rs. v.	Rhus venenata
Rsm.	Rosmarinus
Rub.	Rubia tinctorum
Rum.	Rumex crispus
Rus.	Russula
Rut.	Ruta
Rx. ac.	Rumex acetosa
Sac. l.	Saccharum lactis
Sac. o.	Saccharum officinale
Sang.	Sanguinaria canadensis
Sap.	Saponium
Sars.	Sarsaparilla
Sbd.	Sabadilla
Sbi.	Sabina
Sbl.	Sabal serrulata
Sca.	Scammonium
Sch.	Schinus
Scil.	Scilla maritima
Scir.	Scirrhinum
Scol.	Scolopendra
Scor.	Scorpio
Scro.	Scrophularia
Scu.	Scutellaria
Se. a.	Senecio aureus
Se. j.	Senecio jacobaea
Sec.	Secale cornutum
Sel.	Selenium
Sep.	Sepia
Sfn.	Sulfonal
Sg. n.	Sanguinarinum nitricum
Sg. t.	Sanguinarinum tartaricum

Sga.	Senega	Sol	Sol
Sgn.	Sanguinarinum	Son.	Solaninum
Sgs.	Sanguisuga	Son. ac.	Solaninum aceticum
Sgu.	Sphingurus	Sp. m.	Spigelia marilandica
Sil.	Silica	Spa. u.	Spiraea ulmaria
Sil. m.	Silica marina	Spi.	Spigelia
Sin. a.	Sinapis alba	Spo.	Spongia tosta
Sin. n.	Sinapis nigra	Sprn.	Spiranthes
Siu.	Sium	Sptn.	Septicaeminum
Sko.	Skookum chuck	Src.	Sarracenia
Sl. x.	Salicylicum acidum	Ss. x.	Sulphurosum acidum
Sla.	Slag	Sta.	Stachys betonica
Sld.	Solidago	Ste.	Stellaria media
Sll.	Salol	Sti.	Sticta pulmonaria
Sln.	Salicinum	Stil.	Stillingia sylvatica
Slp.	Silphium	Stm.	Stramonium
Slv.	Salvia	Stn.	Stannum
Smb. c.	Sambucus canadensis	Stn. i.	Stannum iodatum
Smb. n.	Sambucus nigra	Sto. b.	Strontium bromatum
Smp.	Sempervivum tectorum	Sto. c.	Strontium carbonicum
Sna.	Senna	Sto. n.	Strontium nitricum
Snc.	Sanicula	Stp.	Staphisagria
Snt.	Santalum	Strp.	Strophanthus
Sntn.	Santoninum	Sty.	Strychninum
So. a.	Solanum arrebenta	Sty. n.	Strychninum nitricum
So. c.	Solanum carolinense	Sty. p.	Strychninum phosphoricum
So. m.	Solanum mammosum		
So. n.	Solanum nigrum	Sty. s.	Strychninum sulphuricum
So. o.	Solanum oleraceum	Sty. v.	Strychninum valerianicum
So. pc.	Solanum pseudo-capsicum	Su. x.	Sulphuricum acidum
		Suc.	Succinum
So. t.	Solanum tuberosum	Sul.	Sulphur
So. t. ae.	Solanum tuberosum aegrotans	Sul. h.	Sulphur hydrogenisatum
		Sul. i.	Sulphur iodatum

Sul. t.	Sulphur terebinthinatum	Tnn.	Tannin
Sum.	Sumbul	Ton.	Tongo
Sx. m.	Salix mollissima	Tox.	Toxicophis
Sx. n.	Salix nigra	Trac.	Trachinus
Sx. p.	Salix purpurea	Trad.	Tradescantia
Sym. r.	Symphoricarpus racemosus	Trb.	Trombidium
		Trf. p.	Trifolium pratense
Symt.	Symphytum	Trf. r.	Trifolium repens
Syph.	Syphilinum (Luesinum or Lueticum)	Tri.	Triosteum
		Trl.	Trillium
Syz.	Syzygium	Trm.	Trimethylaminum (Propylaminum)
Tab.	Tabacum	Trn.	Tarentula hispanica
Tam.	Tamus	Trn. c.	Tarentula cubensis
Tax.	Taxus baccata	Trp.	Tropaeolum
Tea.	Thea	Trt.	Triticum repens
Tel.	Tellurium	Trx.	Taraxacum
Tep.	Teplitz	Ts. ff.	Tussilago farfara
Ter.	Terebinthina	Ts. fg.	Tussilago fragrans
Teu.	Teucrium marum-verum	Ts. p.	Tussilago petasites
Teu. s.	Teucrium scorodonia	Tt. x.	Tartaricum acidum
Tha.	Thallium	Ttr.	Tetradymite
Ther.	Theridion	Tub.	Tuberculinum
Thev.	Thevetia	Tur.	Turnera aphrodisiaca (Damiana)
Thio.	Thiosinaminum		
Thl.	Thlaspi bursa pastoris (Bursa pastoris)	Ul. f.	Ulmus fulva
Thri.	Thyroiodinum	Up.	Upas
Thu.	Thuja	Ur. n.	Uranium nitricum
Thyr.	Thyroidinum	Ur. x.	Uricum acidum
Til.	Tilia	Ure.	Urea
Tit.	Titanium	Uri.	Urinum
Tnc.	Tanacetum	Urt.	Urtica urens
Tng.	Tanghinia	Usn.	Usnea barbata

Ust.	Ustilago	Vsp.	Vespa
Uva	Uva-ursi		
		Wil.	Wildbad
Vac.	Vaccininum	Wis.	Wiesbaden
Val.	Valeriana	Wye.	Wyethia
Van.	Vanadium		
Var.	Variolinum	Xan.	Xanthoxylum
Vb. o.	Viburnum opulus	Yoh.	Yohimbinum
Vb. p.	Viburnum prunifolium	Yuc.	Yucca filamentosa
Vb. t.	Viburnum tinus (Laurustinus)	Zea	Zea mays, Mais,stigmata maidis or Shucks
Vbn.	Verbena hastata		
Vbs.	Verbascum	Zeash.	Shucks
Ve. n.	Veratrum nigrum	Zeast.	Stigmata maidis
Ve. v.	Veratrum veride	Zin.	Zincum
Ver.	Veratrum album	Ziz.	Zizia
Ves.	Vesicaria	Zn. a.	Zincum aceticum
Vi. o.	Viola odorata	Zn. br.	Zincum bromatum
Vi. t.	Viola tricolor	Zn. cy.	Zincum cyanatum
Vic.	Vichy	Zn. i.	Zincum iodatum
Vin.	Vinca minor	Zn. m.	Zincum muriaticum
Vip.	Vipera	Zn. o.	Zincum oxydatum
Vis.	Viscum album	Zn. p.	Zincum phosphoricum
Voe.	Voeslau	Zn. pi.	Zincum picricum
Vp. r.	Vipera redi	Zn. s.	Zincum sulphuricum
Vp. t.	Vipera torva	Zn. v.	Zincum valerianicum
Vrn.	Veratrinum	Zng.	Zingiber

Part I

A Clinical Repertory

Introduction to
A CLINICAL REPERTORY

PERHAPS the best way for me to introduce the CLINICAL
REPERTORY to my readers will be to quote from the *Dictionary of
Materia Medica* that part of the Preface which describes the
portion here repertorised. Writing the section "Clinical" with
which each remedy is introduced in that work, I said :—

"Clinical"

"Next under the head CLINICAL, I have given an alphabetical list of the diseases
in relation to which the remedy has manifested or seems likely to manifest some
curative power. This list is of no independent authority, many of the items being
merely suggestions of my own. It is not to be regarded either as inclusive or
exclusive, but rather as suggestive. But the list serves further purposes ; and first,
it enables me to save space. If I were to describe the sphere of a remedy in each
of the diseases in which it has been used, i should be obliged to repeat the same
indications many times over in slightly varied form. The main indications of a
remedy same in a any disease, and the fine indications will be found on referring
to the headings under which they occur in the Schema. Further, the list enables me
to relate the *Dictionary* to the *Prescriber*. A number of the names of diseases in the
list will be found printed in italics. This does not mean that the medicine is more
indicated in these diseases than in the others; it is merely to indicate that under that
particular heading the drug will be found mentioned in the *Prescriber*, and that there
its special indications are given and compared with those of other remedies. For
example, under ATROPINUM is the following list: 'Blepharospasm. Convulsions.
Enuresis. Epilepsy. Eyes, affections of. *Gastric Ulcer*. Locomotor ataxy. Mania.
Neuralgia. *Pancreatitis*. Spinal irritation. Tetanus. Vision, disorders of.' On

referring to the *Prescriber*, under GASTRIC ULCER and PANCREATITIS, *Atropinum* will found mentioned along with other remedies. Finally, the lists will be afford a convenient basis for compiling a Clinical index."

THE CLINICAL REPERTORY here presented is the work promised in the last sentence of the above-quoted passage.

It will be noted that the *Dictionary* was linked to the *Prescriber* in the Clinical section of the former. That link is preserved in the CLINICAL REPERTORY. But instead of the names *diseases* being italicised , as in the Clinical headings, the names of the *remedies* an italicised in the CLINICAL REPERTORY. In the example quoted above the words *"Gastric Ulcer"* and *"Pancreatitis"* were printed in italics to show that *Atropinum* under which they occur would be found mentioned under these headings in the *Prescriber* and its indications compared with those of other remedies. In the CLINICAL REPERTORY, under the heading "Gastric ULCER" and "Pancreatitis," among the remedies given *"Atro."* appears in italics. This indicates that under the same headings it is given in the *Prescriber*. Under Locomotor Ataxy *"Atro."* appears but not in italics. This implies that it is not given in the *prescriber* under the heading.

The edition of the *prescriber* to which reference is made in this work is the sixth, which I prepared in the interval between the appearance of the first and second volumes of *Dictionary*. In it will be found an Introductory chapter on "The Place of a Clinical Repertory in Homoeopathic Practice." Having gone fully into this subject there I need say little about it in this connection. The chief problem of scientific therapeutics consists in the discovering of indications for remedies. All ways of finding indications are open to practitioners, and the clinical avenue is one of them. This is not the method which Hahnemann rightly condemned, and which is still the prevailing one in old-school therapeutics, that, namely, of seeking for remedies for *diseases in the abstract*. One result of this last method is that certain diseases come to have certain remedies assigned to them, and all patients who are found to be suffering from any given disease must be dosed with one of the remedies credited to it. Hahnemann delivered all who have accepted his scientific method from the thraldom of this purely academic, artificial practice. He fitly described it as "treating the names of diseases with the names of therapeutic actions."

There will not, I think, be any likelihood of the readers lapsing into this kind of practice through the use of my CLINICAL REPERTORY. The lists of remedies are in no the way put forth as complete lists. In homoeopathy any remedy may be required in any case of nay disease. The occurrence of the name of any remedy under the heading of any disease shows that in its action it has a general correspondence with the most marked features of cases of that disease. This gives a legitimate point of comparison for a start, at any rate, in the work of selection.

It will frequently happen that the prescriber will have in mind a number of remedies which more or less closely correspond to a given case, and when he consults the CLINICAL REPERTORY this knowledge will enable him at once pick out of the list there presented the most similar remedy to his case. Should he still be uncertain, if the *Prescriber* does not help him out of his difficulty, he will still have the *Dictionary* to appeal to, in which each of the remedies in named in the REPERTORY will be found described individually in detail.

Further, if there is any point of *Causation* in the case, or any striking type of *Temperament*, this work may itself provide the determining factor without the prescriber having to go further afield.

The use of the nosological correspondence is, as I have said, one method by means of which a similar, if not the most similar, remedy may be discovered. Another method is by ascertaining the similarity of *Specificity of seat*. Some drugs have a predominant affinity for certain organs, and these drugs will often relieve a great variety of affections seated in, or arising from diseases of these particular organs. In compiling the CLINICAL part of my *Dictionary* I kept this in view. Many general headings such as "Liver, diseases of", "Spleen, affections of," will be found there; and they will also be found in the CLINICAL REPERTORY. The lists of remedies given under these headings will show the drugs which have been observed to hit these organs hardest, and will thereby give a very important point for comparison. The work of Paracelsus and his disciple Rademacher deals largely in Specifics based on this homoeopathicity of organaffinity. The greatest modern exponent of this practice is the late Dr. Compton Burnett, who has brought once more to light vast therapeutic treasures which had been allowed to the lie forgotten in the works of these great masters. Those who understand the value of such indications will find much to assist them in the CLINICAL REPERTORY.

A CLINICAL REPERTORY

[The name of a remedy printed in italics signifies that the same remedy may be found mentioned in the Prescriber under the same heading. The name of a remedy appearing in the brackets signifies that the particular affection under which it appears does not occur in the Dictionary of Materia Medica under to the CLINICAL heading, but has been added to my copy since the Dictionary was published.

Abdomen, COLDNESS in—Phel., Ple.

    DISTENDED—*Cin., Dio., Fil., Ign., Lyc., Sil., Thu.*

    LARGE—*Calc.*

    OPERATIONS on, VOMITING after—Bis. Cep.

    PLETHORA of—Alo.

    SWELLING of—Prf.

    THROBBING in—Bru.

Abortion—Alet,. Asc. s., Fil., Gos., Kou., Lyc., Mur., Nx. M., Prt., Pin., 1. Rhs., Rsm., Rum., Sbi., Tan., Thu.

    AFTER-EFFECTS of—Sbi.

    HAEMORRHAGE after—Thl.

    TENDENCY to.—Act. r.

    THREATENED—Bap., Caul., Cro., Ham., Phyt., Sec., Vb. p.

    See also **Miscarriage.**

Abscess.—Anan. *Aps., Arn., Ars., Bel.,* Ca. s., *Caln., Chi.,* Elt., *Fl., x.,* Gui., *Hep.,* Hpz., Mat., *Mr. Sol.,* Na.sa., Pyro., *Sil.,* Symt., Syph., Thyr.

    COLD ABSCESS.—Ol. J.

Abscesses, MULTIPLE—Vsp.

SUCCESSION of.- Syph.

Acetonaemia.—(Cbl. x.)

Acidity.—*Ag. n.,* Ca. ar. *Calc., Cb. v.* Cham. Lo. s., Lun., Par., Pod., Pr., v., Rob., *Su. x.*

INFANTS, in.—Na. p.

Acne.—Ail., Athra., Ant. s. a., Ar.lp., As. br. As. r., Ast. r. *Bel.,* Bls., *Cb. v.,* Cbl. x., Crb. s., Chm. u., Cop., Dio., Gph., (Ign.), Ind., Jg.c., Jg. r., K. bi. *K. br.,* K. m., Kre., Mld., Pi. x., Pix, Pso., *Pul.,* Sil., Sul., i., Sum. Tub., Uri., Vin.

Acne, NOSE, of.—Caus.

PUNCTATA—Sul. i.

ROSACEA—*Aga.,* Ars., *As. i. Cb. a.* Caus., Eug., *Hyd., Nux,* Oop., *Rhs, Ss. x.*

Acromegaly—Thyr.

Actinomycosis—K. i., *Nt. x.*

Addisons Disease.—Adr., *Ag. n., Bac., Na. m.,* Ol. j., Pet., Van.

Adenitis—Dul.

Adenoids—Agr. n., (Calc.), Ca. fl., Lo. s., *Pso.,* Sg. n., Spi., Stp., *Sul.*

Adhesions—Thio.

PLEURITIC—Ran b.

Adrenal Neuralgia—Adr.

After-Pains—Caul., Cham., Cro., Cup., Hyp., Lach., Opi., Par., Rhs., Sbi., Sec., Vb. o., Xan.

Agalactia—Agn., Caus., Urt., Ust.

See also **Lactation,** DEFECTIVE., **Milk,** ABSENCE of ; *and* **Milk,** SUPPRESSED.

Ague—E. ar., Mlr., Plnt., Sul., Trx., Vbn.

CHRONIC—Vbn.

See also **Brow-Ague**; **Fever,** INTERMITTENT; *and* **intermittent Fever.**

Albuminuria—Ado., Am. bz., Arm., Au., m., Ca. ar., Cnb., Cub., Evm., Ev. a., E. pu., Fe. i., Fe. pi., Hel., Hlon., Hoa., K. chl., Kis., Lc. v., Lach., Li. c., Lyc., Mth. b., Nph., Na. c., Na. hch., Ocm., Ena., Pet., Phas., Phyt., Pilo., Pip. m.

Ric., Smb. c., Sec., Sld., Sfn., Ter., Thyr., Tub., Ur. n.,
Ure., Ves., Z. st., Zng.

PREGNANCY, of—Thyr. (*see also* **Pregnancy,** ALBUMINURIA of.)
See also **Retinitis** ALBUMINURICA.

Alcohol, Effects of—Aln., Aur., Calc., Fe. I., Grna., Sep.

Alcohol Habit—Sul.

Alcoholism—Ana., *Ant. t.,* Apm., Ars., Asr., Avn., Bry., Chi., Ch. m.,
Fl. x. Hdr., Lach., Lo. i., *Nux,* Qer., Rn. b. Rap., Sang.,
Sel., *Strp.,* Syph., *Zin.*

CHRONIC—Su. x.

HEREDITARY CRAVING FOR ALCOHOL—Syph.

Alopecia—All., Asc. t., Bac., Cup. s., Fl. x., Jab., Lo. i., Ol. j.,
Pilo., Ust., Vsp., Vin.

AREATA—K. ph., Pho.

See also **Baldness ;** *and* **Hair,** FALLING OFF.

Amaurosis—*Aco.,* Ant. s. a., Au. m., *Bel.,* Bz. n., Cap., Crd. b.,
Caus., Cen., Dph., Dig., Elp., Fe. mg., Gel., *Hep.,* Hyo.,
Men., *Nux, Pho.,* Pb., Pul., So. n., So. t., Spi., Sty., Sul.,
Tab., Up., Ve. v.

Amblyopia—Anag., Bz. d., Crb. s., *Chi.,* Cich., Chn. s., Crt. h.,
Dph., Drs., Lach., Mrl., Nph., *Nux,* Onos., Oxt., *Ph. x.,*
Pho., Ph. h., Rap., *Rut.,* Sac. I., *Sntn.,* Sga., Thyr., Zin.

POTATORUM—Ter.

Amenorrhoea—Alns., Ars., Aur., Bry., Caul., Epn., Fe. i., Gas.,
Gos., Gph., Gui., Hdm., Hel., Hlon., Ind., K. ca., K. ph.,
Kre., Ln. c., Lo. i., Mgt. n., Ol. j., Ov. g. p., Prt., Pin. l.,
Plat., Pod., Plg., Pul., Pl. n., Rho., Rhs., Snc., Se. a., Sep.,
Sin. n., *Sul.,* Tan., Tep., Thyr., Tur., Ver., Ve. v., Wis., Wye.

Anaemia—Ac. X., Alet., Anil., *Ag. n., Ars.,* Au. ar., Bz. d., *Calc.,*
Ca. p., Crb. s., Csc., *Chi.,* Chl. h., Cin., Cyc., Fer., Fe. as.,
Fe. m., Hlon., Ipc., Ird., K. bi., K. ca., K. ph., Lc. v. d.,
Man, Merc., *Na. m.,* Na. n., Ol. j., Oxg., *Pet., Pi. x.,* Pb.,
Pul., Rub., *Sil.,* Stn., Strp., Sul., Tab., *Thyr.,* Urt., Ver.

ACUTE PERNICIOUS—*Pho.,* Pi. x., *Thyr.*

See also **Brain,** ANAEMIA of; *and* **Malarial Anaemia.**

Anaesthesia—Ctn. ch., Ker., Pb.

Anaesthetics, Antidote to—Ac. x.

Anasarca—Frg., Ver.

    SCARLATINA, after—Stm.

Aneurism—*As. i., Ba. c.,* Ba. m., Cac., Ca. fl., Cb. a., Euc., Gui.,
    K. i., Lach., Li. c., *Lyc.,* Lcs., Mgn. gr., Pb., Rn. s., Spo.

Anger—*Aco., Cham., Cro.*

    EFFECTS of—Bry., Coc., *Ign., Nux.* (*See also* **Asthma,** FROM
    ANGER)

    FITS of—Ce. s., *Stp.*

Angina Faucium—Dul.

    PECTORIS—*Act. r., Aml.,* Ag. cy., *Asi.,* Aur., Au. m., Bis.,
    Cac., Ca. hp.; Cam., *Cb. v.,* Chm. m., Ch. ar., Ch. s., ChI. h.,
    Chr. o., Coca, *Crat.,* Cu. a., *Cup.,* Dig., Dio., Glo., Haem.,
    Hep., *Hy. x.,* Hyo., Jg. c., Klm., Lct. v., Lt. m., *Lil., Li.c.,*
    Lo. i., Lyc., Mgn. gr., Mos., *Naj.,* Na. ns., Ox. x., Pet.,
    Phyt., Sac. l., Smb. c., Smb. n., Scil, Scol., Spi., Spo., Sti.,
    Sto. c., Tab., Trn., Ther., Thu., Thyr., Ver., Wis., Zn. v.

    TONSILLARIS—Fe. m. (*See also* **Quinsy; Tonsillitis;** *and*
    Tonsils, INFLAMED)

Anidrosis—*K. i., Na. c., Pb.*

Ankle, ITCHING ERUPTION about—Sel.

    PAINS in—Trm.

Ankle, PAINFUL—Mn. m.

    SPRAIN of—Sto. c.

    SWELLING of—*Aps.,* Mim.

    WEAK—*Calc., Ca.. p., Ham.,* Man., Mn. m., Na. c., Pin. s., *Sil*

Anorexia—Gn.I., Gn. q., Lo. c., Pr. v.

    See also **Appetite,** LOST

Anosmia—*Am. m.*

    See also **Smell,** Loss of.

Anterior Crural Neuralgia—Gel., Gna., Snc.

 Anthrax, of Sheep—Ther.

Antidote to Poisons—Cf. t.

Antiseptic—Brc. x.

    See also **Sepsis.**

Antrum of Highmore, AFFECTIONS of— Com., *Mag. c., Mr. c.*

    DISEASE of—K. *sc., Pho.*

    INFLAMMATION of—*Chel.*

    PAIN in—Eu. a., Mr. bin., Plg.

    TUMOUR of—Hec.

Anus, ABSCESS of—Ba. m.

    ABSCESS near—Ca. s.,

    AFFECTIONS of—*AEsc.,* Alo., *Alm., Aln., Gam., Gph., Ign.,* Lct.
        V., Paeo., Sin. a.

    BLEEDING from—Csc.; *Sgs.*

    BURNING in—Jg. r., Mr.p.r., Rdm., Sto. c.

    CONSTRICTION of—Nm. x.

    EXCORIATION AND CHAPS of—Agn.

    FISSURE of—Cep., Iris, *Nt. x.,* Paeo., Pet., Pho., Phyt., Pip. n.,
        Rat., Rhs., Sil., Syph., Thu.

    FISTULA of—Au. m., Paeo., Sil., Thu.

    HERPES of—E. pf.

    INCONTINENCE of—Erg., Sec.

    IRRITATION of—*Amb., Ant. c., Cin.*

    ITCHING in—Ca.. ac. Cop., Pin. s., Pso., Rn. s., Rm, f., Rdm.,
        Sin. a., Sla.., Stp., *Teu., Vbs.*

    OPEN —Sec.

    PAIN in—Sti.

    PATULOUS—So. t. ae.

    PRESSURE of—Sep.

    PROLAPSE of—Asr., Ery. a., Eu. a., *Fe. p.,* Ind., *Mu. x.,* Pip. m.,
        Pod., Plp., Rut., So. t. ae., Sul., Tab.,. Trb. .(*See also*
        Prolapsus ANI.)

    PRURITUS of—Pho., Ur. n.

    RHAGADES of—Cnd. (*See also* FISSURE of.)

Anus, SORENESS of—Jal., Sla.

SPASM of—Eu. a.

SWEATING near—Pyro.

Anxiety—*Ign.*

Aorta, Pain in—Sty.

Aortitis—Cb. v., Euc.

Aphasia—Chn. a., Glo., *K. br., Lyc., Stm.,* Syph.

See also **Speech,** Lost

Aphonia—Amm., Anan., Arm., Cb. v., Dul., Fer., Gel., K. chs., Pop. c., Rum., Sang., Sty.

See also **Voice,** Loss of.

Aphthae—*Ant. t., Ars.,* Asi., *Bor.,* Bry., Chi. b., Chi., Chlm., Co. c., Cub., E. *ar.,* Fe. s., Frl., Hel., *K. chl.,* K. m., Merc., *Mr. c., Mu. x.,* Na. m., Ric., Su. x.

Apoplexy—*Aco.,* Ana., Aps., *Arn.,*As. f., Ast. r., Bap., Ba. c., *Bel.,* Bro., Bry., Cac., Cd. br., Cd. s., Crb. h., Crb. s., Caus., Chn. a., Chi., Chl. h., Cof., Crt. h., Cu. a., Fl. x., For., Gas., Glo., Gre., Hel., Jn. v., K. br., K. cy., Lach., Lim., Li. br., Na. ns., Nx. m., *Nux,* CEna., *Opi.,* Rn. g., Sep., Sin. n., So. a., Stm., Sto. c., Tab., Ver., Ve. v.

THREATENED—Lau., Prm. ve.

Appendicitis—Amc., Bap., Clch., Crt. h., (Dio.), Ech. a., Gin., *Ir. t.,* Lc. v. d., Lach., Merc., Mr. c., Pb., Rm. c., Rm. f., Rhs., Sbl., Scro., Tub.

See also **Typhlitis.**

Appetite, DEPRAVED. — *Calc., Pul., Sep., Sil.*

DISORDERED—*Act. r., Cb. a., Chi., Hep., Ign., Iod.*

LOST. — *Pr. s., Rhs.* (See also **Anorexia.**)

Arachnitis—Chlf.

Ardor Urinae—Pix, Pop. t., Rm. f., Rhe., Scu.

Arms, Varicosis of—Lc. c.

Arteries, AFFECTIONS of—Ca. hp.

ATHEROMA of—Cac.

DISEASES of—Bls., *Pho.*

THROBBING of—Fag.

Arterio-sclerosis—Pb. i.

Arthritis—Arb., Icth.

DEFORMANS—Caus.

See also **Gout.**

Ascarides—Ac. x., Anth. n., Ar. m., Grn., Mag. c., Sep.

Ascites—Agn., Apo., Au. m. n., Can. s., Cep., Cinm., Lct. v., Led., Lpt., Pr.s., Sac. o., Se. a., Sga.

Asphyxia—Sul. h.

NEONATORUM—Ant. t., Lau.

Asthenopia—Amc., Cb. v., Cin., Cro., Jab., Lach., LiI., Man., Nic., Rho., Sec.

Asthma—*Aco.,* Amb., Amc., Am. c., Amg., Antf., Ant. i., *Ant. t.,* Aps., Aral., Ag. cy., Arm., *Ars.,* Ar. dm., Ar. m., Asa., Asc. t., Aur., Au. m., Ba. m., Bz. x., Bl. a., Bl. o., Bro., Bry., Cac., Cld., Ca. ar., Ca. hp., Can. s., Cap., Cb. v., Chn. a., Chi., Ch. ar., Ch. s., Chl. h., *Chlm.,* Cin., Coca, Ccs. c., Cof., Clch., Con., *Cup.,* Der., Dgn., Dig., Drs., Erio., Euc., Eu. pi., Fel., Fer., Gad., Ga. x., Glv., Gnd., Hep., Hdr., *Hy. x.,* Hyp., *Ibe.,* Ict., Ipc., Jnc., K. bi., K. br., K. *ca.,* K. chl., K. chs., K. cy., K. n., K. ph., K. sc., Lc. v. d., Lach., Lct. v., Lau., Led., Lmn., Ln. u., Lo. *i.,* Lo. s., Lyc., Mgn. gl., Mnc., Man., Med., Mep., Mr. bin., Mil., Naj., Nph., Na. s., *Nux,* Ol. a., OI. j., Osm., Pec., Phel., Ph. x., Pho., Ph. m., Phyt., Pb., Pop. c., Pso., Ptl., Pmo., Qeb., Rum., Smb. c., Smb. n., Sang., Sg. n., Snc. Sars., Scil., Sga., Slp., Spo., Stn., Sti., Sty., Suc., *Sul.* h., Sum., Syph., Tab., Ter., Thu., Trac., Tri., Tub., Var., Ver., *Ve. v.,* Wye.. Xan., Zin., Zn. v., Zng., Ziz.

ANGER, from—Cham.

BRONCHIAL—Pod.

CATARRHAL—Sbl.

DRY—Scil.

HUMID—Pec.

HYSTERICAL—Nx. m.

MILLARI—Crl., Cup., Gre., Lo. i.

NERVOUS—Val.

PERIODICAL—All.

PITUITOUS—Sin. n.

SPASMODIC—Val.

SPLENIC—Scil.

    See also **Cardiac Asthma;** *and Miner's Asthma.*

Astigmatism—Gel., Lil., Phst.

Atelectasis—Sul.

Atheroma—Lach., Van.

Athetosis—Lth., *Sty.*

Atony—Rs. a.

Atrophic Pharyngitis—Sbl.

Atrophic Rhinitis—K. bi.. Lmn., Sbl.

    See also **Nose.**

Atrophy—*Ars.*, Ba. c., Ca. si., Cet., *Iod.,* K. ph., Na. *m., Pb.,* Pb. i.,
Sbl.

    See also **Breast,** ATROPHY of; **Children,** EMANCIPATED;
Marasmus; *and* **Progressive Muscular Atrophy.**

Aura of Epilepsy—Nct., Vis.

Aural Neuralgia—Cof.

Axilla, ABSCESS in—Hep., Ird.

    INFLAMED GLAND in—Rap.

    ITCHING in—Elp.

    PAIN in—*Jg. c.*

    PERSPRIRATION of—*K. ca.*

    PERSPIRATION of, OFFENSIVE—*Lyc., Nt. x.,* Tel.

    TUMOUR of—Tel.

Axillary Glands, SUPPURATION of—Jg. r.

Back, ACHING of—*K. ca. (See also* **Backache.)**

    AFFECTIONS of— *AEsc.*

    PAINS in—*Act. r., Arn.,* Ca. cs., E. pf., Homa, Lo. S., Nym., *Ox.
x.,* Src.

PULSATION in—Rn. r.

STIFFNESS of—Su. x.

WEAKNESS of—*Ca. p., Chi., Ign., Sil.*

Backache—AEsc., Ccs. c., Glg., Gam., Idm., Inu., Jnc., K. *ca.,* Lrs.. Mns., Pso., Sbl., Stp., Tab., *Ter.,* Thyr., Tri., Var.

SEXUAL EXCESS from—Symt.

Balanitis—*Caln., Mr. sol.,* Thu.

Balanorrhoea—Ja. c.

Baldness—Arn., Ba. c., Rsm., Sep., Tha.

See also Alopecia; and **Hair,** FALLING OFF .

Barber's Itch—Li. c., Phyt., Sul. i., Tel.

Barrenness—Caul.

See also **Sterility.**

Bashfulness—Amb., Stp.

Bathing, EFFECTS of—Phst.

Bazin's Disease—(Bac.), (Tub.), (Sec.)

Beard, ERUPTIONS of—Hep.

SYCOSIS of—*Calc.*

Bearing—down Pains—Caul.

Bed-sores—Arn., Cam., Chl. h., (Fl. x.), Hpz., Lach., Paeo., Pet., Pyro., Sul., Val.

Bee-stings—Snc., Urt.

Beri-Beri—Lth., Rhs.

Bile, Excess of—Mn. s.

Biliary Colic—Ber.

See also **Gall-stone Colic.**

Bilious Affections—Ant. t.

ATTACK. — *Ber., Bry., Chi., Iris, Lpt., Nux, Pod., Trx.*

FEVER —Asc. t., Crt. h., Elt., Ev. a., E. pf., Gel., Lpt., Mlr., Nyc.

HEADACHE—Co. c. (*See also* **Headache,** BILIOUS) .

Biliousness—Aq. m., Ast. f., Bap., Ber. a., Dio., Ev. a., *Fer.,* Frg.. Gn. l., *K. ca., Lyc., Mag. m, Na. s., Nux, Sul.,* Yuc.

Bites—Gnd., Hyp., Led.

RABID ANIMALS, of—Ech. a. (*See also* **Dog-bite.**)

REPTILES, of—Lcs. (*See also* **Snake -bites** and **Tarentula-bites.**)

Black-eye—*Arn.,* Erig., *Ham.,* Led.

Bladder, AFFECTIONS of—Aps., Baro., *Bz. x., Ber., Cth., Caus.. Dul.,* Elt., Euc., Gad., Geu., *Nux.* Ro. a., Sars.

CATARRH of—Hdrn. a., Pop. t., *Prei., Pul.,* Sga., Slp., Trl., Vic. (*See also* **Cystitis.**)

CATARRH of, CHRONIC—*Nt. x.* (See also **Cystitis.**)

HAEMORRHAGE from—Rs. a. (Mil.).

INFLAMMATION of—Con. (See also **Cystitis.**)

IRRITABLE—*Cop.,* Gli., Mit., Onos., Oxt., Pyr. a., *Sga.,* Sep., *Ter.* Trt.

PAINS in—Sty.

PARALYSIS of—Cac., Cia. v., *Fe. p.,* Hyo., Nrn., *Opi., Sec.,* Sty.

(*See also* **Urine,** INCONTINENCE of, ,&c.)

PARESIS of—Mag. m.

PROLAPSEof—Pyr. a.

STONE in—Ca. ren., Epg., Hdrn. a., Lips.

WEAKNESS of—Bel.

Blenorrhagia—Cop., Ja. g., Pip. n.

Blepharitis—Arg., Cham., Ephr., Gph., Hep., Plg., Stp.

CILIARIS—Mr. i. f., Sga.

Blepharo-conjunctivitis—Up.

Blepharophthalmia—Dul.

Blepharospasm—Aga., Atr., Cham., *Cod.,* Cro., Der., Eser., Grna.. Jat., Phst., *Pul.*

Blindness—Acn., Bth., Fil., Hur., Hur. c., Klm., Lc. v., Mnc., Mep., Rus.

DAY—Bth.

NIGHT—*Bel., Hel.,* Hyo., Nux, Pts., Rn. b., Sty., Ver.

SUDDEN—Aco.

Blood-poisoning—Ech. a., Trac.

See also **Pyaemia** and **Septicaemia.**

Blotches—K. bi., Smb. c.

FACE, on—K. ca.

Blow, Effects of—Gam.

Blushing—Aml., Mli.

AFTER EATING—*Carl.*

Body, Odour of, Offensive —*Mr. sol., Pso.,* Sac. 1., So. t. ae., Wis.

See also **Odour of Body.**

Boils. —Abr., Allm., Anan., Athra., *Arn.,* As. r., *Bel.,* Bls., ,Cd. s., Ca. chl., Ca. *m.,* Ca. s., Crt. h., Elt., *Hep.,* Hpz., Hoa., Lach., Led., Mld., Na. sa., Ph. x., *Phyt.,* Pi. x., Pso., Rs. v., Sbi., Sap., Sec., *Sil.,* So. a., *Sul.,* Uri.

BLIND—Snc.

FACE, on—*Ca. p.*

MEATUS, in—Ca. pi.

WRIST, on—Snc.

Bone, AFFECTIONS of—Aran., *Aur.,* Ca. fl., Ca. p., Cis., Coc. i., Fl. x., Gad., Get., Gui., Gre., Hec., Mr. c., *Mez.,* Na. sf., O1. j., *Rut.,* Sars., Tep., Ther. ,

BRUISED—*Rut.*

CANCER of—*Pho.,* Symt.

CARIES of—Sl. x., Tub.

DISEASES of—Asa., *Calc.,* Eub., *Mr. Sol., Pho., Phyt.,* Stp., *Stil.,* Sto. c.

EXOSTOSES on—*K.bi., Pb.*

INJURIES of—Symt.

NECROSIS of—Bth., *Sil*

NODES on—*K. bi., Nux,* Stil.

PAINS in—Ang., (Cinm.), Cyc., *E. pf.,* Homa., Man., Mn. m., *Rho.,* Rhs., *Rut.,* Src., Wil.

SWELLING of—Lc. x.

TUMOURS of—Phyt. ,

See also **Antrum of Highmore; Malar Bones; &c.**

Borborygmi—*Cin., Jat.,* Lo. s., *Lyc.,* Mnc., Mn. m., *Rum.,* Sg.

n., Snc., Src.

Bowels, Looseness of—Su. x.

See also **Diarrhoea.**

Brachial Neuralgia— Calc., Hyp., Ind., Par., Ter.

Brachialgia—Pip. m.

Brain, AFFECTIONS of—*Arn., Ba. c., Bel., Bry., Cu. a.,* Cyp., Dt.
a., For., *Gel., Nux* Oln., *Opi., Pho.,* Se. j., Ziz.

Brain, ANAEMIA of—Tab.

ATROPHY of—Fl. x., Iod.

BASE of, AFFECTED—Hlod.

BASE of,CONGESTED—Pop. c.

BASE of, PAIN in—Pi. x.

CONCUSSION of—Hyp., K. ph., Man., Sil., Su. x.

CONGESTION of—Abs., *Cac.,* Ca. br., Cro., *Fe. py., Glo.,*
Sul.

INFANTILE AFFECTIONS of—Nx. m.

INFLAMMATION of—Ar. t., Chr. o., Merc.

INJURIES of—Na. s.

IRRITATION of—Cap., Scu.

PARALYSIS of—Zin.

SOFTENING of—*Aga.,* Amb., Bap., Bls., Buf., K. ph., Nx.
m., Pho., Pb.

TUMOUR of—Pb.

Brain-fag—*AEth., Ana.,*Anh., Arg., Ar. it., Ca. *p.,* Glv., K. ph., Na.
m., Nct., *Ph. x.,* Pho., *Pi. x.,* Pip. m., *Sil.,* Tab., Zin., Zn.
p.,Zn. v.

Breast,, ABSCESS—Pho.

AFFECTIONS of—*Act. r.,* Au. s., Com., *Con.,* Hal., Hlon., Hep.,
Hyp., Iod., Lpi., Ol. a., Onos., Ori., Prf., Phel., *Phyt.,* Sul.,
Zin.

ATROPHY of—Chm. u., Onos., Sbl.

CANCER of—Bad., Ba. i., Bro., Cb. a., Chm. u., Gph., Lo. e.,
Sars., Scir. (*See also* TUMOUR of.)

ERUPTION on—Pip. n.

ERYSIPELAS of—Cb. v.

FISTULA of—Pho.

INDURATIONS of—Ca. fl., Gph.

INFLAMMATION of—Ac. 1., *Bry.,* Plnt., Sbl.

NODOSITIES in—Caln.

PAIN BEHIND —*Pul.*

PAIN BELOW—Rn. b., Rap. (*See also* **Infra-mammary Pain.**)

PAINS in—Iof., Mrl., Mur., CEna., Pro S., Sty., Sum.

PAINFUL —*Calc.,* Con., Lc. c., Ocm., Sbl., So. t. ae., Sprn.
   (*See also* **Menstruation,** BREASTS PAINFUL during; *and*
   Pregnancy, BREASTS PAINFUL during.)

SCIRRHUS of—Sars. (*See also* CANCER of; and TUMOUR of.)
   SENSITIVE—Syph.

SINUSES in—*Sil.*

SORE. —Symt.

SUPPURATION of— Caln.

SWELLING of—Mri., Pip. n., So. a., So. o.

TUMOURS of—As. i., Bro., Ca. i., Chm. u., Cnd., Fe. i., Hec.,
   Mr. i. f., Phas., *Sang.,* Scro., Sko., Tep.

ULCERATION of—Paeo.

Breasts, Pains between—Rap.

Breath, FETID—*Arn.*

OFFENSIVE—*Aur.,* K. tel., *Mr. sol., Nt. x., Pet.,* Qer., Rat., Rhe.
   So. t. ae., Su x., Zng.

PUTRID. — Sprn.

SOUR—*Nux.*

Bright's Disease—*Aps.,* Brac., Cai., Ca. p., Ch. ar., Dig., Evm., Fe.
   as., Fe. p., Glo., K. as., K. *cit.,* K. i., Klm., Lc. v. d., Lyc.,
   Lcs., Mr. c., Nt. X., Ol. j., Pb., Pyro., Sars., Scil., Sul., Zn.
   m., Zn. pi.

HEADACHE of—Zn. pi.

See also **Kidneys.**

Bronchial Glands, AFFECTIONS of—*Calc.*

DISEASES of—*Bel.*

Bronchitis—*Aco.,* All., Alo., Aln., Amc., Am. c., Am. m., Ant. i., (Ant. s. a.), *Ant. t.,* Arn., *Ars.,* As. i., Asc. s., Asc. t., Avi., Bal., Bl.o., *Bry.,* Cac., *Cb. v.,* Crd. m., *Caus.,* Chl. h., Cin., *Con.,* Cop., Drs., Erio., Eth., Euc., Fe. p., Gnd., Gui., *Hep.,* Hpt., Hpz., *Hyo.,* Ibe., *Ipc.,* Jab., K. *bi.,* K. ca., Ln. c., *Mr. sol.,* Nph., Nrs., *Nt. x.,* Osm., Phel., Ph. x., *Pho.,* Pin. s., Pix, Pod., Pmo., *Pul., Rum.,* Sbl., *Sang.,* Sg. n., Scil., *Sga.,* Slp., Stn., Sti., *Sul.* Ter., Tub., Ver.

    CAPILLARY—Ph. x.

    CHRONIC —Ird., Myo.

    CROUPOUS—*K. bi.*

    MEMBRANOUS —Ca. ac., Pho.

Bronchorrhoea—Ber. a., Fe. i., Teu. s.

Bronzed Skin—Adr.

Brow Ague—*Ars.,* Ced., *Ch. s.,* Cu. a.

Bruises—*Arn.,* Bad., *Con.,* Erig., For., *Ham., Hyp.,* Led., *Rut.,* (Su. x.)

Bubo—Alm., Au. m., Bad., Buf., Ca. s., *Caln., Cb. a.,* Cnb., Hep Hfb., *K. i.,* K. m., Lach., Li. c., *Mr. sol.,* Nt. *x.,* Ocm., Pest., Syph.

Bulimy—Brs., Fe. s.

Bullae—Pop. c.

Bunion—Aga., Ar. Ip., *Bz. x.,* Hyp., *K. i.,* K. m., *Rho., Sil., Ve. v.*

Burning Pains—Ac. f.

Burns—Ac. x., Ca. s., *Caln., Cth.,* Cb. v., Cbl. x., Crb. s., Caus., *Ham., Hep.,* Jab., *K. bi.,* K. m., Na. c., Pas., Pet., Pi. x., Plnt., Sprn., Stm., *Urt.*

Bursitis—Rut. (*See also* **Ganglion.**)

Cachexia— K. bi.

    CANCEROUS—Pic. x.

    QUININE of—Chne., Euc., (Na.. m.)

Caecum, AFFECTIONS of—*Ars.*

GURGLING in — Rm. f.

INFLAMMATION of—*Lach.*, Rhs. *Ve. v. (See also* **Appendicitis**
and **Typhlitis.**)

Calculus—Baro., *Ber., Calc.*, E. pu., Gli., Gas., Jnc., *Prei.*, Priet.,
Sars., Sld.

BILIARY—*See* **Gall-stones**.

PREVENTION of—Urt.

RENTAL PASSAGE of— *Ocm. (See also* **Renal Calculi.**)

URINARY—Epg. *(See also* **Bladder,** STONE in.)

Callosities—Ant. c., Gas., Trn.

Camp Diarrhoea—Pod., Sptn.

> *See also* **Diarrhoea.**

Camp Fever—Mlr.

Cancer—Aln, Anan, Anil., *Ars., As. i., Ast. r.,* Au. ar., Au. m., *Bap.*,
Ba. i., Bro., *Bry.*, Buf., *Ca. i.,* Ca. ox., Clt., Cb. a., Chel.,
Cic. v., (Cinm.), Cis., Cit., Clem., *Con.,* Crt. h., *Cnd.,* Cur.,
Elp., Eps., Eu. ht., Eub., Fe. i., *Gli.*, Gph., *Ham.,* Hpz., Hn.
m., *Hdr., Iod.,* K. as., K. *cy.,* K. *i., Kre.,* Lp. a., Lo. e., *Lyc.,*
Mat., Mth. b., Mil., *Ol. a., Opi.,* Orn., Oxg., *Pho., Phyt.,*
Pso., *Sang.,* Scir., *Sep.,* Sil., SIp., Sol., Suo x., *Thu.,* Trf. p.,
Vi. O.

BONE of——*Pho.,* Symt.

BREAST, of—Gph. *(See also* **Breast,** CANCER of.)

LIP, of—Ant. m., *Hdr., Lyc.,* Tab.

PAINS of—Ca. ac.

STOMACH of—Ac. x., Act. s., Bis., (Cd. s.)., Mag. p., Pt. m.,
Sec.

See also **Carcinoma;** and under **Pancreas; Rectum; Sigmoid**
Flexure; Uterus.

Cancerous Cachexia—Pi. x.

DIATHESIS—Scir.

ULCERS—Ch. s.

Cancrum Oris—*Ars.,* K. chl., K. ph., Merc., *Mr. c.,* Su. x.

Carbuncle—Athra., *Aps., Arn.,* Ars., *Asi., Bel.,* Buf., *Ca. chl.,* Ca.

s., Ca1n., *Cb. v.,* Cbl. x., Crt. h., Ech. a., *Hep.,* Hpz., Hoa., K. ph., Kre., *Lach.,* Sec., *Sil., Trn. c.*

Carcinoma—Au. m. n., Lp. a.., Nec.

    See also **Cancer.**

Cardiac Asthma—Amb., Qeb.

Cardiac Asthma. PARESIS—Jt. u.

    See also **Heart,** PARALYSIS of.

Cardialgia— Cup., Fe. s., Fe. t., Lo. i., Mag. m., Sto. c.

    See also **Heartburn;** and **Pregnancy,** HEARTBURN of.

Caries—Ang., Ank., Arg., As. f., Au. m., Buf., Calc., Cinm., Gui., Hep.,Hpz., K. i., Na. sf., Pt. m., Ther.

Carriage Sickness—(Arn.), Nux.

Cartilages, AFFECTIONS of—(Arg.)

    BRUISES of—Rut.

    PAINS in—(Arg.), Lo. s., Rut.

Caruncle— *See* **Urethra.**

Catalepsy—Ac. c., Aco., Aran., Art. v., *Cn. i., Cic. v.,* Cur., Eth., Fer., Ing., *Lach., Mos.,* Nx. m., *Opi.,* Pip. m., Rap., Spo., Stm., Tab., Thu.

Cataract —Anag., Ag. i., Arm., *Calc.,* Ca. fl., Can. s., Cb. a., Caus., Chm. u., Cin. m., *Clch.,* Col., *Con.,* Eub., Ephr., Hd. h., Jab., K. m., K. sc., Lyc., Nph., *Pho.,* Plts., Pod., Pul., Sac. o., Sntn., Sec., *Sil.,* Sul., Tel., Zin.

Catarrh—Agr. n., All., Aln., Alm., *Ant.* c., Ant. s. a., *Ant. t.,* Apo., Ag. i., *As. i.,* Ar. m., Ard., Asr., Asc. t., Bad., Bal., Baro., Ca. fl., Cb. v., Cen., Cep.; Cet., Cham., Chlm., Cnb., Cop., Crl., Cup., Drs., Dul., Erio., Eug., Fe. i., *Gph.,* Hpt., *Hdr.,* lll., Ict., Ipc., Jnc., K. *bi.,* K. ca., K. sc., .Lo. s., Mag. c., *Mr. sol.,* Mr. k. i., Mr. d., Mr. i. f., My. c., *Na. m.,* Nux, Ov. g. p., Phel., Pho., Pmo., *Pul.,* Rum., Sbl., *Sang.,* Sg. n., Sin. n., Sko., So. o., Sti., *Sul.,* Wil., Ziz.

    CHRONIC— Hpz.

    INTESTINAL—Pho. (*See also* **Diarrhoea;** and **Intestinal Catarrh)**

NASAL—Pho. (*See also* **Colds; Coryza; Nasal Catarrh;** *and* ;
Nose, CATARRH of.)

Catarrhal Affections—Chi.

    FEVER—Asc. s., Eug., Mr. k.i., Mrt.,Pop. c.

    PNEUMONIA—Ant. a., Tub.

Catheter' Fever—Aco., Pts.

Catheterism—Mag. p.

Cauliflower Excrescences—Stp.

Cellulitis—*Sil.*

    See also **Pelvic Cellulitis.**

Cerebellum,PAIN in—Rn. g.

Cerebral Deafness—Chn. a., Mu. x.

Cerebro—*Spinal Irritation*—Se. j.

Cerebro-spinal Meningitis—Act. r., Ail., Ced., Cic. v., Coc. i., Crt. h.,
    Cu. a., Gel., Hlod.

Cervix Uteri, Affections of—Mur.

Chafing,—Su. x.

Chagres Fever—Sul.

Chalazion—Stp.

    See also **Stye.**

Chancre—Ail., *Aps.*, Ag. n., Asc. t., Au. m., Cnb., Crl., Crt. h., Iof.,
    Ja. c., Jg. r., Lc. c., Lach., Merc., Mr. ac., *Mr. c.,* Mr. i. f., *Nt.*
    x., Ph. x., Pt. m., Sul.

Chancroid—Hdr., Ja. g., Mr. p. r.

Change of Life—*Act. r.,* Bls., Hlon., *Ign., K. ca., Kre., Lach.* Nx.
    m., Sang., Sars., *Sep.,* Smp., Ther., Trl., Ust., *Val.*

    See also **Climacteric;** and **Menorrhagia** at CLIMAXIS

Chapped Hands—Lyc., *Na. c., Pet.,* Prm. o., Sars., *Ss. x.*

Chaps—*Gph.,* Pul.

    See also **Anus,** RHAGADES of; **Cracks in Skin; Fissures;**

Hands, CHAPPED **Rhagades.**

Cheloid—Cp. 1., (MId.), *Nt.x .,* *Sil.,* Sul., Vac

Chemosis— Gre., Vsp.

Chest, AFFECTIONS of—*Aco., Arn., Chel.,* Men., *Ox. x.*

OPPRESSION of—*Smb. n.*

PAINS in—*Act. r., Jg. c., K. n., Pul., Rn. b., Sang., Sul.*

SORENESS of. —Kao.

STERNUM, PAIN behind—*Rn. s.*

STERNUM, PAIN in—*Rut. (See also* **Sternum,** PAINS in.)

STITCHES in—Mrt.

Cheyne-Stokes Breathing—Ac. f., Atp., Gnd., K. cy., Prt.

Chicken-pox. Aco., *Ant. t., Mr. sol.,* Rs. d.

Chilblains—Abr., *Aga.,* Aln., Bad., Cd. s., Calc., Ca. s., *Caln.,* Cb. v. Frg., Ham., *Hep.,* Iod., K. ca., K. m., K. ph., Lach., Mu. x., Nt. x., Nx. m., api., *Pet.,* Ph. x., Pho., *Pul.,* Rn. b., *Rhs.,* Rs. V., Sec., Stn., *Sul.,* Su. x., Tam., *Thyr.,* Tub., *Ve. v.,* Zin.

Children, DISEASES of—Ped.

EMACIATED—As. f.

Chilliness— Pim.

Chills—Acn., Ac. f., Aran., Pmt., Pyr. a., Var.

EFFECTS of—Bry.

Chin, AFFECTIONS of—Spo.

ERUPTION on—Sil., (Sul. i.), Zin. (*See also* **Sycosis** MENTI).

Chloasma—Caul., Sep., Sul.

Chlorosis—Abs., Alm., Arg., Au. ar., Bry., Chlm., Cup., Cyc., Fer., Fe. as., Frz., Gph., Hlon., Hep., K. fc., Mil., Na. hch., Pet., Pho., Plat., Sac. o, Sin. n., Zin.

Choking, EASY—Mep., Nt. x.

SENSATION of—Arnt.

Cholera—Aco., Ag. p., Ampl., Anil., Ant. t., *Ars.,* Avn., Bis., Ca. ar., Cb. v., Cbl. x., Ch. s., Clch., Ctn., Cu. as., Cup., Dul., Elt., Evm., Evo., Eu. co., Eu. 1., Gna., Grt., Guac., Hl. f., Hel, Ipc., Jat., Lau., Lim., Ph. x., Phyt., Ple., Ric., Sec., Tab., Zin.

ASIATICA—*Ars., Cam., Cu. a.,* Hy. x., *Ver.*

INFANTUM—Aco., *AEth.,* Cd. s., Ca. p., Cm. br., Cph., Eu. co., Gui., K. br., Kre., Lau., Mnc., Eno., Ox. x., Pas., Pod., Pso., Ric., Sec., Tab.

MORBUS—Ant. t., Caul., Ev. a.

Cholerine—Asr., Ctn., *Cu. as., Dio.,* Eu. co., Jat., K. ph., Nup., Nx. m., *Ver.*

Chordee—Cam., Cm. br., Cn. i., Cth., Ja. c., *K. br.,*Myg., Sin. n., Stm., Ter.

Chorea—*Act.r., Aga.,* Ag. p., Aml., Ant. c., Arn., Art. v., Asa., Buf., Calc., *Ca. p.,* Cast., Caus., Ced., Chel., Chl. h., Cin., Coc. i., Cod., Con., Cro., *Cu. a.,* Cu. as., Cup., Cyp., Dio., Elc., Fer., Fe. s., For., Hpm., Hyo., *Ign.,* K. sc., Lt. k., Lau., Mag. p., Mor., Mu. x., Myg., Na. m., Pho., Phst., Rho., Rus., Scu., Sec., Sep., Sin. n., So. n., *Stm.,* Sul. t., Sum., Tan., Trn., Trn. c., Ter., Thu., *Ve. v.,* Vis., Zin., Zn. br., Zn. cy.

SLEEP in—Ziz.

Choroiditis—Gel., *Pr. s., Rhs.,* Vi. o.

Chronic Rheumatic Arthritis—Sul. t.

See also **Rheumatic** ARTHRITIS **Rheumatic** GOUT; **Rheumatoid Arthritis.**

Chyluria—Iod.

Cicatrix. —*Fl. X., Phyt., Sil., Thio.*

See also **Scars.**

Ciliary NEURALGIA—Am. br., Ced., Col., Crt. h., Hyn., K. cy., Lc. f., Lach., Paeo., Par., Phel., Pho., Phyt., Plnt., Pro s., Rho., Spi., Tax., Ter. (*See also* **Neuralgia** SUPRA-ORBITAL

PARALYSIS—Par.

SPASM—Eser., Hyn., Jab., Phst.

Circulation, Feeble—*Rhs., Sil*

Cirrhosis of Liver—Ca. ar.

See also **Liver,** CIRRHOSIS of.

Clairaudience—Nx. m.

See also **Hearing,** ILLUSIONS of.

Clairvoyance—(Aco.), Cn. i., Dt. a., Hfb., Mgt. n., Nx. m., Pyr. a., Val.

See also **Vision,** HALLUCINATIONS OF; *and* ILLUSIONS of.

Clavus—Aqui., *Ign., K. ca.,* Nic., *Nux, Pul.,* Pl. n., Thu.

Clergyman's Sore Throat—Ar. t., crb. s., Hlt., Sti., Stil.

Climacteric, THE—Hlon., Nt. x., Nx. m., Phst., Sang., Sars., Sl. x., Smp., Ther., TrI., Ust.

  FLUSHINGS of—Aml., Brc. x., Jab., K. bi., Man., Sang. (*See also* **Flushing.**)

  FLUSHINGS AND VERTIGO of—Ph. x.

  SUFFERINGS of—Cyc., Lau., Mur.,Oop., Orc., Sul., Su. x.

  See also **Change of Life;** and **Menorrhagia** at CLIMAXIS

Climaxis—*See* **Climacteric.**

Clonic Spasms—Med.

Clumsiness—(Aps.), (Bov.), K. ohl., Spo.

Coccygodynia—Ant. t., Ca. cs., Cb. a., Ct. eq., *Caus., Cic. v.,* Eub., Fl. x., Gam., Grt., *K. bi.,* Kre., Mez., Ph. x., Pho., Phst., *Sil.,* Trn., Ttr., Xan.

Coccyx, ITCHING of—Bov.

  SORENESSof—Snc.

  ULCER on—Paeo.

Coff'ee, Effects of—Cham., Grna.

Coitus, Complaints after—Ced.

Cold Abscess—Ol. j.

Cold, Sensitiveness to—Mep.

Cold Sores—Ca. fl.

Coldness;—*Aco., Aga., Ars.,* Hlod.

Colds—*Aco., Ars., Calc., Cam., Cep.,* Chlm., Ctn., Dio., *Ephr.,* Gel., Hil., *Hep.,* K. ca., *K. i., Mag. m., Mr. sol.,* Mr. k. i., *Nux,* Pho., *Pul., Sang.,* Spi., Sta., Sti., *Sul.,* Ss. x.

  CHRONIC—Hpz.

  EASILY taken—Gas., Nt. x.

  LIABILITY to—Osm., Pl. n.

Colic—Alet., All., Alo., Aln., Anth. n., Aph., Arm., Ar. it., Asc. t., Ast. f., *Bel., Cham., Cin., Coc. i.,* Cof., Clch., Clcn., *Col.,* Clv. a., Dio., Dir., Elt., Ephr., Fe. p., Gam., Gn. l., Gph., Haem., HI. v., Ill., K. br., K. n., Mag. p., Mnc., Mn. o., Mom., *Nux,* Onis., *Opi.,* Ped., Pb., Pb. chr., Rm. c., Scro.,

Sna., *Stn.*, Vrn., *Ver.*, Vbs. .

FLATULENT —Cham., (Mag. p.), Plg.

FLATULENT IN INFANTS—Sna.

Colic, HORSES, in—Hy. x., (Mag. p.)

See also **Biliary** COLIC; **Hysterical** COLIC; **Lead** COLIC; **Menstrual** COLIC.

Collapse—Hmer., Nct., Ver.

CHOLERA, of—As. h.

Colour Blindness—Bz. d., Onos., Tab.

Coma—Amg., Chi.

Coma Vigil—(Cur.), *Hyo.*, Lon.

Comedo—Eug., *Sel.*

Commissures, Soreness of—Ars.

Compound Fractures—Hyp.

Concussion—(Arn.), Cic. v., Hel.

See also **Brain,**CONCUSSION of; *and* **Spine,** CONCUSSION of.

Condylomata—Au. m., *Ephr.*, K. i., Merc., Mr. d., Mr. n., Na. S., *Nt. x.*, Ph. x., Pi. x., Pt. m., *Sbi.* Snc., Sep., Stp., *Thu.*

Congenital Syphilis—Kre., (Syph.).

Congestion—Ca., hp., Mli., Ve. v.

Conjunctivitis—Chl. h., Ery. a., Ephr., Fe. p. h., Gnd., K. bi., Mrl., Mr. d., My. c., Na. p., Ptv., Snc., Tel., Tha.

PHLYCTENULAR—Scil., Sil

RHEUMATIC—Mim.

See also **Blepharo—conjunctivitis; Eyes,** CONJUNCTIVITIS; **Granular Conjunctivitis;** *and* **Granular Lids.**

Conscientiousness, Morbid—Spa. u.

Constipation—Ab. n., Ac. l., AEs. g., *AEsc.*, Alet., All., Alo., Aln., *Alm.,* Am. m., Amph., Ana., Anag., Ago., Ant. c., Ant. s. a., Aps., Aq. m., As. mt., Ast. r., Az., Bel., *Bry.*, Ca. ar., Cb. a., Cb. v., Cbl. x., Carl., Cas. s., Csc., *Caus.*, Chel., Chn. V., *Chi.,* Chio., Cich., Cim., Chn. S., Cinm., Cit., Cob., Coll., Dph., Dct., Dio., Dir., Ery. a., Eug., Eu. hp., Fecl., Fe. m., Fe. s., Frz., Ga. x., Gas., *Gel., Gph.,* Grt., Gui., Hli.,

Hep., Hmer., *Hdr.,* Hyd., Ind., Iod., *Iris,* K. bi., K. m., Kis., Kre., Lc. v. d., Lct. v., Lpt., Lim., *Lyc.,* Mag. c., Mag. m., Mlr., Mnd., Mn. m., Mez., Mor., Mus., Nab., *Na. m.* Na.n., *Nt. x.,* Nm. x., *Nux,* Ol .j., *Opi.,* Pal., Prol. a., Pet., Pho., Phst., Phyt., Pin. 1., Pin. s., Pip. n., Plat., Pbo., Pb., Plp., Pop. c., Pso., Ptl., Pyro., Qer., Rat., Rm. c., Rhe., Rdm., Rut., Snc., Sap., Src., Sa.rs., Sel., Sga., Sil., Sil. m., Sin. n., Sla., So. t. ae., *Spi,* Spo., Sto. c., *Sul.,* Su. x., Syph., Tab., Tnn., Thu., Thyr., Trf. p., Ul. f., *Ver,* Vbs., Vic., Wis., Wye., *Zin.,* Zn. i., *Zn. m.*

CHILDREN of—Prf., Snc.

CHRONIC—Coca.

NURSLINGS, of—Alm., Aps.

Constipation, SCYBALOUS—Ss. x.

SUCKLINGS, of—Alm., Aps.

See also LABOUR, CONSTIPATION after.

Consumption—*Aco., As. i., (Bao.), Bap., Bry., Ca. ar., Calc., Ca. i., Ca. p., Drs., Fe . ac., Ham., Hep., Iod., Ipc., Jab., K. ca., K. i., Kre., Lyc., Mlr., Mil., Pho., Stn., Sul., Tub.*

See also **Phthisis;** *and* **Tuberculosis.**

Consumption, BLEEDING—*Acal., Aco., Fe. ac., Ham., Ipc., Mil., Pho.*

Consumptiveness— Bac.

Contraction—Gui.

TENDONS of—Caus. Mez.

See also **Dupuytren's Contraction;** *and* **Fingers, Contracted.**

Convulsions— (Abs.), Acn., Aco., *AEth.,* Alet., Amb., Art. v., Ast. r., Atr., Ba. m., *Bel.,* Bz. n., Cam., Cbn., Cast., Caus., *Cham.,* Chn. a., Chlf., Chlm., Cic. v., Cin., Coc. i, Cof., Crt. h., *Cup.,* Cyp., Dt. m., Eth., Evo., Frg., Gel., Glo., Hel., Hy. x., Hfb., Ign., Ipc., Ir. fl., Jas., Jn. v., K. ox., Ker., Lab., Lau., Ln. u., Lon., Mag. p., Mor., Nx. m., *Nux,* CEna;., Ox. x., Pas., Plat., Pb. chr., Pyre., Rx. ac., Rus., Sntn., Scol., Sec.,

Siu., So. c., Spa. u., Stn., Sul. h., Thu., Up., Ve. V., Zn. cy.,
Zn. m., *Zn. s.*, Ziz.

PUERPERAL—Pilo., Thyr. (See also Puerperal CONVOLSIONS)
STRAMONIUM AND OTHER POISONS, from—Cit.

URAEMIC—Hy. X., Pilo., (Urt. u.)
See also **Labour,** CONVULSIONS in; and **Pregnancy,**
CONVULSIONS of.

Coprophagia— Ver.

Cornea, OPACITY of—Cd. s., Ca. fl., *Can. s.,* Cin. m., Ctn., Hep., K.
bi., Mag. c, Sac. o., Sga., Trn., Tub., Zn. s.

SPOTS on—Ant. s. a., Arm.

ULCERATION of—Ca. si., Ca. s., Hep., Na. c., Pod., Pso., Snc.,
Corns Tub. —Ac. x., An. oc., Ant. c., Arn., Bor., Bov., Ca.
cs.Chi: b., Cur., Fe. pi, *Hdr.,* Hyp., Kis., Lyc., Med., Na.. c.,
Nt.x., Ph. x., Pim., Rn. b., Rn. S., Rum., (Sl. x.), Sul., Su. x.,
Wis.

PAIN in—Hfb.

Corpulence—Am. br., Aur., *Ca. ar., Calc.,* Fuc., *Pho., Phyt.,* Ts. fg.
See also **Obesity.**

Coryza—Ail., Abrs., Am. br., Am. m., Antho., Aph., Apo., As. mt.,
Ar. m., Ard., Asp., Bad., Bry., Calc., Cnt., Cep., Chi. b.,
Cyc., Eug., Fe. i, Homa., Iod., Jal., Jg. c., K. bi., K. chs., Lo.
s., Lrs., Mr. bin., Mrt., Nrs., Na. as., Na. c., Na. i., Nym.,
Ol. a., Ol. j., Osm., Ov. g. p., Oxg., Pnt., Phel., Ph. m., Pop.
c., Rn. s., Rho., Rob., Rum., Sbd., Sl. x., Sg. n., Snc., Scil.,
Se. a., Sil., Sin. n., Sprn., Sul. i., Tel., Up., Yuc., Zn. o.

Coryza, DRY—Smb. n.

Costiveness—Pbo.
See also **Constipation.**

Cough—*Ab. n.,* Acal., *Aco., AEs. g.,* AEsc., *AEth., Aga.,* All., Alo.,
Aln., *Alm., Amb.,* Am. br., *Am. c.,* Am. m., Ana., (Ant. s. a.),
*Ant. t.,*Aph., Aral., Ag. cy., Arg., Ars., Asc. t., Ast. f., *Bel.,*
Bis., Bro., Bry., Cai., *Calc.,* Ca. fl., Ca. s., *Cap.,* Cb. a., *Cb.*
v., Csc., *Caus.,* Cep., Cham., Chel., Chi., Chr. o., Cim., *Cin.,*

Coca, Cod., *Clch.,* Clcn., *Con.,* Cop., *Crl.,* Ctn., Cup., Cur., Dph., Dio., Dir., Dol., *Drs.,* Erig., Ery. a., Ery. m., Eth., Eug., E. pf., Eub., Ephr., Epn., Fer., Fe. p., For., Gad., Gui., *Hep., Hyo.,* Ict., Ill., Ind., Inu., *Iod.,* Iof., *Ipc.,* K. ca., K. i., K. pm.,_Lach.,_ Lchn., Lct. v., Lau., Lpi., Ln. c., Lip. m., *Lo. i.,* Lo. s., Lyc., Lcs., Mag. c., Mag. p., Mag. s., Mgt. s., Man., Mli., *Mr. sol.,* Myo., Mrt., Nrs., *Na. m.,* Nic., *Nt. x.,* Nx. m., *Nux:,* CEna., Ol. j., Oxg., Oxt., Phel., Ph. x., Pho., Phyt., Pip. n., Plg., Pso., *Pul.,* Rap., *Rum., Smb. n.,* Snc., Sntn., Se. a., *Sga., Sil.,* Sin. n., *Spo.,* Stp., Sti., (Stil.), Strp., *Sul.,* Ther., Trf. p., Ts. ff., *Vbs.,* Wye., Zn. i.

CATARRHAL—*Scil.*

DAY, by—Vi. o.

DRY—*Mth. pi.*

EXPLOSIVE—Sty.

PREGNANCY, of—Vb. o.

PREGNANCY of, MORNING—*Bry.*

REFLEX—Cer. o.

SPASMODIC—*Osm.,* Vi. o.

TICKLING—Slv.

See also **Measles,** COUGH of; and **Whooping-cough.**

Coxalgia—All., Ars., Calc., Col., Drs., Hyp., Ph. x., Src., So. m., Thu., Val.

See also **Hip—joint Disease.**

Cracks in Skin—Ank., Bal., Bz. x., *Cnd.,* Mag. p., *Na. m., Pet.,* Zin.

See also **Chapped Hands; Chaps; &c.**

Cramp—*Aga.,* Ag. p., Amph., Ag. cy., *Arn.,* Asi., Crb. o., Carl., Cham., *Clch., Cup.,* Dio., Elt., Epn., Fer., Fe.m., Grt., Inu., Ird., Jat., K. ox., Lau., Lyc., Mag. p., Men., *Nux,* Pau., Ple., Pb. chr., Sec., So. t., Stn., Sto. c., Sty., Sfn., Ver., Vb. o., Zn. m.

STOMACH, in—AEs. g.

See also **Diaphragm,**CRAMP in; **Feet,** CRAMP in; **Palms,**

CRAMP in; **Writer's Cramp.**

Cravings, Morbid—Sto. n.

Cretinism—Ca. p., Lp. a.

Croup—Ac. x., *Aco., Ant. t., Ars.,* Ar. dm., *Bel., Bro., Calc.,* Cham., Chlm., Cub., Cu. a., *Cup.,* Dphn., Fe. p., *Hep., Ign., Iod.,* K. i., K. m., Kao., Lc. c., Lo. i., Mos., Pho., *Smb. n.,* Sang., Sgn., Sld., *Spo.,* (Suc.), Ss. x.

Crusta Lactea—Calc., Ca. s., Dul., Eub., Iris., K. chl., Mlt., Mr. i. f., Mez., Pb. i., Pso., Vin., Vi. t.

Crusta Serpiginosa—Pso., Sul.

Crying of Infants—Syph.

Cyanosis—Antf., Bz.n., Cup., Dig. Lach., Lau., Na. ns., Phen., *Rhs.,* Sfn,

Cynanche Cellularis—Athra.

Cystitis—Aco., Bis., Can. s., Chm. u., Cnb., Con., Cop., Equ., E. pu., Fe. p., Hel., K. chl., K. m., Lyc., Mth. b., Mus., Pts., Pch., Pip. m., Pb., Pr. s., Sbl., Sbi., Sep., Trn., Tax., Ter., Uva.., Ves., Z. st.

CHRONIC—Sntn.

Cysts—Ba. c., Bov., Ca. s., Stp.

See also **Sebaceous Cysts; Tarsal Cysts;** *and* **Wens.**

Dandruff—All., *Ars.,* K. sc., Pho., Snc., *Sep.*

Day-blindness—Bth.

Deafness—Acn., Agr. n. (All.), *Amb.,* Ba. m., Caj., Caln., Cb. v., Caus., Chei., Chi., Ch. sal., Coca, Elp., Fe. pi., Gel., Gph., Ipc., K. as., Led., Lo. e., Lo. i., Mag. c., Mag. m., Mr. d., Na. c., Pet., Pilo., Pl. n., Rhe., Sln., Sang., Sg. n., Scro., Sld., Syph., Ul. f., Vbs., Vb. t., Vis.

CATARRHAL—Man., Mu. x.

CEREBRAL—Chn. a., Mu. x.

Debility—Ac. x., Adr., Alet., Als., *Ana.,* Ar. sc., *As. i.,* Avn., *Calc., Ca. p., Cb. v.,* Carl., Chne., *Chi.,* Chio., Coca, Coc. i., Clch., Clcn., Cur., Dir., Ery. m., Eu. a., Fer., *Fe. p.,* Frz., Glg., Ga. x., Gas., Gn. l., Gin., Hlon., Her., *Ign., Iod.,* K. ca., K. fc., K

i., Lev., Lo. c., Lo. i., Lyc., Mag. c., *Na. m.,* Na. n., Na. sa.,
Na. s., *Nx. m.,* Onos., Orc., Prt., *Ph. x.,* Pi. x., *Pso.,* Rs. g.
Sbd., Snc., Sel., *Sil.,* Stn., Trx., *Ver.,* Wye., Zn. o.

DRUNKARDS, of—Na. s.

NERVOUS—Cur., Cyp.

SLEEPLESSNESS, With—Cyp.

See also **Nervous Debility.**

Decemetitis—K. bi.

Decubitus—Fl. x. (*See also* **Bedsores.**)

Delirium—AEth., Anh., Ar. t., Chi., Ch. s., Dt. f., Dt. m., Dbn., Ga.
x., Hyn.. Iof., Ir. fl. *Nux,* Pyre., Rho., Sul. h., Zea.

Delirium Tremens—Act. r., Aga., *Ant. t.,* Ars., *Bel.,* Bis., Calc.,
Cn.i., Cap., Chlf., Cri. r., Crt. h., Cyp., Dig., Eth., Fe. p.,
Hyo., Lach., Lol., Pas., Pst., Rn. b., Scu., *Stm.,* Tea., Tn. p.

Deltoid, PAIN in—Zn. o., Zn. v.

RHEUMATISM of — Lrs. Nx. m., Ox. x., Syph., Urt., Zng.

RIGHT, PARALYSIS of— (Cur.)

Delusions— *Cn. i., Plat.*

Dementia—Crt. h., Lil.

Dengue Fever—*Aco., E. pf., Gel., Rhs.*

Dental Fistula—Caus., Stp., Sul.

Dentiotion—*Aco.,* Ard., Bor., Bry., *Calc., Ca. p.,* Caus., *Cham.,*
Chlm.,Cin., Cup., Dol., Gel., Ign., *Kre.,* Mag. p., Mil., Pas.,
Phst., plat., Ple., Pod., Scu., *Sil.,* Stn., Stp., Syph., Ter., Til.,
Tub., Zin., Zn. br.

ABNORMAL— *Mr. sol.*

DIFFICULT—Hec., Phyt., Rhe. (*See also* **Wisdom-teeth.**)

Depression of Spirits—*Ars., Aur., Bel.,Con., Hel., Ign., Na., m.,*Na.
sa., *Plat.,* Pb., Se. j., *Spi., Trn.*

Desquamation—Pix.

Diabetes—Ac., x., All., Aln., Am. ac., Ank., Arg., (Ag. n.),
Ari., *Arn.,* As. br., Asp., Bov., Calc., Ca., p., Cbl. x. Carl.,
Chm. u., Cod., Clch., Col., Cur., E. pu., Fe. i., Fe. m., Fe. p.
Hlon., Hdrn. a., Mag. s. Med., Mos., *Mur.,* Na. m., Na. p.

Na. s., Oxg., Phas., Phlo., *Ph. x.,* Pi. x., Plnt., Rat., Rs. a.,
Sac. l. Sac. o. Snc., *Scil.,* Sec., *Sil.,* Sti., Sul., Su. x. Syz.,
Trx., Tri., Trl., Ure., Vic.

INSIPIDUS—Apo.,K. n., Scil, *Ur. n.*

MELLITUS—*Opi., Ur. n.*

PANCREATIC—Iris, Pan.

Diaphragm, AFFECTIONS of—Ver.

CRAMP in—Sec., Vb. t.

NEURALGIA of—Zn. o.

PAIN in—Homa., *Stn.*

PARALYSIS of—Sta.

RHEUMATISM of—*Act. r. Bry., Cac., Sti.,*

SPASM of—CEna., Sty.

STITCHES in—Spi.

Diaphragmitis—Bis., Hep., Prf., Stm., Ve. v.

Diarrhoea—Acal., Ac. l., Aco., AEth., Ag. p., Agr. n., All., *Alo.,*
Als., Aln., Am. m., Ang., *Ant. c.,* s.a., Aph., Aps., Ap. a.,
Apo., Aral., Arn., *Ars.,* As. mt., As. f. As. r. Ard., Asa., Asr.,
As-ct. Asi., Ast. f., Az., Bel., *Bz. x.,* Bis., Bo. la., Bor., Bov.,

Diarrhoea *(continued)*—

Bry., Calc., Cap., Cb. v., Cbl. x., Crd. b., Csc., Cst. v., Cean.,
Cen., Cnt., Cep., Cet., *Cham.,* Chp., Chel., Chm. m., *Chi.,*
Ch. ar., Ch. s., Chr. o., Cin., Chn. s., Cinm., Cis., Cit., Cof.,
Cchn., *Clch.,* Coll., Clcn., *Col.,* Clost., Cvl., Clv. a., Co. c.,
Cto., *Ctn.,* Cub., Cu. a., Cu. as., Cu. s., Der., Dgn., Dio.,
Dir., Dor., *Dul.,* Elae., Elt., Eps., Ere., Ery. a., Euc., Eug.,
Evm., Evo., E. pf., Eu. a., Eu. co., Eu. l., Fag., Fel., *Fer.,* Fe.
mg., *Fe. m.,* Fe. Pn., Fe. p., Fe. s., Frl., For., Frz., Glv.,
Gam., Gas., Gel., Gen., Gn. c., Gn. l., Ger., Gna., Grt.,
Guac., Gui., Grna., Haem., Hel., Hl. o., Hl. v., Hep., Hur. c.,
Hfb., Hyo., Hyp., Ilx., Ind., Iod., *Ipc.,* Ir. fl., Ir. g., *Iris,* Jab.,
Ja. g., Jal., Jat., K. ac., K. as., K. m., Kis., Kre., Lct. v., Lau.,
Lpt., Lia., Lil., Lim., Lina., Ln. c., Lips., Lo. i., Lrs., *Mag.
c.,* Mag. m., Mag. s., Mlr., Mn. o., Mla., *Mr. sol., Mr. c.,* Mr.

d., Mil., Nph., Nrs., Na. ss., Nt. s. d., Nup., *Nux*, Nym.,
Ocm., CEno., Ol. j., Onos., Opu., Pan., Pau., Ped., Pnt.,
Pet., Ph. x., Pho., Ph. h., Phst., Phyt., Pin. s., Pix, Plnt., Ple.,
Pb. chr., *Pod.,* Plg., Prin., Pso., *Pul.,* Pl. n., Pyro., Qer., Rn.
b., Rap., Rm. c., Rm. f., *Rhe.,* Rho., Rs. g., Rh. s., Rs. v.,
Ric., *Rum.,* Sl. x., Sx. n., Sx. p., Sll., Snc , Sntn., Sap., Src.,
Sca., Sch., Sec., Sin. n., Sla., Sti., Sto., c., *Sul.,* Su. x., Sum.,
Tab., Thev., Thu., Thyr. Trb., Vrn., *Ver.,* Wis., Wye., Yuc.,
Zn. a., Zn. v., Zng.

CAMP—Pod., Sptn.

CHRONIC—Rs. a., Rhs.

MEMBRANOUS—Bo. s.

NERVOUS—Zin.

NIGHT, at—Caj.

PHTHISIS, of—Pul.

STUPOR, with—Zin.

See also **Cholera; Intestinal Catarrh; Menstruation,**
DIARRHOEA BEFORE; and **Tubercular Diarrhoea.**

Digestion, DISORDERED—Cast.

TOO RAPID—Tax.

SLOW—Frl., Nm. x., Par., Snc.

WEAK—Par.

See also **Dyspepsia;** and **Indigestion.**

Diphtheria—Ac. x., Ail., Amg., Aps., *Ars.,* Ar. t., Bap., Bro., Cth.,
Cap., Ch. ar., Chlm., Crt. h., Dphn., Dor., *Ech. a.,* Ech. p.,
Gel., Gui., Hpz., Ign., *Iod.,* K. chs., K. m., K. pm., K. ph.,
Kao., Lc. c., *Lach.,* Lchn., Lc. v. f., *Lyc.,* Mnc., *Mr. bin., Mr.
cy.,* Mr. i. f., Mr. scy., *Mu. x.,* Na as., *Phyt.,* Rn. s., Rhs.,
Sbd., Sl. x., Sang., Ss. x., Sa. x. Trn., Zin., Zn. m.

Diphtheria, AFTER-EFFECTS *of*—Pso.

See also **Throat,** DIPHTHERITIC.

Diphtheritic Paralysis—Caus., Con., Dphn., Rho.

See also **Paralysis,** DIPHTHERITIC.

Diplopia—Cyc., Eug., Ger., Iof., Onos., Phyt., Pb., Spo., Strp.,

Syph., Ve. v.

Direction, Sense of, Lost—Cm. br.

Disappointment, Effects of—Alm.

> *See also* **Love, Disappointed.**

Dislocation—Agn., For., Rut.

> EASY—Mgt. s.
>
> PAINS from—Am. c.

Dissection Wounds—Aps.

Distension—Cb. v., *Lyc.*, Na. n., *Pul.*

> *See also* **Abdomen,** DISTENDED; and **Stomach,** DISTENSION of.

Distortions— Sec.

> *See also* **Face,** DISTORTION of.

Diuresis—Ank., Bz. n., Thyr., Yoh.

Dog-bite—Lach.

Dreams—Epn., *Opi.*

> ANNOYING—Rs. g.

Dropsical Swellings—Cld.

Dropsy—Ac. x., *Aco.*, Ado., Am. bz., Ampl., Anag., *Aps.*, Ap. a., *Apo., Ars., As. i.,* Asc. s., Asp., Au. m., Bl. a., Brs., Bry., Buf., Cac. Cai., Caj., Ca. ar., *Calc.,* Ca. s., Crd. m., Csc., Chn. a., Chm. u., Chi., Ch. s., Chl. h., Cit., Clch., *Dig.,* Dul., Elt., Equ., Ery. a., Evm., E. pu., Fl. x., For., Gph., Grt., *Hel.,* Ibe., Ict., Ir. g., Jnc., Jn. c., K. ac., K. as., K. ca., K. i., K.m., Klm., Lc. v. d., Lach., Lia., Lyc., Mr. s., Na. m., Oxd., Phas., Pho., Pb., Prm. vg., Pr. s., Rn. b., Sac. o., Snc., *Scil.,* Se. a., *Strp., Ter.,* Thl., Thyr., Ure., Uri., Ves., Z. st., Zng., Ziz.

> CARDIAC—Coll., *strp.*
>
> PREGNANCY, during—Snc.
>
> SPLENIC—Qer., Scil.
>
> WANDERING—Prm. vg.
>
> *See also* **Ovaries,** DROPSY of; and **Renal** DROPSY.

Drowsiness— Dbn.

> *See also* **Sleepiness.**

Dumb Ague—Chne.

Duodenum—*Ars.*

    CATARRH of—Ber., *Pod.*, Rhe., Ric.

    ULCER of—*K. bi., Ur. ,n.*

Dupuytren's Contraction—Ar. lp., *Gel.*

Dwarfism—Mr. p. a., Ol. j.

Dysentery—Aco., *Alo.,* Als., Aln., Alm., Ago., Arn., Asc. t., Bap., Bel., Bnz., Bo. la., Bo. s., Ca. s., Cth., Cap., Cb. v., Cbl. x., Chp., Cnb., Cit., Clch., Coll., *Col.,* Cop., Co. c., Cub., Cph., Cu. s., Der., Dio., Dor., Dul., Elt., Euc., Evm., Eu. a., Eu. l., Fe. m., Fe. p., Gel., Ger., Hfb., Ipc., Iris, K. chl., K. m., K. n., K. ph., Leo., *Lpt., Lil.,* Lyc., Mag. s., Merc., *Mr. c.,* Mr. cy., *Nt.* x., *Nux,* Pel., Phyt., Picr., Plnt., Pod., Plg., Ptl., Pyre., Pyro., Rat., Rhe., Rs. g., *Rhs.,* Ric., Sll., Sptn., Stp., *Sul.,* Ter., Thl., Trl., Trb., Urt., Vrn., Zin., Zn. m., Zn. s.

    CHRONIC—Rs. a.

Dysmenia, or **Dysmenorrhoea**—Aco., Aga., Alet., Ana., Atp., Aran., Art. v., Asr., Asc. s., Ber., Brac., Bro., Cast., Caul., Cer.o., Cham., Ch. s., Chl. h., Coll., Col., Cro., Crt. h., Cur., Dio., *Gel.,* Gna., Gos., Gph., Gui., Haem., Hdm., Hlon., Hyo., Ign., Inu., Iris, Jab., Jn. c. K.ca., K. fc., K. n., Klm., Lc. c., Lc. f., Lp. a., Lau., Lo. i., Lyc., Mac., Mag. m., Mag. p., Mag. s, Man., Med., Mli., Mrl., Mil., Mit., Mom., Mur., Naj., Na. c., Nic., Nx. m., Opi., Pet., Phyt., Plat., Pb., Pod., Plg., Pop. c., Pul., Rap., Rhs., Sbl., Sbi., Sang., Sap., Sars., Se. a., Sep., Sul., Syph., Tan., Trn., Ter., Ther., Thu., Thyr., Tur., Ust., Ver., Ve. v., Vb. o., Vb. p., Wye., Xan.

    MEMBRANOUS—Bor., Ca. ac., Con., Gas., Gui., Hlt., Mag. p., Vb. o.

    NEURALGIC—Vb. o.

    SPASMODIC—Vb. o.

    See *also* **Menstruation,** ABNORMAL, &c.

Dysparunia—Fe. m., Na.. m., Sprn., Stp., Thu.

    NEWLY-MARRIED WOMAN in—Stp.

Dyspepsia—*Ab. n.,* Abs., Act. r., AEth., All., Alm., *Ana.,* Anth. n.,

Ant. c., Ant. t., Aran., *Ag. n.,* Ari. s., *Ars.,* Asa., Ba. m., *Bry.,* *Calc.,* Ca. p., *Cb. v., Cbl. X.,* Cham., Chel., Chi., Coll., Co. fl., Crt. h., Cyc., Dio., Dir., Euc., Fe. i., Fe. m., Fe. p., Frz., Fuc., Gn. c., Gn. l., Hpt., Her., Homa., *Hdr.,* Hy. x., Iris, *K. bi., K.* ca., K. fc., K. sc., Lach., *Lpt.,* Li. c., Lo. i., Lo. s., Lup., *Lyc.,* Mag. c., Mag. m., *Mr. sol.,* Na. c., *Na. m.,* Na. p., Na. s., Nt. x., Nup., Nx. m., *Nux,* Prt., Pep., Pet., Ph. x., Phst., Picr., Pod., Pop. c., Pr. V., Pso., Ptl., *Pul.,* Pl. n., Pyr. a., Rhs., Rs. V., Rob., Rum., Rut., Sbd., Sac. l., Sac. o., *Sang.,* Sars., Scro., Sep., Stn., Sto. b., Su. x.

ATONIC—Rat.

CALOMEL, from—Pod.

DRUNKARDS, of—Na. s.

Dyspepsia, FLATULENT—Sl. x.

NERVOUS—K. ph.

PREGNANCY, of—Sbd., Sin. a.

See also **Digestion,** DISORDERED, &c.; **Indigestion;** **Lactation,** DYSPEPSIA of.

Dysphagia—Epl., Gn. c., Gre., Ple., Ph. chr., Pop. c., Rs. v., Sec., Vis.

Dyspnoea—Acn., Ac. f., Cit., Cup., Cur., Mr. ac., Mos., Rn. b., Rn. g.

Dysuria—Alet., Apo., Epg., Erig., Euc., Lup., Mr. ac., Mr. s., Mit., Prei., Pts., Pin. s., Pip. m., Pip. n., Pb., Plg., Pr. s., Ro. c., Sbl., Sntn., Sars., Se. a., Sld., Tax., Thl., Trt., Uva., Vrn., Zin.

FLATULENT—Pr. s.

See also **Urination.**

Ear, AFFECTIONS of—*Aco., Ars.,* Ar. dm., Aur., *Bel., Calc., Cap., Ch. s.,* Clch., Com., *Ctn.,* Cur., Elp., *Fe. p., Gph., Hep., Hdr., K. m.,* Kre., *Man., Mr. sol.,* Mez., Nt. x., Prt., *Pet.,* Phyt., Sil., *Sul.*

BOILS in—Pi. x.

DEAFNESS—Chi. *(See also* **Deafness.)**

DISCHARGE from—AEth., Ard., *Bor.,* Crt. h.

DISEASES of—Fe. pi.

ECZEMA behind—Lyc., Sto. n.

ECZEMA *of—Bov., Rhs.*

ERYSIPELAS of—*Aps.*

INFLAMMATION of—Cac., K. ca., Led., *Plnt. (See also* **Otitis.)**

INFLAMMATION of INTERNAL and EXTERNAL—K. bi.

INFLAMMATION of,PERIFOLLICULAR——Ca. pi.

MIDDLE, AFFECTIONS of—Thyr.

NOISES in—Acn., *Chi.,* K. i., Kis., Lach., Lct. v., Lo. d., *Na. sa.,* Sfn., Sul. i. *(See also* REPORTS in; **Headache,** with TINNITUS; *and* **Tinnitus Aurium.)**

OTALGIA—K. i. *(See also* PAINS in; **Earache;** *and* **Otalgia.)**

OTORRHOEA—Caus—(See *also* **Otorrhoea.)**

PAINS in. —K. bi., Rdm. —*(See also* OTALGIA; **Earache:** *and* **Otalgia.).**

PAINFUL—Vb. o.

POLYPUS *of—Hep.,* Lach., Lyc., *Sang.,* Tax., *Thu.*

REPORTS in—Itu.

RING-HOLES, ULCERATION of—Stn.

SENSITIVE TO AIR—Mez.

THICKENING in—Rhe.

TINNITUS in—K. i—*(See also* **Headache,** with TINNITUS; *and* **Tinnitus Aurium.)**

WAX in—*Elp.,* Lach.

Ear, WAX in, EXCESSIVE— Wis.

Earache—*Cham.,* Gen., Gui., K. bi., K. i., Lo. e., Na. n., *Plnt.,* Pr. s., *Pul.,* Rn. s., Rdm., Rho., Sbd., Sac. l., Spi., Vis., Xan., Zin.

See also under **Ear;** *and* **Otitis.**

Ecchymosis—Arn., Crt. h., *Pho.*

See also **Extravasation.**

Eclampsia—Cast.

Ecstasy—Cof., Cyp., Ker., Stm.

Ecthyma—Ank., *Ant. t.*, Eu. pp., Jg. c., Jg. r., *Mr. sol.*, Pop. c., *Rhs.*

Eczema—*Aln.*, Alm., Ana., *Ant.* c., Arb., *Ars.*, As. r., Au. m., Ber. a., *Bov.*, Bry., Ca. s., Cth., Cbl. x., Ce. b., *Cic. v.*, Cod., Com., Co. a., Co. c., *Ctn.*, Cur., Fag., Fe. s., *Gph.*, *Hep.*, Iof., Iris, Jg.c., K. as., K. m., K. sc., Led., *Lyc.*, Merc., Mr. bin., *Mr. c.*, Nph., *Oln.*, Osm., *Pet.*, Pip. m., Pix, Plg., Prm. o., Prm. ve., Pso., Pyro., Rn. b., Rs. d., *Rs. v.*, Snc., *Sep.*, Sko., Sprn., Stp., *Sul.*, Sul. i., Tel., Thyr., Vac., *Vin.*, *Vi. t.*, Zin.

CAPITIS—Mlt.

FACIEI—Mr. p. a.

GOUTY—Ure., Ur. x.

IMPETIGINOIDES—Ank., Hdr.

MARGINATE—Ss. x.

PUSTULAR—Hoa.

RUBRUM—Anil., Pso.

SERPIGINOSUM—Ar. lp.

VACCINAL—Sko.

WEEPING—Sul i.

See also **Ear,** ECZEMA behind, *and* of; **Irritation** in ACUTE ECZEMA; *and* Scalp,ECZEMA of.

Egotism—Pal.

Elbow, PAIN in—Zn. o.

OLECRANON, in—Rap.

Elephantiasis—*Ana.*, Hpz., Sil., Stil.

ARABUM—(Ars.), Elae., *Hyd.*, Mst. s.

Emaciation—Amb., Caus., Ce. b., Dul., Gui., Iod., K. bi., K. i., Merc., Ol. j., Pb., Rap., Smb. n., Snc., Sto. c., Sul., Zn. m., Zn. v.

LIVER DISORDER, with—Chio.

LOWER LIMBS, of—Pin. s.

SCOFULOUS—Cet.

See also **Atrophy.**

Embolism—K. m.

Embolus—Ca. ar.

Emissions—*Ca. p., Cth., Chi., Cup.,* Dgn., *K. br., Nux., Ph. x., Pi. x.,* Plnt., Sx. n. *(See also* **Seminal Emissions.)**

Emissions, NOCTURNAL—Iris, Mag. m., Thu.

Emotions, Effects of—Gel.

Emphysema—Am. c., Ant. a., Bro., Cb. v., Cur., Gnd., Hep., *Lo. i.,* Sty., Ver.

Emptiness, Sensation of—Astg.

Empyema—Cb. a., Chi.

Enchrodroma—(Conc.), *Sil*

Endometritis—Alet., *Ars.,* Vis.

Enteralgia—(Cast.), Cu. as., Cyc., Dio., Na. p., Sntn.

    See also **Gastro-enteralgia.**

Enteric Fever—*Aga., Ars., Bap.,* Bel., *Bry., Ech. a., Ham., Hyo.,* Iod., Iof., *Ipc.,* Lach., *Mr. c., Mr. cy., Mu. x., Ph. x., Pho., Pyro., Rhs., Ter.*

    See also **Typhoid Fever.**

Enteritis—Aco., sntn.

    See also **Gastro-enteritis.**

Entropion—Bor., Gph., Tel.

Enuresis—Am. c., Atp., Apo., Atr., Au. s., Bz. x., (Brac.), Ca. p., Caus., Ce. s., Chn. v., Chl. h., Cin., Cub., Equ., E. pu., K. n., K. ph., Kre., Lina., Mag. s., Mil., Na. s., Nt. o., Ox. x., Ph. x., Pi. x., Pix, Plnt., Pso., Rs. a., Rus., Rut., Sbl., Snc., Sntn., Sars., Scro., Sel., Se. j., Sga., Sil., Stm., Sto. c., Sty., Sul., Thu., (Thyr.), Til., (Tub.), Vbs., Vsp., Vi. t., Zin.

    DIURNAL—Fer.

    NOCTURNAL—Arg., Ur. n.

    WHEN WALKING—Sap.

    See also **Urine,** INCONTINENCE of.

Ephelis—Lyc., Mu. x., Pho. *See also* **Freckles.**

Epidydimitis—Vb. o. *(See also* **Orchitis;** and **Testicles.)**

Epiglottis, Affections of—Wye.

Epilepsy—Abr., Abs., *Act. r.,* CEth., Am. br., Amg., Aml., Anag.,

Atp., Arg., Ag. n., Art. v., Ast. r., Atr., Au. br., *Bel.,* Bz. n., *Buf.,* Caj., Ca. ar., *Calc.,* Ca. p., Cam., Cn. i., Ct. eq., Caus., Chn. a., Ch. ar., Cic. m., *Cic. v.,* Crt. h., Cup., Cur., Cyp., Dt. m., Drs., Fgs., Glv., Gel., Glo., Hel., Hl. v., Hy. x., Hyo., *Ign.,* Ind., K. bi., K. br., *K. cy.,* Lach., Lau., Li. br., Lun., Med., Mli., Mil., Mos., Na. m., Na. s., Nct., Nt. x., Nt. o., Nux, *CEna.,* (Onis.), Onon, *Opi.,* Pas., Pho., Phst., *Pb.,* Plg., Pul., Rn. b., Sntn., Sec., *Sil.,* So. c., Spa. u., Stn., *Stm..* Sfn., Sul., Sum., Syph., Tab., Tan., Ter., Thu., Ver., Vbn., Vis., Zn. cy., Zn. v., Ziz.

Epilepsy, GREAT EXERTION OF STRENGTH with—Aga.

MENSTRUAL—Ced.

TRAUMATIC—Na.s.

See also **Hystero-epilepsy; Petit Mal;** *and* **Status. Epilepticus.**

Epiphora—Mrl., Scil.

See also **Lachrymation.**

Epistaxis—Abr., Amb., Anag., Ant. s. a., Atp., Bal., *Bry.,* Can. s., *Cb.v* V., Crd. m., Ce. s., Chel., Chn. s., *Cop., Cro.,* Crt. c., Elp., Epn. *Fe. p.,* Fe. pi., Glo. *Gph., Ham.,* Hli., Hpt., Hyo., Ind., Idm., K. bi., K. n., Lap., Lyc., *Mil.,* Mli., Onon., *Pho.,* Pi. x., Pim., Pul., Rap., Rat., Rho., Rs. g., Rum., Rut., Sbd., Sntn., Sec., Se. a., Sep., So. t. ae., Stn., *Sul.,* Trn., Tep., Til., Vip., Wis.

MENSTRUAL—Na. S.

Epithelial Tissue, Affections of—Arg.

Epithelioma—Ars., As. i., Cic. V., Cnd., Jeq., K. as., K. chl., K.sc., Kre., Lp. a. *Lyc.,* Mag. s., Mth. b., Nec.

LIP, of—*Ars.,* Kre.

Epulis—Calc., Lc. c., *Pb., Thu.*

Erections—Osm.

Erethism—Aur.

Erotomania— *Ca. p., Coth., Hyo., Nux, Ori., Pho., Pi. x., Plat., Stm., Trn.*

Eructations—*Ab. n., Ag. n., Cb. a., Cb. v., Cbl. x., Cham.,* K. Pi., Kre., Mn. m., *Nx. m., Sul.*

Eruptions—Ac. c., Ar. lp., Arm., *Bry.,* Crl., *Cu. a.,* Cup., Kre., Pix, Pso., Rs. v., Ric., Sars., Sil., Sid., *Sul.,* Tax., Tep., Zin.

ITCHING—PSQ.

MOIST—PSO.

SCROFULOUS—Src.

SUPRESSED—Cam., Zin. (See also **Suppressed Eruptions, Effects of.**)

   See also **Ankle; Beard; Chin, &c.,**ERUPTIONS on; **and Smart- ing Eruptions.**

Erysipelas—Am. c., An. oc., Anan., Athra., **APS.,** Ag. n., Ars., Aur., Bel., Bor., Cam., Cth., Cb. v., Cbl. x., Cham., *Chi.,* Chl. h., Cis., Com., Con., *Crt. h.; Cu. a.,* Cup., Dor., Elt., Eu. cy., Eu. pp., Eub., *Fe. p.,* Frg., *Gph.,* Gno., *Hep.,* Hpz., Inu., Jab., Jg. c., Lach., *Na. m.,* Na. p., Pas., Plnt., Ptl., Rn. a., Rs. d., *Rhs., Rs. v.,* Tep., Tub., *Ve. v.,* Zn. a.

BULLOSA— Ter.

Erysipelas, VESICULAR—Urt.

   See also **Breast.** ERYSIPELAS of.

Erythema—Atp., *Bel.,* Brc .x., Gnd., *Mez.,* Pi. x., Plnt., pb. chr., Ter., Tub., Urt.

FACE, of—Gph.

NODOSUM—*Aco.,* Aps., Jg. c., K. br., K. i, Led., Phyt., *Rhs.,* Rs. v., Su.x.

Ethmoiditis—Na. sf.

Eustachian Tubes, AFFECTIONS of—Mr. d., Phyt.

CATARRH of—K. sc., Lo. s., Sg. n.

OCCLUSION of —K.m.

Examination Funk—Ana..

Excitment—*Aco., Bel., Cham., Cof.*

   See also **Mental Excitement; and Nervous Excitement.**

Excoriation—*AEth.,* Arn., *Cham., Lyc., Mr. sol.,* Snc.

Excrescences—*Sil.*

See also *Urethra.*

Exhaustion—*Arn.,* Sna.., Zn. pi

Exophthalmic Goitre—(Atp.) , Ca.c., Eph., Fer., Fe. i, Hal., (Lcs.). Spi., Spa., Thyr., (Tub.)

> See also **Goitre.**

Exophthalmos—Aml., Dgn., K. as., Lcs., Pa.s., Pho., Sg. t., Sap., Scu., Spo., Sty.

Exostosis—Arg., Ca. *fl.,* Dph., Dul., *Hec., K. bi.,* Mez., Pho., *Pb.,* Rhs., Rut.

> See also **Bone.**

Extravasations—Ari.

See also **Ecchymosis.**

Exudations—Bls.

Eyes, AFFECTIONS of—*Aco.,* AEth., *Aln.,* Alm., Amc., *Aps.,* Ar. sc., *Ag. n.,* Arm., *Arn., Ars.,* As. mt., Asr., Atr., *Aur.,* Bap., *Bel.* Brc. x., Bar., Cd. s., *Calc.,* Crd. b., *Caus.,* Chr. o., *Cin., Clem.,* Cob., *Clch.,* Com., *Con.,* Crt. h., Ctn., *Cyc.,* Dph., Dt. m., Dir., *Ephr.,* Fag., Fe. pn., *Fl. x.,* For., *Gel., Gph.,* Grt., Gre., *Hep.,* Homa., *Hyo.,* Ilx., Iof., Ipc., Jab., K. as., K. *i.,* K. m., Lab., Lc. c., *Lach.,* Lil., Li. c., Lrs., Mac., Mnc., Mep., *Mr. sol.,* Mr. ac., *Mr. c.,* Mr. n., Mez., *Mor.,. Na. m., Nt. x., Nux,* Onos., *Ox. x.,* Pho., *Phst.,* Rho., Sars., Scil., *Sep., Sil., Stm., Sul., Zin.*

> BLEPHARITIS—Cham.
>
> > See also **Blepharitis.**
>
> CHOROIDITIS—Gel., *Pr. s., Rhs.,* Vi. o.

Eyes, CONJUCTIVITIS CATARRHAL and PURULENT—Cu. s.

> See also **Blepharitis; and Conjunctivitis.**
>
> CONVULSIONS of—Crb. h.
>
> CONVULSIONS, LIDS, of—*See* **Blepharospasm.**
>
> CORNEAL OPACITY—*Can. s.*
>
> > See also **Cornea,** OPACITY of.
>
> CYSTS ON LIDS—K. i.
>
> > See also **Stye; Tarsal Cysts;** *and* **Tarsal Tumours.**

GRANULAR INFLAMMATION of—*Thu.*

GRANULAR LIDS—Cu. S., Na. as., Zin. (*See also* **Granular Lids.**)

GRANULR OPHTHALMIA—*Pul.*

HAEMORRHAGE into—Lach.

HEAVY —Cnn.

HYPEROPIA of—Jab.

INFLAMMATION of—*Am. m., Ant. t.,* Caln., Cth., Cnt., Cham., Cic. v.,. Cnb., Clv. d., Der., Eub., Gam., Hph. v., Ja. g., K. ca., K. Ox., Lyc., Mag. c., Mnc., Med., Mr. bin., Na. as., Pbo., Pb., Prm.o.,. Rn. r., *Rhs.,* Tel.

INFLAMMATION of, GOUTY—Merc., *Nux.*

INJURIES of—Phst., Symt.

IRITIS—K. bi. (See also **Iritis;** and **Kerato—iritis.**)

IRRITATION of—Per.

KERATITIS—K. bi.

   See also **Keratitis.**

LACHRYMAL SAC, INFLAMMATION of—*Pul.*

LIDS, AFFECTIONS of—Spa. u.

LIDS, MARGINS of, BLISTERS on—Pal.

LIDS, MARGINS of, INFLAMED—Jat.

LIDS, TUMOURS of — Teu.

LIDS, TWITCHING of—Grna. (*See also* **Blepharospasm.**)

MUSCAE VOLITANTES—Itu. (*See also* **Muscae Volitantes;**)

NEURALGIA of—Ce. b., Ch. m. (*See also* **Ciliary Neuralgia.**)

ŒDEMA around—K. ca.

OPERATIONS on—Aln., Ars., Jab.

OPHTHALMIA—Cham. (*See also* INFLAMMATION; GRANULAR OPHTHALMIA; **Granular Lids; Ophthalmia; and Phlyctenular Ophthalmia.**)

OPTIC NERVE, SCLEROSIS of—*Sty. n.*

OPTIC NEURITIS—*Aps.,* Tab., Thyr.

PAINS in—Bad., Chr. o., Gnd., Mag. s., Rut., *Spi.,* Symt.

PAINS over—Jg. r.

    PARALYSIS of—Sntn.

    POLYPUS OF CANTHUS—Lyc.

      See also **Polypus.**

Eyes, PTERYGIUM—*Rat.*

    PUPILS DILATED —Dbn., So. pc.

    SCLEROTICA INFLAMED—Tan. (*See also* **Sclerotitis.**)

    SCROFULOUS AFFECTIONS of—Scro.

    SCROFULOUS INFLAMMATION of—Fe. i. (*See also* **Ophthalmia.,**
    SCROFULOUS ; and **Scrofula.**)

    SIGHT WEAK—Mep., *Nx. m., Rhs., Rut.*

    SMARTING of—Rn. r.

    STRAIN of—Na. m., Phst.

    STAPHYLOMA—Ephr., Ilx.

    SWELLING OVER—Cen.

    SYPHILITIC AFFECTIONS of—Mr. i. f.

    TENSION in—Jab.

    TUMOURS of—*Bz. x., Stp., Tku.,* Zin.

    TWITCHING of—Jn. v.

    WATERING of—Mrl., Scil. (*See also* **Lachrymation.**)

    For other Affections of the Eye, *see* **Amblyopia; Asthenopia;**

Black-eye; Intra—ocular Affections; &c.

Eye—teeth, Pains in—Ther.

Face, BLOTCHES on—*K. ca.*

    BOILS on—Ca. p.

    BONES of, PAINFUL—Astg. (*See also* **Antrum; and Malar
      Bones.**)

    CHAPPED —Nic.

    COMPLEXION UNHEALTHY—*Na. m.*

    DISTORTION of—Crt. h. (*See also* **Distortions.**)

    ERUPTION on—*Ars., Cb. a., Cic. v., Crt. h., Lyc.,* Phen.

    ERYTHEMA of—Gph.

    FLUSHING of—Aco.

NEURALGIA of—Chi., Ccn. s., K. ph. (*See also* **Neuralgia; and Prosopalgia.**)

PARALYSIS of—(Aco.), Am. p., Cd. s., Caus., Cep., Cur., For., k. *chl.,* Mr. k. i.,O1. a., Pet., Sga., Zn. pi.

PARALYSIS of, from COLD —Rut.

PIMPLES on—*Amb., Clem.,* Ind., *Led.*

ROUGHNESS of—Ber. a.,*Pet*

YELLOW—Sep.

Fag—(Mag. c.), (Pi. x.), Zin.

Fainting—(Aco.), Amg., Antf., *Ars.,* Cro., Cup., Cur., *Ign.,* Jal., Lach., Lina.., Mgt., Mgn. gl., Merc., Mos., Na. ns., Nx. m., Oln., Pho., Prt., Se. a., Spo., Sum., Tax., Ther., Thyr., Ver., Vsp.

FITS— Cham.

FLOODING, with—Trl.

SPELLS—Lc. v. d.

FAINTNESS—*Act. r.,* Arnt., Coc. i., *Hdr.,* Lt. k., Lo. i., Rap., Sars., *Sul.*

False Conception—Caul., Nux.

See also **Pregnancy,** IMAGINARY.

Farcy—K. bi.

Fatigue—Bls., Cai., Fe. pi., Tur.

Fatty Degeneration—*Pho.,* Van.

Fatty Tumours—*Aga.,* Thu., Ur. k.

Favus—Hyd., Jg. r., Med., Mr. ac., Ss. X., Vin.

FEAR—*K. ca.,* Mli., *Plat., Pul.,* Suc.

EFFECTS of—*Aco., Bel.,* Coc. i., *Ign.,* opi. (*See also* **Fright,** EFFECTS of.)

TRAINS and CLOSE PLACES, of—Suc.

Feet, AFFECTIONS of—*Caul., Gph.*

BURNING in—*Aps., Clcn., Sec., Sil., Sul.*

COLDNESS of—*Cb. v., Sec.,* Sto. c.

CRAMPS in—Sec.

FETID —Thu.

FIDGETY—K. ph., Pl. n.

GALLED EASILY—Cep.

HEELS, PAINS in—*Ca. cs. (See also* **Heel,** PAIN in.)

HORNY and SORE—*Ant.* c.

PAINFUL—*Clch.*

PAINS in—Am. m., *Bro.,* Cltr., *Led., Rn. b., Rhs.*

PERSPIRING—*Lyc., Nt. x., Sil., Sul. (See also* SWEAT.)

SOLES, PAINFUL—*Pet., Pul.*

SOLES PAINS in—*Mu. x.*

SORE—*Arn., Ph. x.*

SWEAT of—Ba. c, Idm., Lc. x., Mag. m., Snc., *Sil.,* Zin. *(See also* PERSPIRING.)

SWEAT of, CHECKED, CONSEQUENCE of—For.

SWEAT of FETID—Tel.

SWEAT of SUPRESSED—Sl. x., Sil., Zin.

TENDER—Led., Rum.

WEAKNESS of—Rn. r.

Femur, CARIES of—Sto. c.

PAINS in—Src.

Fester—*Sil.*

TENDENCY to—*Hep., Pet.*

Fever, BILIOUS—Nyc.

See also **Bilious** FEVER

GASTRIC—Bap., K. s., Tri.

HECTIC—Lo. e. *(See also* **Hectic Fever.**)

Fever, INTERMITTENT—Calc., Fer. *(See also* **Ague;** *and* **Intermittent Fever.**)

REMITTENT—Nyc. *(See also* **Infantile Remittents;** *and* **Remittent Fever.**)

Fevers—Ac. x., *Aco.,* Alet., All., Als., Am. ac., Ant. c., *Ars.,* Ar. it. Asi., Ast. f.,. Aur., Bnz., Bzn., Ber., Bo. la., Caln., Cltr., Crd. b., Crd. m., Cnt., Cham., Chm. u., Chn. s., Coca, Cchn... Dph., Dig, Dor., Epl., Ery. m., Fe. p., Glv., *Gel.,* Gn.l., Gui., Gno., Hfb., Hyn., Ir. t., Lim., Mlr., Merc., Na. sa., Ol. j., Oxt., Prt., Phen., Pim., Psc., Ple., Pbo., Pod., Prm. ve., Prin.,

Pyre., Qeb., Rn. a., Rap., Rho., Rut., Sx. n., Sx. p., Sll., Sap., *Sul.,* Tri., Var., Wye.

See also **Catarrhal** Fever; **Catheter Fever; Chagres Fever;.**

Fibroma—*Hnn. m., K. i.* Lp. a. Lil., Lyc., *Sec., Sil.,* Trn., Ter., Teu., Thl., Thyr., Ust., Xan.

HAEMORRHAGE from—Trl.

Fidgets—Api. g., Asr., Men., Scil. (*See also* **Feet,** FIDGETY.)

Finger—joints, Ulcers on—Bor.

Fingers, Contracted—Can. s.

Fissures—Alm., Gph., Merc., Rat.

Fistula—Alm., Au. m., (Bac.), Ba. m., Ber., Cac., Calc., *Ca. p.,* Ca. s., *Caln., Caus.,* Cop., Cnd., Euc., *Fl. x.,* Hdr., Iris, Mld., Nt. x.. Ol. j., Pet., Pho., Pyro., Qer., *Sil.,* (Tub.).

DENTALIS—Caus., Stp., Sui.

LACHRYMAL—Aga., Bro., Chel., Lach., Mil., Nt. x., Sil., Stn.

See also **Anus,** FISTULA of; *and* **Breast,** FISTULA of.

Fistulous Abscess—Na. s.

Flatulence—Acal., *Ag. n.,* Ari. s., Asa., Ca. fl., *Ca i., Cb. v., Cbl. x.* Cast., Cham., Dct., Dio., Dir., Fe. mg., Homa., Ign., Jg. r., Jnc., *Lach.,* Lo. s., *Lyc.,* Mrl., Mom., Nph., Na. n., *Nx. m.,* Orn., Ph. x., Pho., Pt. m. n., P. od., Rap., Rm. f., Rob., Sl. x. Scu., Sin. a., Sla., Tep., Zng.

INCARCERATED—(Rap.), Rho., Thu.

OBSTRUCTED—Ign., (Rap.)

ODOURLESS—Y. uc.

See also **Dyspepsia,** FLATULENT

Flatulent Colic—Cham., Plg.

Flushing—Aml., Kre., Oop., Rap., Sl. x., Su. x., Vsp. CLIMACTERIC—Jab., Sang. (*See also* **Climacteric,** FLUSHINGS of.)

See also **Indigestion,** with FLUSHING.

Foetus, MAL-POSITION of—Pul.

Foetus, MOVEMENTS of EXCESSIVE—(Cro.), Opi., (Thu.)

Follicular Pharyngitis—Cis. (*See also* **Throat.**)

Foreign Bodies, Expulsion of—(Lo. i.), Sil.

Fracture—*Ca. p.*, E. pf., *Rut., Sil., Symt.*

NERVOUS—Symt.

NON-UNION of—Symt., Thyr.

See also **Compound Fractures.**

Freckles—(Adr.), Ir. g., *K. ca.*, Lyc., Mu. *x., Nt. x.*, Nx. m., Pho., Pul., *Sep.*, Sol., Sul., Tab.

Fretfulness—Ca. br.

Fright—Gel.

EFFECTS of—*Aco.*, Act. s., Glo.

See also **Fear**, EFFECTS of.

Frontal Sinuses, CATARRH of—(Mg. m.), (Na. m.), Thu.

Frost-bite—*Fe. p.*, Mgt. s., Nt. x., Nx. m., Pet.

Frowning— Rhe.

Fungus Haematodes—Lach., Pho.

Furuncles—As. r.

See also **Boils.**

Gagging—Pod.

Galactorrhoea—Con., Iod., Ust.

See also under **Lactation;** *and* **Milk.**

Gall-bladder,AFFECTIONS of—Bap., Bo. la., Dio.

PAIN in—Fe. s.

Gall-stone Colic—Ber., Chi., Chio., Ipc., Lyc., Ter.

Gall-stones—Ber., Calc., Crd. m., Chel., Chlf., Chlst., Evm., Ev. a., Evo., Fel., Lach., Li. c., Lo. i., Man., Nt. s. d., Nux, Pch., Pod., Ptl., Trx., Tbl., Vic.

Ganglion—*Bz. z.*, Bov., Fe. mg., Ph. x., Pb., Rut., Sil;., Sul., Thu.

FOOT, of—Ped.

Gangrene—Aga., Athra., Aps., *Ars.*, Bis., Bth., Brs., Cb. a., *Cb. v.*, Cbl. x., (Cep.), Chr. o., *Ech. a.*, Erg., Eub., K. ph., *Lach.*, Rn. a., Ric., Sec., Su. x.

AMPUTATION, after—Hyd.

HOSPITAL—Cis.

SENILE—(Cep.)

Gangrenous and Fetid Suppurations—Ch. s.

Gastralgia—Ac. f., Bis., Ch. ar., Cod., Dph., Dio., Grn., Gph., Grt.,
K. ca., Klm., Li. c., Lo. i., N. ap., Nx. m., Ptl., Rn. b., Rum.,
Stn., Stp., Su. x., Zin.

Gastric Affections— Cro., Dor., Elae.,
See also under **Stomach.**

CATARRH—Cm. br., Cry., Hdr., Pod., Sil., Spi., Ver.

DISORDERS—Mu. x.

DISTURBANCES—Cup.

FEVER—Bap., K. s., Tri.

IRRITATION—Per.

ULCERS—*Ag. n., Ars., Atr.,* Ca. ar., *Ham., Ipc., K. bi.,* K. ph.,
Orn., Pet., Rat., Sin. a., *Ur. n.*

Gastritis—Ag. e., Ag. p., Ags., Ars., As. i., As. r., Bis., Cth., Ch. m.,
Chlm., Cop., Eu. co., Eu. i., Fe. p., Fe. s., Gau., K. n., K.
pm., K. s., Mn. s., Pho., Rx. ac., Sl. x., Snc., Sec., Sin. a.,
Tt. x., Zn. a.

Gastrodynia—*Ars., Nux, Ox. x.* (See also under *Stomach.*)

INTERMITTENT— Iris.

Gastro-enteralgia— Phal.

Gastro-enteritis—Bry., Na. ns., Rhs., Ric., Sntn., Sca.

Gastromalachia—Kre., Mr. d.

General Paralysis—Aga., Equ., Iof., Phst., Ver.

INSANE, of—K. br., *Pho.*

Genital Weakness—Per. (*See also* **Sexual Weakness.**)

Genitals, MALE, CONGESTION of—Clcn.

MALE, PAIN in—Clcn.

SWEAT of OFFENSIVE—Fag.

German Measles—Atp. (*See also* **Roseola.**)

Giant Urticaria—Sntn.

Giddiness—Bls., Qer. ,

See also **Vertigo.**

Glanders—Hpz., *K. bi., Lach.*

Glands, Affections of—AEth., Amc., Ar.lp., Bad., Fe. pn., Hec.,
    Sbl.,Stp., Sul.

    Cervical Ulceration of—Rs. v.

    Enlargement of—Ac. l., Alns., Am. m., Ast. f., Ba. i., Bro.,
    Chm. u., Fe. i., Hal., Ign., Lp. a., Mez., Phyt., Pb. i., Sars., Scir.,
    Scro., Sil. m., Symt., Tab.

    Induration of—Ca. fl., Cb. a.

    Induration of Parotid Glands—Bro.

    Inflammation of—Anan., Crl., Hpz., Rhs.

    Inguinal, Swelling of—Pin. s., Ter.

    Parotid—See **Mumps; Parotid Glands; and Parotitis.**

    Scrofulous, Swelling of—Na. p.

    Submaxillary, Swelling of —Pin. s.

Glands, Suppuration of—Ig. r., Sec., Sil. m.

    See also **Axillary Glands,** Suppuration of.

    Swelling of—Aco., K. m., Li. c., Lyc., Sec., So. a., So. o., Sti.
    (See also **Glandular Swellings.**)

    See also **Bronchial Glands; Inguinal Glands; &c.**

Glandular Swellings—*Ars., Ar. t., Ba. c.,* Ba. m., *Bel., Calc., Ca. i.,*
    Ca. m., Ca. s., *Caln.,* Cap., Crb. s., Cis., Ephr., Epn., Gph.,
    Hep., K. i., Mr. sol., Nt. x., Sil.

    See also **Glands,** Swelling of.

Glaucoma—Ced., Col., Eser., Gnd., Osm., Pho., Phst., Ppz., Pr. s.,
    Spi., Wis.

Gleet—Alns., Ala., Aln., Ba. m., Bov., Cld., Calc., Ca. p., Chm. u.,
    Cnb., Cub., Dor., Equ., Ery. a., Erig., Fl. x., Gph., K. bi., K.
    sc., Med., Mez., *Nph.,* Na. m., Nt. x., pts., Pho., Phyt., Pso.,
    Sbl., Sang., Se. a., Sep., Suo., Tel., Ter., Thu., Ves.

    Chronic—Pop. t.

Globus Hystericus—Arnt., (Asa.), (Ign.),Klm., (Lach.), Lct. v.,
    (Lyc.), Na. hch., Rap., Suc., Sul.

    See also **Hysteria.**

Glossitis—Aco., (Aps.), Cth., Crl. h., Kre., (Merc.), Phyt., Rn. s., Su. x.

    See also **Tongue.**

Glosso-pharyngeal Paralysis—Na. m.

Glottis, Spasm of—Vsp.

Goitre—Au. s., *Bel.,* Bro., *Calc.,* Crb. s., Caus., Crt. c., *Fer., Fl. x.,* Fuc., *Glo.,* Hal., *Iod.,* Lp. a., Lyc., Mr. i. f., Na. *c., Na. m.,* Na. p., Ol. j., Pod., Sec., *Spo.,* Thyr., Thri., Vip.

    EXOPHTHALMIC—Cac., Fer., Spo., Thyr. (*See also* **Exophthalmic Goitre.**)

Gonorrhoea—Aco., Agv., Alo., Aln., Anag., Ar.lp., Ag. n., Arm., As. f., Aur., Au. m., Ba. m., Bz. x., Calc., Ca. p., Ca. s., Cam., Cn. i., *Can. s., Cth.,* Caul., Chel., Chm. u., Cnb., Clem., Cob., Ccs. c., Cop., Cub., Cp. a., Dig., Dor., Eps., Equ., Ere., Ery. a., Erig., i Euc., Eu. pi., Fer., Fe. i., Fe. p., Fe. s., Fl. x., Frg., Gel., Hdy. Hdr., Hyd., Icth., Ja. c., Ja. g., K. i., K. sc., Lc. c., Lct. v., Lup., Mr. n., Mr. p. r., Mth. b., Mez., Myg., *Nph.,* Na. m., *Na. s.,* Ol. a., Prei., Par., Pet., Pts., Phyt., Pch., Pip. m., Plg., Pso., Pul., Rat., Sbl., Sbi., Sx. n., Sll., Snt., Sars., Se. a., Sep., Sill m., Sul., Sul. i., Ter., Thl., *Thu.,* Trad., Ts. p., Ves.

    CHRONIC—Zea st.

    SECONDARY—Agn.

    SUPPRESSED—*Med.,* Vi. t.

Gonorrhoeal Ophthalmia—Hdy.

Rheumatism—Dph., Ja. c., *Med.,* Phyt., Pul., Sars., *Sul., Thu.*

Gout—Abr., Am. bz., Am. p., Anag., Ank., Aps., Arb., Ar.lp., Arb., Bel., Bls., Bz. x., Caj., Ca. ren., Crb. s., Carl., Ced., Cham., Chr. o., Cnb., *Clch., Cup.,* Dph., Euc., E. pf., For., Gas., Gn. l., Gna., Grt., Gui., Her., Hyd., Ird., Jal., K. bi., K. i., Klm., Kis., *Led.,* Li. c., Lrs., *Lyc.,* Lys., Mlr., Man., *Mr. sol.,* Na. l., Na. m., Na. p., *Nux, Ox. x.,* Pan., Ph. x., Phyt., Pin.s., Ppz., Plat., Pb., Pso., *Pul.,* Pyr. a., Qer., Rn. s., Rks., Sbi., Sac. l., Sars., Sld., Ste., *Sul.,* Tax., Tep., Ure., Ur. x., *Urt.,*

Vic., Vi. t., Wis., Wil.

See also **Arthritis.**

Gouty Concretions—Na. l.

See also **Joints,**CONCRETIONS in.

Joints—Agn.

Swellings—Calc.

Granular Conjunctivitis— Phyt.

Granular Lids—(Ch. m.), Cu. s., Ephr., Fag., Jeq., Mrl., Na. as., Sang., Zin., Zn. s.

See also **Eyes.**

THROAT—Homa., Phyt., Yuc. (*See also* **Throat.**)

Gravel—Arm., Baro., *Ber.*, Ca. ren., *Ch. s.*, *Cas. c.*, Epg., Equ., E. ar., E. pu., Gli.,*Gph.*, Hdrn. a., *Lyc.*, *Nm x.*, Ocm., *Ox. x.*, Pts., *Ph. x.*, Plg., *Sars.*, Sep., Sto. b., Urt., Ves., Vic.

WHITE and RED—Na. hch.

Groin, Pain in—Epn.

Growing Pains—Gui.

Growth, Defective—Bac. (Thyr.).

Gum-boil—*Mr. sol.*, Snc.

Gumma—K. *i.*

Gum-rash—*Ant. c., Aps., Cham., Rhs.*

Gums, AFFECTIONS of—*Mr. c.*

BLEEDING of—Lach.

ITCHING of—Rho.

NEURALGIA of—Doi.

SENSITIVE—Am. c.

SORE— *Nt .x.*

ULCERATION of—Agn., *Pho.*

UNHEALTHY—*Mr. sol.*

Gun-shot Wounds—Hyp., Symt.

Haematemesis—*Arn.,* Crd. m., Cup., Fe. p., *Ham., Ipc.,* Mil., Stn. Zn.m.

Haematocele—Erig.

Haematoporphyrinuria—Sfn.

Haematuria—Adr., *Arn.*, Cac., Ch. s., Crt. h., Equ., *Ham.*, K. chl., Lyc., Mez., Mil., Na. hch., Nt. x., Phas., Sec., *Ter.*, Thl., Tub., Uva., yes.

Haemoglobinuria—Ch. s., *Pho., Pi. x.*, Sntn.

Haemoptysis—Acal., (*Aco.*), Cac., Ca. fl., Crd. m., Csc., Chel., Chlm., Cro., Fe. p., Hlx., Hep., Hyo., Ill., Led., Lips., Lcs., Mli.,Mil., Na. as., Onis., Pho., Pb., Sang., So. m., Stn., Strp., Tub.

See also **Consumption,** BLEEDING; *and* **Phthisis.**

Haemorrhage—Ab. n., Aco., Alns., Aln., Aran., Aur., Au. m., Bth., Bov., Bry., *Cac.*, Ca. s., Cb. v., Crd. m., Csc., Chi., Ch. s., Cinm., Cit., Cob., Ccs. c., Coll., Cro., Drs., Dul., Elp., Ere., Erg., Erod., Epn., Fer., Fe. m., Fe. p., Fe. s., Fic. r., Ga. x., Ger., *Ham.*, Hyo., *Ipc.*, Jn. c., K. ca., K. chl., K. i., Kre., Lach., Leo., Mgt., Mr. cy., Mil., Nt. x., Nx. m., Plat., Pso., Rat., Rs. a.., Rs. g., Rhs., Rut., Sgs., Scir., Sec., Se. a., Thl., Thu., Trl., Urt., Vip., Wis.

ANTE-PARTUM—Trl.

POST-PARTUM—Can. s., Sec., Trl.

WATERY—Lt. m., (Sgs.)

See also **Typhoid Fever,** HAEMORRHAGE in.

Haemorrhagic Diathesis—(Adr.), Aran., Bov., Chl. h., *Crt. h., Ham.*, Kre., *Pho.,* Sec.

Haemorrhoidal Discharge—Lo. i., Mu. u.

Haemorrhoids—Abr., *Aco.*, AEs. g. *AEsc.*, Alet., Alo., Am. c., *Am., m.,* Ana., Anag., Ant. c., Aral., As. mt., Aur., Au. m. n., Bad., Ba. c., Bel., *Cap., Cb. a., Cb. v.,* Crd. m., Caus., Chel., Chi., Chr. o., Cim., Coca, Coc. i., *Coll.,* Cop., Dio., Dul., Ery. a., Erig., Eu. a., Frl., *Fl. x.,* Glv., Gas., Gph., Grt., *Ham.*, Hli., Hep., Hdr., Hyp., *Ign.,* Iod., Ipc., K. ac., K. br., K. ca., K. chl., K. m., Kis., Lach., Lam., Lpsa., Lim., Lina., Ln. c., Lips., Lyc., Mag. m., Mr. bin., Mu. u., *Mu. x.*, Mus., *Nux,*

Paeo., Pnt., Pet., Phst., Phyt., Pin. s., Pip. n., Plnt., Plat., Pb., Pod., Plg., Plp., Pso., *Pul.,* Rn. fi., Rn. s., Rat., Rdm., Rhs., Rs. v., Sin. n., Sla., Stil., Sto. c., *Sul.,* Tep., Ter., Thu., Ul. f., *Vbs.,* Wis., Wye, Zn. v.

STRANGULATED—*Aco.*

Hair, ABNORMAL GROWTH of—Ol. j.

AFFECTIONS of—Jab., *K. ca.,* Thu., Wil.

BEARD,of, FAlling off—Sgu.

DRY—Pso.

FALLING OFF—Au. m., Au. m. n., Cb. v., Chn. s., *Fl. x.* For., Hl. f., Lyc., Mnc., Ped., *Ph. x.,* Sel., Sgu., Su. x., Tax., Thyr., Wis. (*See also* **Alopecia;** *and* **Baldness.**)

Hair, GREY—Su. x.

GROWS DARKER —Wis.

GROWTH of, NEW—Thyr.

GROWTH of, RAPID— Sac. o., Wis

HEAD , OF, FALLING OFF—Sgu .

OILINESS of—Bz. n., Hfb.

TANGLING—Pso.

Hallucinations—Anh., Cu. a.

 See also **Clairaudience; Clairvoyance;** *and* **Vision,** HALLUCINATIONS of.

Hands, AFFECTIONS of—*Caul.*

CHAPPED—Lyc., *Na. c., Pet.,* Prm., O., Sars., Ss. x.

ERUPTIONS on—Pix.

HOT—Gad.

PAINS in—Cltr., *Led., Pul., Rhs., Rut.*

PERSPIRING—Fag., *Fl. x.,* Pi. x.

RED—Chi. b.

SWELLING of—Aps., *Ag. n., Bry., Fe. p.*

 See also **Palms,** CRAMP in; *and* **Psoriasis** PALMARIS

Hangnails—K. chl., Up.

Hay Asthma—*Ars.,* Lo. i., *Nph., Sbd.,* Sul. i.

Hay Fever—Abrs., Antho., Aral., As. i., Ard., Asc. s., Bad.,

Cep.,. Dul., Eub., Gel., K. bi., K. i., Lach., Ln. u., Lo. s., Mlr.,. Mr. k. i., Naj., Na. i., Pso., Rn. b., Ro. d., Sg. n., Sga., Sin. n.. Sko., Sti., Suc.

Head, CONFUSED—Ath.

CONGESTION of—Pso.

CONVULSIVE MOVEMENT of—(Lyc.), Nx. m.

EMPTY SENSATION in—Cn. br.

ENLARGED SENSATION of—Antf., Pip. m.

NODDING of—Au. s.

NUMB—Ost.

PAINS in—Lpi., Pan.

RUSH OF BLOOD to—Paeo., Sul.

Headache—Ac. c., *Aco., Act. r., AEsc., .AEth.,* Ail., All., Alm., Am. pi., Amph., Amg., Aml., Ana., Anag., Anh., Anth. n., Atp., Aph., Api. g., Ag. m., Aran., Ar. sc., Ag. n., Arm., Arn., Ars.,. As. mt., Ar. it., Ar. t., Asa., Asr., Asc. s., Asc. t., Ast. r., Astg., Ath., Arnt., Au. ar., Au. m. n., Bap. c., *Bel.,* Bls., Bnz., Ber. a., Bis., Bo.la., Brc. x., *Bov.,* Bru., Brcn., *Bry., Cac.,* Caj., Ca. ac., Ca. ar., Calc., ca. hp., Ca. i., Ca. p., *Cn. i.,* Can.s., *Cap.,* Cb. a., *Cb. v.,* Crb. o., Crd. b., Caus., Cen., *Cham., Chel.,* Chn. a., Chm. m., *Chi.,* Ch. m., *Ch. s.,* Chio., Cich., Chn. s., Cinm.

Headache (*continued*)—

Clem., Cob., Coc. *i.,* Cof., Clcn., Col., Clv. d., Cro., Crt. c., Crt. h., Cnd., Cp. a., Cur., Cyc., Dig., Dio., Dir., Drs., Dul., Elae., Elp., Elc., Eph., *Eps.,* Eser., Evo., E. pu., Eu. hp., Eub., Epn., Fag., Fgs., Fel., Fe. br., Fe. m., *Fe. py.,* Fe. s., Fe. t., Fl. x., For., Fnc., *Gel.,* Gen., Gn. l., Gin., *Glo.,* Gph., Grt., Grna., Gno., Haem., Hel., Hlod., *Hep.,* Her., Homa., Hfb., Hyp., Ign., Ind., Idm., Iod., Iof., Ir. fl., Ir. foe., Ir. t., *Iris,* Jg. c., Jg. r., Jnc., K. bi., *K. ca.,* K. cy., K. n., Klm., Lc. c., Lc. f., Lc. V., Lc. v. d., *Lach.,* Lchn., Lam., Lap., *Lpt.* Li. c., Lo. c., Lo. d., Lun., Lrs., Lcs., Mac., Mag. m., Mag. p., Mnc., Man., Mli., Mns., Mth. pi., Mth. pu., Mor., *Naj.,* Na.

c.. Na. hch., *Na. m.,* Na. s., Nic., Ni. s., Nup., Nx. m., *Nux,* Oln., ol. j., Onon., Onos., Osm., Paeo., Pal., Par., Prt., Pnt., Pet., Phas., *Phel.,* Phen., *Ph. x.,* Pho., Phst., Phyt., Pim., Pip. m., Pip. n., Pb., Pr. p., Pso., Pyro., Rn. g., Rap., Rhe., Rdm., Rs. g., Sbd., Sbl., Sac. l., Sll., *Sang.,* Sg. n., Snc., Sap., Sars., Sel., Se. j., *Sil.,* Sin. a., Sol, So. n., So. t. ae., *Spi.,* Sta., Stn., Sti., Stm., Sto. c., Sto., n., Sty., *Sul.,* Syph., Tr., Ther., Thu.. Tri., Tub., Ts. p., Up., Val., Var., Ver., Ve. n., Vb. o., Wye., Xan., Yuc., Zin., Zn. p., Zn. pi., Zn. s.

BILIOUS—Bap., Co. c., Pod., Ptl., Tri.

CATARRHAL—Smb. n., Stil.

CHLOROTIC—Zin.

CONGESTIVE—Sto. c., Usn.

DULL—Ost.

DULL, HEAVY —Sin. n.

FRONTO-OCCIPITAL—Ore.

GASTRIC—Ptl., Rob., Trx.

HAEMORRHOIDAL—(Coll.)

INTERNAL and EXTERNAL—Gui.

MENSTRUAL—Coc. i., K. ph., Ust.

MERCURIAL—Stil.

NERVOUS—Nic., Scu., Ver., Ve. v., Zin.

NEURALGIC—Med.

NOSE, EXTENDING to—Prt.

OCCIPITAL—Ore., Pet., Var.

PERIODIC—Nic., Sac. o.

PHOTOPSIA, with—(Cyc.), (Iris), (K. bi.), Tax.

PRESSIVE—Men.

SCHOOL-CHILDREN, of—Ph. x. (*See also* **School-headache.**)

SCHOOL-GIRLS, of—(Ca., p.), (Na. m.)

SICK—Chlf., (Iris), Pod., (Sang.), Sti., Ver., Ve. v.

STUDENTS, of—Pi.x.

Headache, SUN, FROM—Gel., Glo., K. bi., KIm., Stm.

SYPHILITIC—(Au. ar.), Stil., Syph.

TEMPORAL—Yuc.

TENSIVE—Sto. c.

TINNITUS, WITH—Sfn.

> *See also* **Bright's Disease,** HEADACHE of; **Influenza,** HEADACHE of; **Hemicrania; Megrim; Migraine; Snow-headache.**

Head-lice—Sbd.

> *See also* **Pediculosis; and Phthiriasis.**

HEARING ALTERED—Phyt.

ILLUSIONS of—Cnn., Rdm.

> *See also* **Clairaudience.**

Heart, AFFECTIONS of—Aco., *Act. r.,* Ado., Amc., AmI., Ana., Aps., Apo., Arg., *Arn,* Ars., *As. i.,* Asa., Asc. t., Ast. r., Au., br., Au. m., Bad., *Ba. c., Bel.,* Bov., Buf., *Cac.,* Cam., Caus., Cen., Ce. b., Ccs. c., Clch., Coll., Cvl., Cty., *Crat.,* Cro., Crt. h., Dgn., *Dig.,* Dir., Fag., Fer., Glo., Gnd., *Ibe., Ign.,* Iod., Iof., Jab., K. ca., K. m., K. n., Lc. v. d., *Lach.,* Lau, Lpi., Liz., *Li. c.,* Lo. i., Mag. m., Mgn. gr., *Mr. sol.,* My. c., *Naj.,* Na. i., *Na. m., Nux,* Phas., Phst., Phyt., Plg., Pop. c., Pr. p., Pr. s., Pyr. a., Rum., *Spi.,* Sto. c., Strp., Sum., Tax., Tub., Ve. v.

CONSCIOUS ACTION of—Ibe.

CONSCIOUSNESS of—Pyro.

DEGENERATION of—*Pho.*

DISEASES of—Asp., Bro., Ca. ar., *Cb. v.,* Coca, Gel., Klm., Lyc., Lcs.

DISORDERED —Cean.

FAILURE of—Crat., Hlod., *Mos.,* Phas., Pyro., Thyr., Zea st.

FATTY—Phyt.

FATTY DEGENERATION of—K. fc.

Heat in—Lchn., (Rho.)

HYPERAESTHESIA of—Cof.

HYPERTROPHY of—Bro., Cac., Chl. h., Crat., Eth. n., Iod., Phyt., Pr. v., Spo.

INFLAMMATION of—*Bry.*

INFLUENZA HEART—Ibe.

INTERMITTENT— Tab.

IRRITABLE—Pr. v.

JARRING, EFFECTS of—Glo.

MURMURS of—Pho.

OPPRESSION of—Ov. g., p.

PAIN in—Ari., Ce. S., Lchn., Li. m., Men., Pau., Pod., Rum.

PALPITATION of—Fer., Fe. p., Glo., *Lil.*, Mgt. s., Ol. j., Phas., Pin. s., *Pul.,* Rap., Scil., Sec., Tub., Up., Val., Yoh. (*See also* **Palpitation.**)

Heart, PALPITATION of, NERVOUS—Sum.

PARALYSIS of—Atp., Chl. h., Erg., Jt. u., Lo. p.

PRESSURE at—Prm. vg.

RAPID ACTION of—Pyro.

SLOW—Lt. k.

VALVULAR DISEASE of—Thyr.

WEAKNESS of—Pr. v.

See also **Dropsy,** CARDIAC.

Heartburn—Api. g., *Ag. n.,* Cd. br., Caj., *Cap.,* Crb. s. Chn. s., Eub., Fag., Fe. i., Lach., Lct. V., Li. m., *Lyc.,* Mag. m., *Pul.,* Sin. a., Sin. n., So. n., Su. x., Vic., Zn. s.

See also **Cardialgia;** *and* **Pregnancy,** HEARTBURN of.

Heat, Effects of—Gel.

Heat-spots—*Aps.*

Hectic Fever—Abr., *Ars.,* Au. m. n., Bal., *Bap., Chi.,* Ch. ar., Fer. Hep., Lo. e., Ph. x., *Pyro.,* Stn.

Heel, BLISTER on—Caus., Na. c.

PAIN in—*Ca. cs.,* Cyc., Rap., (Sbi.), Tt. x., Up., Val., Zin.

RHEUMATISM of—Man.

SENSITIVE—J at.

Helminthiasis—Arec., Cic. v., Fe. s.

See also **Lumbrici; Tape-worm; Thread-worms; Worms.**

Hemicrania—Acn., Chn. a., Ch. ar., Mth. b.

See also **Headache; Megrim;** *and* **Migraine.**

Hemiopia—*Aur., Li. c., Lyc., Mu. x.,* Na. m., Tit.

Hemiplegia—Crb. s., Chn. a., Cnn., Elp., Hy. x., Lach., Pi. x., Stn., Sty., Xan.

LEFT—Phst., Sntn.

RIGHT—Ird., Ir. fl.

See also **Paralysis.**

Hepatitis—Act. s.

See also **Liver,** INFLAMMATION of.

Hernia—*Aesc.,* Alm., Amph., Bry., *Calc.,* Ca. p., Cap., Crb. s., Cast., Cep., Cham., Coc. i., Cof., Cub., Eug., Gn. c., Gui., Gre., Hel., Ir. foe., (Itu), Lach., Lam., Li. c., Lyc., Mag. c., Mag. s., Mgt. n., Mgt. s., Mez., Na. m., *Nux,* Osm., Ox. x., Phas., Picr., Pr.s., Pso., Rap., Rhs., Sars., *Sil.,* Spo., Symt., Tab.,Ter., Thu., Ver.

FEMORAL— Wis.

INCARCERATED—Opi.

INGUINAL—Grn., Spi., Su. x., Wis., Zin.

STRANGULATED—Pb., Ter.

UMBILICAL—Grn.

Herpes—AEth., Alns., Ank., Ber. a., Ber., Bor., Calc., Ca. fl., Com.. Con., Col., Crt. h., Cup., Dul., Ery. m., Gph., Ict., Jg. c., Jg. r., Kre., *Mr. sol.,* Na. c., Na.m., *Nt. x.,* Pet., Ph.x., Rn. s., *Rhs.* Rs. v., Src., *Sars.,* Sep., So. o., SuI., Tel., UI. f.

CIRCINATUS—Na. c., Na. m., Sep.

FACIALIS—Lach.

IRIS—Na. c., Osm.

LABIALIS PUDENDI—Ter.

MERCURIAL and VENEREAL—Mos.

NEURALGIA AFTER—Klm., (Mez.), (Sti.)

PHLYCTENOIDES—Crb. s.

PREPUTIALIS—Hep., Jg. r., K. n., Nt. x., Pet., Phls., Phst., Bars.

ZOSTER—Ag. n., *Ars.,* Bor., *Cth.,* Crb. o., Caus., Cis., Com., Dol Gph., Iris, K. as., K. m., Klm., *Mez., Pr. s.,* Rn. b., Rn. s. *Rhs.,* Thu., Var., Zn. p.

See also **Anus,** HERPES of; **Neuralgia** of HERPES; **Pharyngitis,** HERPETIC; and **Throat,** HERPETIC.

Herpetic Dyscrasia—Crb. s.

Hiccough—*AEth.*, As. h., Bry., Caj., *Cic. v.*, (Cur.), *Cyc.*, Eth., Eug., E. pf., (Gin.), *Hy. x.*, Hyo., *Ign.*, Iod., K. s., *Mos.*, *Na. m.* Nic., Nx. m., Par., Phst., Rn. b., Rat., Sars., Scu., Sec., Sin. n.. Stm., Sto. c., Suc., *Su. x.*, Tab., Trn., Teu., Ve. v., Wye., Zin.. Zn. m., Zn. o.

Hip DISEASE—Caus., Get., Hpz. (*See also* **Hip-joint** DISEASE.)

LEFT, PAIN in—Ov.g. p.

PAIN in—Ton., Trb.

RHEUMATISM of—All.

Hip-joint DISEASE—*Aco.*, *Arg.*, Caus., *Chi.*, Cis., Get., Hep., Hpz.. K. *ca.*, *Ph. x.*, Sil., Stp., Stil., Sul.

PAIN in—Ton., Trb. (*See also* **Coxalgia.**)

Hoarseness—All., Aln., Ampl., Ag. i., Ar. dm., Ar. it., Ar. t., Au. m., Ca. cs., Col., E. pf., Gn. c., Hlt., Hep., Lach., Man., Mth. pi., Nx. m., Par, Sbl., Sac. o'1 5mb. n., Sel., Sto. c., Stp., Syph.. Tel., Vi. o.

BEFORE MENSES—Syph.

See also **Voice.**

Hodgkin's Disease—Ac. 1., *Aco.*, *.Ars.*, *Ca. fl.*, *K. m.*, *Na. m.*

Home-sickness—*Cap.*, Cb. a.,Cnt., E. pu., Hel., Ir. t., *Mag. m. Ph.x.*, Pl. n., Se. a., Sil.

Hordeolum. *See Stye.*

Hospital Gangrene—Cis.

Housemaid's Knee—*Aps.*, (Arn.), *K. i.*, *Rhs.*, *Sil.*, *Sla.*, *Sti.*

Hydraemia—Na. s.

Hydroa—Na.. m., Pop. c., Rs. v.

Hydrocele—Abr., Amc., Ampl., *Aur.*, *Bry.*, Ca. p., Dig., Fl. x., *Gph.*, Hel., Nux, Pho., Pso., *Pul.*, Rn. b., *Rho.*, Rhs., Smb. n., *Sil.*, Sul.

CONGENITAL—Pul.

Hydrocephaloid—Cin., CEno., Pod., Ver.

Hydrocephalus—*Aps.*, Apo., Art. v., Bac., *Bel.*, *Bry.*, *Calc.*, Cbl. x., Cu. a., Dig., Fer., Glv., Grt., *Hel.*, Iod., Iof., Lab., *Pho.*, So. n., *Sul.*, Zin., Zn. br., Zn. m.

CHRONIC—Hd. h.

Hydrogenoid Constitution—Aran., Caus.

Hydropericardium—Lyc.

Hydrophobia—Ac. x., Acn., Agv., Anan., *Bel.*, Cth., Ced., Chl. h., Ccn. s., Crt. h., Cur., Fgs., Guac., Hoa., Hfb., Hyo., Hyp., *Lach.*, Merc., Scu., Spa. u., *Stm.*, Tan., Ter.

Hydrosalpingitis—Gel.

Hydrothorax—*Aps.*, *Ars.*, *As. i.*, Jg. c., K. ca., Mr. s., Phas., Rat., Scil., Sga., *Sul.*

Hygroma—Ca. p.

Hyperaemia—Adr., *Bel.*

Hyperaesthesia—Cof., Oln., Ph. h., Pb.

See also **Hypersensitiveness; and Sensitiveness.**

Hyperchlorhydria—Rob.

Hypermetropia—Jab.

Hyperpyrexia—*Aco.*, *Act. r.*, *Aga.*, *Cam.*, *Ve. v.*

NERVOUS—Zin.

Hypersensitiveness—Asa., *Bel.*, *Cham.*, Cof., Hfb., Hyp., *Ign.*, (Ther.).

See also **Hyperaesthesia.**

Hypertrophy—Cb. a.

Hypochondriasis—Ab. n., *Act. r.*, Ana., Anag., *Ars.*, Calc., *Con.*, Grt., *Hyo.*, K. ph., Lyc., Mil., Mos., Na. c., *Na. m.*, *Nux*, *Stn.*, *Stp.*, *Sul.*, Ter., *Val.*, Vb. t., Zin., Zn. o., Zn. v., Ziz.

Hypopion—Ctn., Pb., Sga., Sil.'

Hysteria—Act. r., Alo., Amb., Am. c., Aml., Ana., Anag., Aqui., Art. v., Asa., Asr., Ast. r., Bap., Caj., Calc., Cm. br., Can. s., Cast., Ced., Cic. v., Cinm., Cof., Crl., Cty., Cro., Cup., Elc., E. pu., Gel., Grt., Hur., Ict., *Ign.*, Ind., Ipc., K. ca., K. ph., Lach., Lct.v., Lil., Lo. i., Lyc., Mag. m., Mil., *Mos.*, Na. c.,

Na. hch., Nt. o., Nx. m., Ori., Pal., Par., Pho., Phst., *Plat.*,
Plg., Pul.,

Hysteria *(continued)*—Pyr. a., Rap., Sac. l., Scu., Sec., Se. a., Sep.,
Sprn., Stn., Sti.,. Stm., Suc., Sum., *Trn.*, Ther., Thyt., *Val.*,
Ver., Vb. o., Vi. o., Xan., Zin., Zn. cy., Ziz.

See also **Globus Hystericus** ; **Perspiration,** HYSTERICAL;
and **Urine,** RETENTION of, HYSTERICAL

Hysterical Colic—Alet.

JOINTS—*Arg., Cham., Jgn.*

VOMITING—*Kre.*

Hystero-epilepsy—Mos., CEna., Opi., Thyr., Zn. v.

Ichthyosis—*Ars.,* Chi., *Hyd.,* Lc. c., *Na. c.,* Pip. m., Plts., Pb., *Thu.,*
Thyr.

Idiocy—AEth., Bac., Ba. m., Tab., Thyr.

Ileus—Cast., Clch., Opi., Smb. n., So. t. ae., Tnn.

Imaginary Diseases—Sbd.

Imbecility—An. oc.

Impetigo—Alns., Ank., *Ant. t.,* Ag. n., Brc. x., *Ca. m.,* Crb. s., *Cic.
v.* Iris, Mld., *Mez.,* Rs. v., *Vi. t.*

FIGURATA—Jg. c.

Impotence—Agn., Ar. lp., *Arn.,* Ar. dm., Au. s., (Bls.), Bz. d., Buf.,
Cld., Calc., Caus., Ce. s., Chi., Chlm., Cob., Ccs. c., Dig.,
Eug.,. E. pu., Hlon., *Hyp., K. br.,* Lth., Lyc., Mos., Mu. x.,
Nup., *Nux,* Oxt., Phas., *Ph.x.,* Pho., Phyt., Plnt., Pso., Rdm.,
Sbl.,. Sx. n., Sec., *Sel.,* Stp., Sul., Su. x., Tur., Ur. n., Yoh.,
Zn. p.

Inactivity—Cn. br.

Indian Continued Fever—Pyro.

Indigestion—Ab. c., Abr., Alet., Am. bz., Ant. s. a., Ars., As. f.,
Asc. s., Ath., Bls., Cac., Cd. br., Cd. s., Ca. ar., Evm. E. pf.,
E. pu., Fel., Haem., Hl. o., Lc. x., Lpi., Lo. d., Lo. e., Ox. x.,
Prf., Rum., Snc., Vsp., Vic., Wis., Wil., Wye.

FLUSHING, with— V. sp.

NOCTURNAL—Rob.

See also **Digestion,** DISORDERED, &c.; **Dyspepsia;**
Lactation, DYSPEPSIA of; *and* **Nervous** DYSPEPSIA.

Indurations—Au. m., Bad.

Infantile Leucorrhoea—Ca.n. s., Syph. (*See also* **Leucorrhoea.**)

Paralysis—AEth.

Remittents—Sntn.

Inflammation—(Aco.), Cup., Fe. p.

Influenza—*Aco.,* As. r., Ar. dm., Asc. s., Asc. t., Avn., Avi., *Bap.,*
Bel. Bry., Cam., cm. br., Cnu., Cb. v., Cbl. x., Crd. m.,
Caus., Cnt.. Cep., Cham., Chel., Chi., Dul., Erio., Ery. o.,
Eug., *E. pf.* Eub., Ephr., Gel., *Gph.,* K. i., Lo. p., Lo. s., Lyc.,
Mth. pi. Mr. k. i., Na. s., Oxg., Phel., Phyt., *Pso.,* Pyro.,
Rhs., Sbd., Sln., Sll., *Sang.,* Sg. n., Snc., Src., Sga., Sti.,
Stil., Sty., Sul., Sul. i ., Ss. x., Tri., Tub., *Ver.,* Ve. v., Wye.,
Ziz.

HEADACHE of—Lo. p.

See also **Heart,** INFLUENZA

Infra-mammary Pain—(Act. r.), Caul., Na., hch., *Rn. b.,* Rap.,
Rat., Sum., Tri., Zin.

Ingrowing Toe-nails—K. m., *Mgt. s.,* Nt. x., Stp., Teu.

Inguinal Glands, Disease of—Bac. t.

Injuries—Ang., Aps., Fe. p., Lach., Pso.

EFFECTS of—Ca. s.

See also **Bone,** INJURIES of; **Eyes,** INJURIES of; *and* **Wounds**

Innutrition—Sbl., Van.

Insanity—Ana., Ba.c., Ce. b., Mli., Ter.

Insomnia—Bnz., K. ph., Rap.

See also **Debility,** with **Sleeplessness** *and* **Sleeplessness.**

Intercostal Neuralgia—(Asc. t.), *Mag. p.,* Zin.

Intermenstrual FLOW—(Ham.), Lun., Mgn. gr., Sbi.

HAEMORRHAGE—K. i., Mag. s.

Intermittent Fever—AEsc., Ang., Ant. t., *Aps.,* Aran., *Ars.,* Ast. f.,

Az., Bry., Buf., Cac., Ca.. ar., Calc., Cnu., *Cap.,* Cb. v., Cbl. x., Crd. m., Csc., Caus., *Cean., Ced.,* Cnt., Chm. u., *Chi.,* Ch. ar., Ch. m.,*Ch. s.,* Cim., Ctn., Coc. i., Cof., Clch., Co. a., Co. c., Co. fl., Elt., Euc., *E. pf., E. pu.,* Fer., Fe. p., Gel., Gn. q., Gre., Ign.,.Ilx., *Ipc.,* Ir. t., K. bi., Lach., Lyc., Men., *Na. m.,* Nx. m., *Nux,* Ol. j., Ost., Pts., Phel., Phls., Ple., Pb., Plp., Pod., Ptl., *Pul.,* Qua., Qer., Rhs., Rob., Sbd., Snc., Sars., Sin. n., *Sul.,* Su, x.. Trn., Trn. c., Urt., Ver., Vic.

    See also **Ague.**

Interscapular Pain—Na. as.

Intertrigo—Cb. v., Caus., Fag., Lyc., Na. p.

Intestinal Catarrh—Cchn., Clch., Pho.,Phyt., Vrn.

    See also **Dirrhoea.**

Haemorrhage—Crt. h.

Sand—(Snc.)

Intestines, NEURALGIA of—Vrn.

    OBSTRUCTION of—Opi., Pb., Pyro.

    ULCERATION of—*K. bi., Mr. c.,* Pyro., Sl. x., Ter.

Intoxication— Led.

lntra-ocular Affections—Mr. i. f.

Intussusception—Mr. c, Pho., Pb., Thu., Ver.

Iris Prolapse of—Ant. sa., Phst.

Iritis, Prolapse of—Ant. s. a., Phst.

    Iritis—Asa., Ch. m., Ephr., Gnd., Iod., *K. bi.,* Mr. c., Sbl., Sl. x., Sga., Spi., Stp., Syph., Ter.

    RHEUMATIC—So. t.

    SYPHILITIC—*Nt. x.,* Stp.

Irritability—Ca. br., Ln. p., So. m., So. t. ae.

Irritation—Alm., *Aps., Ars., Ber., Cld., Cb. v., Cbl. x., Ccs. c., Coll., Dul., Gph., Kre., Lyc., Mez., Mar., Nt. x., Ped., Pet., Rs. v., Rum., Sep., Sil., Sul., Su. x.*

    ACUTE ECZEMA, in—Cm. br.

    See also **Cerebro-spinal Irritation;** *and* **Jaundice,** IRRITATION of.

Itch—Bal., Crb. s., Cu. s., K. sc., Man., Phyt., *Pso.*, Snc., Sul.

SUPPRESSED—Snc.

    See also **Scabies.**

Itching—Aga., An. oc., Ant. s. a., As. mt., Ar. it., (Cur.), Gnd., Mns., Prm. O., Pso., Rat., Snc.

Itching Eruptions—Fag.

Jaundice—Aco., AEsc., Aga., Amb., Ars., Ast. f., Aur., Au. m. n., Au. s., Ber., Bl. a. Bov., Bry., Caln. Crd. m., Cean., *Cham.,* Chel., Chne., Chm. u., *Chi.,* Chio., Chlst., Con., Co. c., *Crt. h.,* Dig., Dol., Elt., E. pl., Fe. pf., Gel., Hep., Hdr., Ilx., Iod., K. m., K. pi., Lach., Lpt., Lips., Man., *Mr. sol.,* Mr. c., My. c., *Pho.,* Pi. x., Pb., Pod., Ptl., Rn. b., Rhe., Ric., Sep., Sul., Trx., Ter., Vip.

ANAEMIA, of—Pho.

IRRITATION of—*Dol.*

MALIGNANT—Pho.

PREGNANCY, of—Pho.

Jaw-joint,CRACKING in—Nt. x. (*See also under* **Jaws.**)

PAIN in—*Ar. t.,* Sgu., Spi., Spo., Xan.

Jaws, AFFECTIONS of—Ca. cas.

CARIES of—*Sil.*

CLENCHED—Mor. (*See also* **Lock-jaw;** *and* **Tetanus.**)

CRACKING in—*Grn.,* Nt. z., *Rhs.*

DISEASE of—Pho.

DISLOCATION of, EASY—*Pet.,* Stp.

GROWTH on—*Thu.*

Jaws, PAIN in—Amph., Dol.

SNAPPING in—Vrn.

TUMOUR of—Hec., Pb.

Jealousy—(Aps.), K. as., (Lach.)

EFFECTS of—Aps.

Jerkings—Men.

Joints, AFFECTIONS of—*Aco., Arg.,* Bac., *Bz. x., Ber.,* Bov., *Calc., Ca. p., Hep., Iod., K. i., Led., Mr. sol., Pho.*

CONCRETIONS in—Am. p., Na. 1. (*See also* **Gout.**)

CRACKING in—Ca. fl., Crd. b., K. m., Led., Thu.

CRACKING in—*Zin.*

FISTULAE and ABSCESS around—Ol. j.

NODOSITIES on—Ca. ren.

PAIN in—*Bry.*

SCROFULOUS—*Ph. x.*

STIFFNESS of—Ol. j., Pin. s., Sty., Tri.

SUPPURATION of—Mst. S.

SYNOVITIS of—*Aps., Pul., Sil* (*See also* **Synovitis.**)

See also **Gouty** JOINTS; *and* **Hysterical** JOINTS.

Joy, Ill Effects of—Cof.

Keratitis—Ch. ar., Ch. m., Chl. h., Crt. h., Ctn., *K. bi.,* Klm., Lc. f., Pho., Sang.

INTERSTITIAL—Lo. e.

See also **Cornea;** *and* **Eyes.**

Kerato-iritis Syphilitica—Mr. cy.

See also **Cornea;** *and* **Eyes.**

Kidneys, ACHING IN—Glg., Snt., (ves.)

AFFECTIONS of—*Bel., Ca. ar., Cth.,* Ce. b., *Fer.,* Fe. i., K. ca., Mth. b., Pb., Rhe., Tax.

BRIGHT'S DISEASE of—*Aps., Fe. p.* (*See also* **Bright's Disease.**)

CONGESTION of—HeI., Sto. n., *Ter.*

DISEASESof—*Ars.,* Euc., Jnc., Ocm.

DISORDERS of—Chm. u.

GRANULAR—Pb.

HAEMORRHAGE from—Rs. a.

INFLAMMATION OF—*Mr. c.,* Se. a.

IRRITABLE—Zn. p.

NEURALGIA of—Ter.

PAIN in—Am. br., Cai., Hlon., Lap., Lo. s., Mit., Pin. S., Pbo,
Sprn., Sul. i. (*See also* **Renal Calculi;** *and* **Renal Colic.**)
PYELITIS—*Ars.,* Zea st.
Kleptomania— Trn.
Knee, ABSCESS of—Tax.
AFFECTIONS of—K. ca.
COLDNESS of—Agn.
CRACKING in—*Coc. i.*
CREAKING of— Wil.
PAIN in—*Bz. x., Ber., Dio.,* Elp.
RHEUMATISM of—Pl. n.
WEAKNESS of—Coc. i.
WHITE SWELLING of—K. ca..
See also **Housemaid's Knee.**
Knock -knee— Mld.

Labia, ABSCESS of—Gos., Tan. .
INFLAMMATION of—*Aps., Ccs. c.*
SORENESS of— Sac. l.
Labour—*Aco., Arn., Ca. fl., Caln., Chi., Coll.,* Gel., *Pyro.*
(*See also* PAINS after.)
CONSTIPATION AFTER—*Ver.*
CONVULSIONS in—*Hy. x.*
DISORDERS of—Cham.
EFFECTS of—Hyp.
FALSE PAINS of—Caul., *Pul.,* Vb. o.
PAINS—Cof., of. t:
PAINS, ABNORMAL—Lyc., Opi.
PAINS AFTER—Cham., *Lach. (See also* **After-pains.**)
PUERPERAL—*Mr. c., Pyro. (See also* **Puerperal Fever.**)
SLOW—Vis.
See also **Puerperal Convulsions, Puerperal Mania, &c.**
Lachrymal Duct, INFLAMED—Gph.

Fistula—Aga., Chel., Sil., Stn. (*See also* **Fistula,** LACHRYMAL.) **Sac.**

SUPPURATION of—Stn.

Lachrymation—Cro., Ephr., Mrl., Scil., Tax.

Lactation—*Aco., Chi.,* Glg., Lct. v., Ric., *Sil.,* Urt.

ABNORMAL—Mds., Phyt. (*See also* **Milk,** ABNORMAL.)

DEFECTIVE:—*Calc.,* Lc.v.d., Ph. x., Sbl. (*See also* **Agalactia;** *and* **Milk,** DEFICIENT.)

DISORDERS of—*Asa., Bry.,* Chm. u., Iod., *Pho., Pul.*

DYSPEPSIA of—Sin. a.

EFFECTS of—Cb. a.

EXCESSIVE, EFFECTS of—Als., (Chi.)

PROFUSE—Con., Iod., Pip. n., So. o., Spru., Ur. n., Ust.

Lactation, SORE MOUTH of—Sin. a.

See also under **Milk.**

Landry's Paralysis—Acn., Con., Hfb.

Laryngeal Crisis—K. br., (Nux), Sty.

Phthisis—As. f., Chr. o., Man., Na. se.

Laryngismus—Ar. dm., Bro., Chel., Chlm., K. br., Lach., Mep., Mos., Phyt., Pt. m., Smb. n., Spo.

Laryngitis—*Aco.,* (Ant. S. a.), *Ant. t., Aps.,* Arg., *As. i., Cb. v., Caus.,* Cep., Drs., Ery. a., *Hep., Iod., K. i., Lach.,* Ln. c., *Man.,* Mr. bin., Na. i., *Pho.,* Plg., Sg. n., *Spo.,* Sti., *Sul.*

CATARRHAL—Sbl.

CHRONIC—*Na. se.*

SCROFULOUS—Sel.

TUBERCULAR—Sel.

Larynx, AFFECTIONS of—Epl., Stil.

CATARRH of—Am. br., K. ca.

DRYNESSS of—Smb. c.

PAIN in—Osm.

SPASM of—Au. i., Cup.

Laughter—*Cro.,* Ker.

INVOLUNTARY—Zn. O., Zn. s.

Lead Colic—*Aln., Opi.*

Paralysis—Ppz.

Poisoning—Caus., Kao., Plat.

Legs, JERKING of—Tab.

PAINS in—*Cb. a., Dio.*

SWELLING of—Sto. b.

Leprosy—Cbl. x., Com., Dph., Elae., Hoa., Hur., Hyd., Lach., Pip. m., *Thyr.,* Tub., *Vac.*

TUBERCULAR —Cltr .

Leucaemia—Na. s.

Leucocythaemia—*As. i., Calc., Cean., Na. m., Pi. x.*

SPLENICA—Qer., Suc.

Leucocytosis—Na. p.

Leucoma—Pod.

Leucorrhoea—(Adr.), Agn., Alet., Alns., Als., Aln., Alm., Aral., Ar. lp., Arm., Ars., Aur., Baro., Ba. m., Ber. a., Ber., *Calc.,* Ca. o.t., Ca. p., Cb. a., Caul., Caus., Cean., Cen., Chn. a., Chi., Chl. h., *Cin.,* Cinm., Cro., Dct., Ery. a., Eu. pi., Epn., Fe. br., Fe. i., Ger., Grn., Gph., Guac., Ham., Hdm., Hlt., Hlon., Hep., *Hdr.,* Hyd., Hfb., Inu., Iod., Jab., Ja. g., K. ca., K. fc., K. m.,

Leucorrhoea (continued)—

Klm., *Kre.,* Lc. c., Lc. v. d., Lc. v.f., Lam., Lap., Lp. a., Lips., Lrs., *Mag. m.,* Mag. s., Mli., Merc., Mr. i. f., Mez., Mom., Mur., My. c., *Na. m.,* Na. p., Ori., Ov. g. p., Pal., Prf., Prei., Phst., Phyt., Pr. s., Pso., *Pul., Sbi.,* Snc., Sap., *Sep.,* So. o., Sld., Sto. c., *Sul.,* Syph., Tep., Thl., Til., Tub., TuT., Urt., Vi. t.,Zig.

CHILDREN , in—Cub., Mr. i. f., Mil.

INFANTS, in—Can. s., Syph.

LITTLE GIRLS, in—Merc.

Levitation, Sensation of—Asr., Ev. a., Jg. r., Lct. v., Mgt. s., Pas., Ph. x., Pho., Phst., Sti., Strp., *Trn.,* Tel., Thu., Val., Vis., Xan.

Lichen—Aga., Ank., *Aps., Ars., As. i.,* Dul., Jg. c., Man., Phyt.,

Rum., Sul., Til.

PLANUS—Sul. i.

TROPICUS—Lo. p.

Lienteria—Abr., Als., Cham., *Chi.,* Fer., Fe. pn., Gam., *Oln.,* Ph. x., Pho., Pso., Rap., Rho.

Lightning, EFFECTS of—Pho.

Lightning-stroke— Mor.

Lipoma—Ur. x. (*See also* **Fatty Tumours.**)

Lips, AFFECTIONS of—Zin.

CANCER of—Ant. m., *Hdr., Lyc.,* Tab.

CRACKED—Gph., Ver.

EPITHELIOMA of—*Ars.,* Kre. (*See also* **Epithelioma.**)

ERUPTION on—*Na. m.*

ERUPTION round—*Srs.*

SORE —*Rs. v.*

STIFFNESS of—Ephr.

SWELLING of—*Hep., Rs. v.*

UPPER, ERUPTION on—Sul. i.

Lisping—Na. c., Nux.

Lithaemia—Sko.

Lithiasis—Lys.

Liver, ABCESSof—Med., Rap., Rhs., Ther.

AFFECTIONS of—AEsc., *Am. m., As. i.,* Au. m., Ca. ar., Ca. fl., Crb. s., Crd. m., *Chel.,* Evm., Ev. a., Fag., Gel., *Hep., Hdr.,* Iod., *Iris,* K. *ca.,* Kis., Lach., Lct. v., Lau., *Lpt., Mag. m.,* Mlr., Mn. s., *Mr. sol.,* My. c., Ost., Phyt., Pch., Pb., Pod., Plp., Pso., Rap., Sac. o., Sel., Stil., Su. x., Trx., Thl., Up., Vic. (*See also* DERANGEMENT; DISEASES; DISORDERS &c.)

Liver, ATROPHY of, ACUTE YELLOW—*Pho.*

CANCER of—Chlst.

CIRRHOSIS of—Ca. ar., Chi., Ure.

COMPLAINTS of—Ast. f., cim.

CONGESTION of—Anth. n., Pi. x., Ptl.

CONTRACTION of—Hyd.

DERANGEMENT of—Co. c., *Lyc., Sul.*

DISEASES of—Bo. la., Chne., *Chi.,* Chio., Chlst., *K. i., Ol. j., Pho.*

DISORDERS of—Ab. c., Ac. 1., *Ber., Bry.,* Chm. u., Cob., Crt. h., *Dio.,* Evo., Fe. pi., *Nux,* Ther.

ENLARGEMENT of—Acn., Con., Fe. as., Fe. i, Hpz., Na. s., Pin. s., Pop. c., Sec., Vip. (*See also* HYPERTROPHYof.)

FATTY:—Pi. x.

HYPERAEMIA of—Ver.

HYPERTROPHY of—Chio. (*See also* ENLARGEMENT of.)

INDURATION of—Fl. x., Gph.

INFLAMMATION of—Aco., Act. s., Mn. s., Ste.

INFLAMMATION of, CHRONIC—Pso.

PAIN in—Gnd., Homa., Prt., Prm. o., Pl. n., *Rn. b., Rn. s.,* Scro.,Trb.

PAIN in, GRIPING—Sch.

RASH OVER REGION of—Sel.

SORENESS of—*E. pf.,* Snc.

SYPHILIS of—Mr. bin.

TORPID—*Sep.*

Liver-cough—Sang.

Liver-spots—Cur., Gre., *Lyc., Sep.*

Location, Sense of, Lost—Glo.

Lochia, FETID—Sec.

OFFENSIVE—Stm.

TOO PROFUSE—Mil.

PROLONGED—Hlon.

SUPPRESSED—Hyo., Mil., Zin.

Lock-jaw—Mor., Pb., Ver.

See also **Tetanus.**

Locomotor Ataxy—*Aln.,* Alm., *Ag. n., Ars.,* Atr.,*Aur.,* Caus., Cnd., Cur., Der., Dbn., *Fl. x.,* Gel., Hlod., *Ign.,* Iof., K. br., *K. i.,* KIm., Lach., Lth., *Lyc., Mfag. p.,* Nx. m.,*Nux,* Onos., Oxt., Ph. x., *Pho.,* Ph. h., Phst., *Pi. x.,* Picr., Pb., Sil., Stm., Sty., Sfn., Trn., Tha.

See also **Laryngeal Crisis.**

Loquacity—(Hyo.), (Lach.), Pst., Pyre.

Love, Disappointed—Ph. x.

Lumbago—*Aco., Act. r., .AEsc., Aga.,* Alo., *Ant. t., Arn., Ber., Bry., Ca. fl.,* Ca. p., Cb. a., Chr. o., Cob., *Clch.,* Dio., *Dul.,* Gin. Gna., *Hdr., K. bi.,* K. ca., K. i., K. ox., Klm., Lth., Lo., s., Mac., Mag. s., *Mr., Sol.,* Nt. m., *Nux.,* Ol. j., Ost., Phyt., *Pi. x.,* Pim., Rn. a., *Rho., Rhs.,* Rs. v., Sbl. Smb. c., Snc., Src., Sec., Se., a., S1a., Sprn., *Sul.,* Ter., Ts. p., Vb. o.,Vis.

Lumbar Abscess—Stp.

Lumbrici—(Cin.), Pin. s., Ple.

See also **Worms.**

Lungs, Affections of—*Aco., Ant. t., Ars., As. i., Bel., Cap., Crt. h., Hep.,* Ill., *Lyc.,* Myo., *Sul.*

Catarrh of—Pmo.

Congestion of—Ant. s. a., Bth., *Cb. v., Dig.,* Nt. o.

Haemorrhage from—*Cac., Pho. (See also* **Consumption,** Bleeding; and Haemoptysis)

Hepatisation of—K. i.

Cedema of—Am. c., Arm., K. i., K. ph., Lach., Na. m., Pho., Pmo., Tub., Ver.

Paralysis of—Hfb., Lo. p., Mos., Pho., Son.

Lupoid Warts—Fe. pi.

Lupus—*Ars.,* Au. ar. *Calc.,* Cltr., Chr. o., Cis., Fe. pi., Gre., *Hep., Hdr., Hyd.,* Jeq., *K. bi.,* Kre., Phyt., Sol., *Sul.,* Thio., Tub.

Excedens—Hpz.

Lymphatic Glands, Enlarged—Thio.

See also **Glands; and Glandular Swellings.**

Lymphatic Swellings—Iod.

Lyssophobia— Hfb.

Malar Bones, Neuralgia in—(Act. r.), Zin.

Pain in—Ca. cs., Plp., Sty.

See also **Antrum of Highmore.**

Malaria—Chio., Mlr.., Mr. bin., Mr. n., Na. s., Ost.

CHRONIC—Zea sh.

Malarial Anaemia—Ost.

CACHEXIA—Aran., Mlr.

FEVERS—Ab. n., Mth. b., Ve. v.

Malignant Pustule—Athra., *Ars., Bel.,* Buf., *Lach.,* Scol.

Mammae, Affections of—Au. s.

See also **Breast,** AFFECTIONS of.

Mania—*Aco.,* Anag., Atr., Ba. m., *Bel., Cn. i.,* Cth., Cri. r., Cro., Crt. c., Cu. a., Cup., Dt. f., Dt. m., Der., Eth., Gel., Glo., Grt., Hfb.. Hyn., *Hyo.,* Iof., Ir. t., Merc., Par., Sbd., Se. a., Sil., So. n., Sp. m., Stp., *Stm.,* Sul., Sul. h., Trn., Tea., Thyr., Tub., *Ver.*

HOMICIDAL—Tea.

SUICIDAL—Tea.

See also **Puerperal Mania.**

Marasmus—Abr., Fe. m., Hep., Nx. m., Opi., Ph. o., Sars.

See also **Atrophy.**

Mastitis—Cham., Crt. h.

Masturbation—Bls., Calc., Grt., Med., Nux, Ph. x., Plat., Sx. n., Trn., Thu., Ust., Zin.

EFFECTS of—Alo., Cob., Sars., Stp., Tab.

See also **Self-abuse.**

Measles—*Aco.,* Am. c., *Ars., As. i.,* Avi., *Bel., Bry., Cam.,* Cap., Cb. V., Cop., Crl., Crt. h., *Cu. a.,* Cup., Drs., Dul., Elt., E. pf., *Ephr.,* Fe. p., Gel., K. as., *K. bi.,* Lach., Mld., *Mr. sol.,* Mr. c., Mu. x., *Opi., Pul.,* Pl. n., *Rhs.,* Rs. v, Scil., *Sul.,* Ver.,Ve. v.

COUGH of—Sti.

PROPHYLAXIS of—Pl. n.

Megrim—Anh., Idm., Tea.

See also **Migraine;** *also* **Headache;** *and* **Hemicrania.**
Melaena—Ham.

Melancholy— *Act. r.,* Am. m., *Ars.,* Aur., Cac., Calc. (Cm.br.),
Con., Hel., Hpm., *Ign., Iod.,* K. as., K. ph., Lo. s., Mac.,
Mli., *Mr. sol., Opi., Plat., Pb.,* Sbd., Snc., Sars., *Ver.*
RELIGIOUS—Pso.

Melanosis—Aur.

Membranous Dysmenorrhoea—Bor., Ca. ac., Con., Gas., Gui.,
Hlt., Mag. p., Vb. o.
See also **Dysmenorrhoea.**

Memory, DEFECTIVE—*Ba. c.*
LOSS of—*Ana., Cam.,* Crb. s., Cri. r., *Dig.*
WEAK—*Coc. i., Rho., Sul., Zin.*
WEAKENED—Oln.

Mendacity— V er.

Meniere's Disease—Crb. s., Caus., *Chi.,* Ch. sal.,*Ch. s.,* K. n.,
Lach., Led., *Na. sa.,* Onos., Pilo., Rhe., Sln., Tab., Trn.,
Ther.

Meningeal Headache—Lo. i.

Meningitis—*Aco., Act. r., AEs* g., Aga., *Aps.,* Arn., *Bel., Bry.,* Buf.,
Cd. s., Cbl. x., *Cic. v,* Crt. *h.,* Cup., Dig., Dul., Eth., *Gel.,*
Glo., *Hel.,* Hyo., Hyp., Iof., Mag. p., Merc., Mr. d., Opi.,
Ox. x., Sil., So. n., Stm., SuI., Ver., Ve. v., *Zin.,* Zn. cy.
See also **Cerebro-spinal Meningitis..**

Menopause—Hlon., Nx. m.
See also **Change of Life; Climacteric;** *and* **Menorrhagia,**
at CLIMAXIS

Menorragia—Alet., All., Apo., An. i., Cen., Cinm., Ccs. c.,
Epn., Fe.s., Fic. r., Hlon., Hep., Hdr., Jg. r., K. ca., K. fc., K.
n., Lc. v.f., Lips., Mag. c., Mag. s., Mgt. s., Mom., Mur., Nx.
m., Prf., Pho., Plat., Pr. s., Rap., Rhs., Rs. v., Se. a., Su. x.,
Trl., Urt., Vb. p., Vis.
CLIMAXIS at—Ust.

Menstrual Colic—Col.
HEADACHE—Coc. i., K. ph., Ust.

Menstruation—*Bel., Nt. x.*

ABNORMAL— *Pul.*

ARRESTED—Symt.

BREASTS PAINFUL DURING—(Calc), (Con.), *Sang.*

DELAYED—*Mag. c.,* Sbl., *Se. a.*

DIARRHCEA BEFORE—*Ver.*

DISORDERS of—*Aco., Act. r.,* All., Am. m., Aps., *Ars.,* Bov., Caj., *Calc., Caul., Caus., Cham., Chi., Con.,* Cyc., *Fer., Gph., Ham., Ipc.,* K. i., *Kre., Li. c., Lyc., Na. m.,* Sep., Sto. c., *Sul.,* Voe.

EARLY, TOO —Lam., Rsm., Tub.

EARLY AND PROFUSE—Se. a.

EXCESSIVE—Nt. x., *Sbi., Sec., Ust*

INTERRUPTED—So. t. ae.

IRREGULAR—*Amb.,* Aran., Ov. g. p., Pip. n.

LATE—Mrl.

NAUSEA before—*Ver.*

OBSTRUCTED—Se. a.

PAINFUL—Cac., *Coc i., Gel., Mag. m., Mag p., Vb. o., Xan. (See also* **Dysmenorrhnoea.)**

PAINFUL, MEMBRANOUS—*Bor.*

PREMATURE—Sin. n., Sol.

PROFUSE—*Cro.*

PROTRACTED— Ve. n.

RETARDTED—Pl. n. (Pul.)

SCANTY—Pip. n. (Pul.), Sto. n.

SUPPRESSED—As. h., Cean., Chn. a., Gel., Glo., Lc. v. d., Nx. m., Plat., Smp., Ve. v., Ziz.

Menstruation,SYMPTOMS BEFORE—*Pho.*

VICARIOUS—*Bry.,* Epn., *Ham.,* Pul., Se. a., Ust. (*See also* **Epistaxis,** MENSTRUAL.)

See also **Amenorrhoea; Dysmenorrhnoea ; Hoarseness** before MENSTRUATION; **Inter-menstrual** FLOW, &c.

Mentagra—Gph. (*See also* **Chin,** ERUPTION on; *and* **Sycosis** MENTI.)

Mental Alienation—Arn.

Mental Apathy—Cn. br.

Mental Derangement—Atp., Cyc.

Mental Despondency—Cyp.

Mental Excitement,EFFECTS of—Coc. i.

See also **Nervous Excitement,** EFFECTS of.

Mental Weakness—.AEth., *Ana.,* Anh., *Ph. x., Zin.*

See also **Delusions; Hallucinations; Insanity; Mania; Mind.**

Mercurial Syphilis—(Aur.),. Dph., (Ni. x.), Ph. x.

Mercurial Ulceration—Mu. x.

Mercury, ABUSE of—(Hep.), (Ni. x.), Pt. m., Sars.

EFFECTS oF—Asa.., Chi., Gui., Lach., Mez., Phyt.

POISONING from—Aur., K. chl.

> *See also* **Dyspepsia,** from CALOMEL; **Headache,** MERCURIAL; **Herpes,** MERCURIAL; AND VENEREAL; *and* **Tremors,** MERCURIAL

Mesenteric Glands, AFFECTIONS of—Grt., Kis.

DISEASE of—Bac. t.

Metritis— Mit.

Metrorrhagia—Apo., Arnt., Bov., Crd. m., Cinm., Cof., Cro., Crt. c., Dct., Elp., Ere., Fic. r., Gel., Hlon., Hnn. m., Hdr., K. ca., Lau., Lrs., Lyc., Mag. c., Mur., Na. hch., Nt. x., Nx. m., Pb., Pr. s., Rap., Rat., Rhs., Sec., Sil., Su. x., Tep., Thl., Trl., Vis., Zn. s.

Migraine—Au. br., Bro., Cf. t., Iris., Jg. c., Na. s., Nic., Ol. a., Prm. ve., Sti., Trn., Ton., Tur., Ziz.

> *See also* **Megrim;** *also* **Headache;** *and* **Hemicrania.**
> **Miliaria**—*Aco.,* Bry., Cac., Eu. cy., *Jab.*

Miliaria ERUPTIONS—Am.c., Ars., Cham:

RASH—K. as.

Milk, ABNORMAL—Rhe. (*See also* **Lactation,** ABNORMAL.)

ABSENCE of—Mil. (*See also* **Agalactia.**)

ALTERED—Stn.

DEFICIENT—(For.), Hec., Thyr., Zin. (*See also* **Lactation,**

DEFECTIVE.)

Milk, EXCESSIVE—Pip. n., Sprn., Ur. n. (*See also* **Galactorrhoea;** *and* **Lactation,** EXCESSIVE EFFECTS of.)

INCREASED— Prt.

SCANTY—Sti.

SUPPRESSED—Sec., Zin., (*See also* **Agalactia**)

THIN —Snc.

See also **Lactation.**

Milk, INTOLERANCE of—Lc. v., Pst.

Milk-fever—Bry., Calc., Cham..

Milk-Ieg—Crt. h.

Millar's Asthma—Crl., Cup., Gre., Lo. i.

Miller's . Phthisis —Calc.

Mind, AFFECTIONS of—*Dio., Hyo., Hyp., Lach.,* Nx. m., *Plat., Sep.*

DERANGED—Atp., Cyc.

WEAKNESS of—AEth. (*See also* **Mental Weakness.**)

See also **Delusions; Hallucinations; Insanity; Mental Alienation, &c.**

Miner's Asthma—Na. as.

Miscarriage—*Aco., Arn., Calc., Cham., Mr. c.,* Rat., *Sbi.,* Sec., *Sil., Sul.,* Vb. o.

PREVENTS— Wis.

See also **Abortion.**

Moles—Na. c., Pul.

EXPULSION OF , TO PROMOTE—Sbi.

Mollities Ossium—*Ca. i.,* Iod., Merc., *Pho.*

Molluscum—Sul.

Contagiosum—*Calc., Sil.*

FIBROSUM—*Sil.*

Morning Sickness, OF DRUNKARDS—Lo. i.

PREGNANCY, of——Iris, Lo. i.

Morphia HABIT—Lo. i.

POISONING—Oxg.

Morphinomania—Na. p.

Morphoea— *Ars., Pho., Sil.*

Morvan's Disease—Au. m., *Lach.,* Sec., *Sil., Thu.*

Mountain Sickness, or Veta—Coca.

Mouth, AFFECTIONS of—*Bel., Mr. c.*

    APHTHAE of—Mu. x. (*See also* **Aphthae.**)

    CANKER SORES in—Oxg.

    COMMISSURES OF, ULCERATED—Chi. b., (Cnd.)

    CRACKS of—(Cnd.), E. pf.

Mouth, DRYNESS of—Dbn.

    INFLAMMATION of—K. chl., Lc. f., *Na. m.,* Sin. a. (*See also*

Stomatitis.)

    MUCUS in—*Rhe.*

    PSORIASIS OF TONGUE—Mu. x.

    SORE—*Ar. t., Hep.,* Hdr., Lach., Nt. s. d., *Nt. x.,* Nm. x., Snc.

        (*See also* **Commissures, Soreness** of; **Lactation,** SORE

        MOUTH of; *and* **Nursing Women,** SORE MOUTH of.)

    ULCERATED—Agn., *Cap., Hn. m.,* J. at., Mu. x., Phyt., Rs. g.,

        Rum., Sin. a., Syph.

    See also **Aphthae; Stomacace;** *and* **Stomatitis.**

Mucous Fever—Sin. n.

Mucous Membranes,ULCERS of—Co. c.

Mucous Patches—Merc., Mr. n., Mr. p. r., *Nt. x, Thu.*

Mumps—*Aco.,* Ail., Bap., Ba. m., *Bel.,* Cb. v., Cham., Fag., Fe. p.,

    Jab., K. bi., K. m:, Lach., Merc., *Mr. c.,* Pan., Phyt., Pilo.,

    Pul., Trf. p., Trf. r.

    See also **Parotitis.**

Muscae Volitantes—*Chi.,* Chlf., (Cur.), Itu, Lct. v., *Nt. x., Nux,* Prf.

    Pho., Thu.

Muscles, Contraction of—Cim.

Muscular Rheumatism—Ja. c.

    See also **Lumbago; Myalgia;** *and* **Rheumatism.**

Music, Intolerance of—Amb.

Myalgia—*Aco., Act. r.,* Alet., *Ant. t., Bry., Caus., Clch., Dul., Gel.,*

    Mac., Ve. v.

See also **Rheumatism.**

Mycosis—Sars.

Mydriasis—Bls., Sg. t.

Myelitis—*Aco., Ars., Cic. v.,* Dphn., Dul., *Nux, Ox. x.,* Pi. x., *Pb.,* Sec.

    CHRONIC—Abr.

    DIFFUSE—Sec.

    See also under **Spine.**

Myopia—Aga., Ang., Arec., Man., Nt. x., Pet., *Phst.,* Pilo., Rap., Spo., Su. x., Syph., Thu.

Myxaedema—Dor., *Thyr.*

Naevus—Ac. x., *Calc.,* Fe. p., Fl. x., *Lyc., Pho.,* Thu., Vac.

Nails, AFFECTIONS of—*Alm.,* Ct. eq., *Hdr., Nt. x.,* Up., Ust. (*See also* **Toe-nails,** AFFECTIONS of.)

    BITING of—Am. br.

Nails, BLUE—Ox. x.

    BRITTLE—Se. a.

    CRIPPLED—Caus.

    DEGENERATION of—*Ant. c., Sec.*

    DISEASED—*Ars.,* K. sc., *Sil.*

    DISORDERS of—*Gph.*

    FALLING off—Hl. f.

    INGROWING—Ttr. (*See also* **Ingrowing Toe-nails.**)

    PAINS under—*Sep.*

    PULP of, INFLAMED—*Caln.*

    SHEDDING of—Brs.

    SOFT—Wil.

    SPLITTING—Stn.

    ULCERATION of—Sang., Ttr.

    ULCERS round—*Pho.*

Narcotics, Antidote to—Ac. x.

Nares, Affections of—Hur.

See also **Nostrils, Cracked.**

Nasal Cartilages, ULCERATION of—Hpz.

Nasal Catarrh—Ephr., Nic., Pho.

    See also **Colds;** *and* **Nose,** CATARRH of.

Nasal Obstruction—Hli.

Nasal Polypus—Ar. m., Cd. s., Lyc.

    See also **Nose,** POLYPUS of.

Naso-pharyngeal Catarrh—Aur.

Naso-pharyngitis—Elp.

Nausea—Ap. a., Apo., Drs., Eth., Fag., Opu., Ther.

    PREGNANCY, of—Lc.v.c. (*See also* **Pregnancy,** NAUSEA of.)

    See also **Menstruation,** NAUSEA before.

Navel, INFLAMMATION of—Phst., Sac. 1.

    PAINS in—Ph. x., Prf.

Neck, CRACKING in—Nic., Thu.

    STIFF—Vic., Vin. (*See also* **Stiff-neck.**)

Necrosis—(Bac.), Sl. x., Sil., Ther.

    See also under **Bone;** *and* **Caries.**

N ephralgia— Ves.

    See also under **Kidneys.**

Nephritic Scarlatina—Na. s.

    See also **Anasarca;** *and* **Scarlatina.**

Nephritis—Aco., Amm., Bry., Can. s., Chel., Chm. u., Ccs. c., K.
    chl., Na. hch., Pb., Plg., Sbi., Tub., Vac.

Nephritis, RHEUMATIC AND GOUTY—Clch.

    See also **Bright's Disease;** *and* **Kidneys.**

Nerves, Injured—(Hlon.), Xan.

Nervous Affections—Ana., Frz., Mnc.

Debility—Cur., Cyp. (*See also* **Debility.**)

Dyspepsia—K. ph.

Excitability—Cm. br. (*See also* **Excitement.**)

Excitement, EFFECTS of—Cf.t. (*See also* **Mental Excitement,**
    EFFECTS OF)

Fever—Calc.

Nervousness—Abs., Amb., Hfb., Hyn., Mag. c., Sac. 1., Se. a., Tea., Wye., Xan.

CLIMACTERIC—Oop.

Nettle-rash—*Ant. c., Aps., Ars.,* Ar. ds., *Ast. f., Dul.,* E1t., Fe. S., K. sc., Lt. k., Mds., Na. m., *Sul.*

See also **Giant Urticaria;** *and* **Urticaria.**

Neuralgia—Acn., Ac. c., Ac. f., *Aco.,* Act. r., Aga., Am. pi., Anag., Apo., Aran., Ag. n., *Ars.,* As. r., Asa., Ast. f., Atr., Arnt., *Bel.,* Cac., Calc., Ca. cs., Cth., Cap., Cb1. x., crd. m., Caus., *Ced.,* Ce. b., *Cham., Chel., Chi.,* Ch. m., *Ch. s.,* Cin., *Cof.,* C1cn., *Col.,* Com., Ctn. ch., Ctn., Cup., Cur., Cyp., Dio., Dir., Dol., Dul., Elt., Epn., Fer., Fe. m., Fe. p., Gau., Gel., *Glo.,* Grt., Gui., Hec., H1od., Hfb., Hyo., Hyp., Icth., Ird., Iris, K. as., *K. bi.,* K. chl., K. cy., *K. i., Klm.,* Kre., Lc. c., Lach.,.Mag. c., *Mag. p.,* Mag. S., Mlr., Mth. b., *Mez.,* Mor., Ox. x., Par., Pau., *Pho., Phyt.,* Pmt., Pip. m., Pip. n., *Plnt., Plat.,* Plc., P1g., Prm. ve., Pr. s., *Pul.,* Rn. a., *Rn. b.,* Rn. s., Rho., Rhs., Rob., Sbd., Sbl., Sac. l., Sll., Sang., Snc., Sec., Sep., Sil., *Spi., Stn., Stp.,* Sti., *Sul.,* (Su. x.), Sum., Syph., Trx., Ter., Tea., Thu., Til., Trac., *Val.,* Var., Vrn., *Vbs.,* Xan., Zin., *Zn. p.*

CRURAL—Xan. (*See also* **Anterior Crural Neuralgia.**)

FACE, of—Ap. a., Ton.

HERPES, of—Plnt.

INTERCOSTAL—(Asc. t.), *Mag. p.,* Zin.

ORBITALIS—Asa., Hyd.

PALPEBRALIS— Ver.

PERIODIC—Ni. s., Prt., Tox.

SUBCOSTAL—Zin.

SUPRA-ORBITAL—(Acn.) , Mr. c., Ter., Vi. o. (*See also* **Ciliary** NEURALGIA.)

See also **Adrenal Neuralgia; Aural Neuralgia; Earache; Malar Bones.** NEURALGIA **in; Prosopalgia; Toothache; &c.**

Neurasthenia—Anh., Avn., Chio., E. ar., K. as., K. ph., Lack., Mag. c., Mth. b., Onos., Ox. x., Ph. x., Pi. x., Pip. m., *Plat.*, Sbl., Snc., Se. a., Stn., Sty. p., Thyr., Vip., Zin.

Neuritis—Ars., Oed.

    MULTIPLE—(Tha.)

        See also **Eyes,** OPTIC NEURITIS; *and* **Peripheral Neuritis.**

Night-blindness—*Bel.*, Hel., Hyo., Nux, Pts., Rn. b., Sty., Ver.

Nightmare—Au. s., Cen., K. bi., *K. br.*, *Nux, Paeo.*, Priet., Pho., Ptl., Rho., Su. x.

Night-sweat—Epn., Picr., Rn. g., Sx. n., Slv., Sec., Stp., Syph., Trx., Ts. p.

Night-terrors—Au. br., Aur., Calc., Chl. h., K. ph., Snc., Scu., So. n., Tub.

Night-watching, EFFECTS of—Zn. a.

Nipples, CRACKED—Ct. eq.

    FISSURES of—Rat.

    IRRITATION of—Ori.

    PAIN in—Rhe. ,

    PAINFUL—*Ctn., Phel.*, Phyt.

    RETRACTED—Sars.

    SORE—*Arn.*, Bor., *Caln., Ham.*, Hep., Hdr., Lpsa., Mil., Pho., Phyt., Sul., Ss. x., Zin.

    ULCERATED—Ct. eq.

Nitrogenous Waste—Sna.

Nocturnal Emissions—Iris, Mag. m., Thu.

    See also **Emissions;** *and* **Seminal Emissions.**

Nodes—Ca. fl., For., *K bi., K. i., Sil.*, Stil.

    See also **Rheumatic Nodes.**

Noises IN THE EARS—K. i., Kis., Lach., Lct. v. (*See also* **Ear,** NOISES in; **Headache,** with TINNITUS; *and* **Tinnitus Aurium.**)

    HEAD, in—*Crb. s., Ch. s.*, Dig., Gph., Ham., Hdr., .Mr. sol., Na. sa.

Noma—Aln., K. ph., So. t. ae.

    PUDENDI—*Ars.*

Nose, ACNE OF—Caus.

    AFFECTIONS of—Am. c., *Arn., Bel., Bor., Cap., Cb. a., Gph.,*
        Lmn., Li. c., Na. as., *Nux, Ox. x.*

    ATROPHIC RHINITIS—K. bi., Lmn., Sbl.

    BLEEDING FROM—Abr., Ant. s. a., *Bry.,* Can. s., *Cb. v., Chel.,*
        Cop., *Cro.,* Crt. c., *Fe. p.,* Fe. pi., Gph., *Ham.,* K. n., .i1Jil.,
        (Na. m.), *Pho., Sul. (See also* **Epistaxis.**)

    CANCER of—Ephr.

Nose, CATARRH of—Pho., Teu., Ther., Trb. (*See also* **Colds** and
    Nasal Catarrh.)

    CATARRH OF, CHRONIC—Thu.

    CRUSTS in—(Cd.s.), Caus. (K. bi.), Fag., Snc., Syph.

    DISEASED BONES of—Mr. bin.

    DRYNESS of—Onos.

    ERUPTION on—*K. br.,* Na. c., Tax.

    EXTERNAL, SENSITIVE—Cnb.

    INFLAMMATION of—*Fl. x.,* Sep., *Sul.,* Ust.

    PAIN in—Rhe.

    PAIN IN ROOT of—Na. as,

    POLYPUS of—(K. n.), Lyc., Mr. bin., Mr. k. i., Thu. (*See also*
    Nasal Polypus.)

    PRESSURE AT ROOT of—*K. bi.*

    REDNESS of—*Aps.,* Na. c., Pso., Vin., Zin.

    REDNESS OF TIP of—*Sil.*

    SCROFULOUS INFLAMMATION of—Fe. i.

    SORE—Fag., *K. bi.,* Kao., Li. m., *Pet.*

    STUFFED—Elp.

    SWELLING of—Au. s., Na. c., Sep.

    ULCERATION of—Rn. s.

    See also **Rhinorrhoea;** *and* **Rhinoscleroma.**

Nostrils, Cracked—Ank.

Numbness—Ac. f., *Aco.,* Aga., *Ars., Cic. v., Cod.,* Cnn., *Con.,*
    Hlod., *Ign.,* Ird., Oln., *Ox. x., Pho., Plat., Pb., Rap.,* Sec.

Nursing, Painful—Phyt.

Nursing Women, AFFECTIONS of—Chio., Oln.

SORE MOUTH of—Hdr.

Nurslings, AFFECTIONS of—Rhe.

Nyctalopia—*Bel.,* Hel., Hyo., Nux, Pts., Rn. b., Sty., Ver.

Nymphomania—Amb., Ba. m., Bel., Cld., Ca. p., Cth., Frl., Fl. x., Grt., Hyo., K. ph., Lach., Lyc., Mur., Nux, Ori., Ph. x., Pho., Plat., Pul., Rap., Sbi., Sx. n., Stp., Stm.,Zin., Zn. pi.

Nystagmus—Aga., Bz. n., Gel., K. i.

Obesity—Asa., Ca. ar., Cap., Gph., Lc. v. d., Li. c., Lrs., Sbl., Thyr., Thri.

See also **Corpulence.**

Odour of Body, ABNORMAL—*K. i.*

CHANGED—*Pho.*

FETID—*Pso.*

OFFENSIVE—*Mr. sol.,* Sac. l., So. t. ae., Wis.

OEdema—Brc. x., Hpz., Homa., Jt. u., K. chl., Lt. k., Lun., Na. sa., Ped., Thyr., Tox., Vsp

GLOTTIDIS—K. i., Sang., Tub.

LUNGS, of—K. ph., Lach.

See also **Lungs,** OEDEMA of.

OEsophagitis—Aco., Amm., Cb. v., K. s., OEna., Rx. ac., Sec., Su. x.

OEsophagus, AFFECTIONS of—*Ign.,* Rap., Sin. a.

CATARRH of—Sga.

CONSTRUCTION of—Na. as., Rhe., Sul.

DRYNESS of—Sch.

INFLAMMATION of— *See* OEsophagitis.

PAIN in—*Pho.*

SPASM of—Acn., Ag. cy., Ba. c., Stm., *Ve. v.,* Zin.

STRICTURE of—Alm., Bap., Caj., Cap., Crd. b., Cic. v., *Gel.,* Hfb., Mnc., *Mr. c.,* Mr. scy., OEna., Pt. m., Pb., Sbd., Sga, (Slp.), Spa. u., Tab., Vrn., Ver., Zn. s.

STRICTURE OF, SPASMODIC—*Naj.*

Olecranon, PAIN in—Rap. *See also* **Elbow.**

Onanism—Trn., Thu.

    EFFECTS of—Alo.

        See also **Masturbation;** *and* **Self-abuse.**

Operations, EFFECTS of—Aps., Cro., Hyp.

        See also **Teeth,** OPERATIONS on; *and* **Traumatism.**

Ophthalmia—AEps., All., Ant. a., Asc. t., Au. m., Bad., Ber., Cai., Cham., Ch. ar., Chs. x., Cro., Ctn., Dul., E. pf., Fag., Jeq., K. bi., Lina., Nab., Na. s., Nic., Ph. m., Pod., Rs. V., Sang., Snc., Syph., Ur. n., Uri., Vsp., Xan.

    ACUTE—Sul.

    NEONATORUM—Ag. n.

    RHEUMATIC—Sul.

    SCROFULOUS—Am. br., As. i., Fe. i., Na. s.,Ol. j., Pso., Sid., Sul.,Vi. t.

    TARSI—Snc.

        See also **Phlyctenular Ophthalmia.**

Opisthotonos—Stn.

Opium Habit—Apm., Avn., Ipc.

Oppression—Bap. c.

Optic Neuritis—*Aps.,* Tab., Thyr.

Orbital Neuralgia—Asa., Hyd.

    See also **Neuralgia.**

Orchitis—Cb. v., Cub., Ere., Mgt., Phyt., Pip. m., Plg., Trad., Ust., Ve. v., Vi. t., Vis.

    See also **Testicles.**

Os Uteri, DILATED—Snc.

Ossification of Arteries—Li. c.

    TOO EARLY—Snc.

Osteitis—Conc.

    DEFORMANS—Hec.

Osteoma—Mez.

Osteomalachia—Gui., Hec.

Osteomyelitis—Ph. x.

Osteosarcoma—Hec.

Otalgia—K. i., Na. n., Spi., Vis.

    See also **Ear,** PAINS in; *and* **Earache.**

Otitis—Cac., Cur., Eug., Gui., K. ca., Led., Na. n., Pi. x., *Plnt.*

    See also **Ear.**

Otorrhoea—Abs., AEps., Alm., Api. g., As. i., Ba. m., Cb. a., Cb. v., Caus., Fl. x., Lach., Lyc., Pet:, Pso., Syph., Vi. o., Vis., Zin.

    FETID—Pso.

    SUPPRESSED— Vi. o.

    See also **Ear.**

Ovaries, ABSCESS of—*Pyro.*

    AFFECTIONS of—*Act. r.,* Am. br., Arg., Bov., *Cth., Col., Con.,* Crt. h., *Ham., Hep., Iod., K. br.,* Kre., Lc. c., *Lach., Lil.,* Merc., *Naj.,* Na. hch., *Pal., Plat.,* Sbl., Sbi., Sac. 1., Stp., Syph.

    CYST of—Rho.

    DISEASE of—Oop.

    DROPSY of—Fe. i., Iod., Lil., Ter.

    ENLARGEMENT of—Trn.

    INFLAMMATION of—*Aps.,* Cac., Gui., *Pul.,* Vis.

    LEFT, AFFECTIONS of—Ust.

    LEFT, PAIN in—Thu., Vsp.

    NEURALGIA of—Caul., Mli., Rn. b.

    NEURALGIA OF INTERMITTENT—Ziz.

    NUMBNESS in—Pod.

    PAIN in—*Aps.,* Cen., Gos., Mea., Ov. g. p., Oxt., Pod., *Pul.,* Ter. Vb. o., Vb. t., Wye.

    TUMOURS of—*Aps.,* Gph., Oop., Pod., Bhs., *Sec.*

Ovaritis—Cac., Vis.

    See also **Ovaries,** INFLAMMATION of.

Over-exertion—Sac. 1.

Over-lifting, Complaints from—For.

Over-sensitiveness—Cof.

See also **Hyperaesthesia;** and **Hypersensitiveness.**

Over-strain, Bodily or **Mental**—Coc. i.

Over-work—Bls.

Oxaluria—*Ber.,* Lys., *Nm. x., Ox. x.*

Ozaena—Alm., Asa., *Aur.,* .Au. m., *Cd. s.,* Ca. fl., Crt. h., Cur., Der., Elp., Hpz., *Hn. m., Hdr., Iod.,* K. bi., K. pm., K. sc., Lmn., Mag. m., Mr. i. f., Na. c., *Nt. x.,* Pho., Phyt., *Pso.,* Snc., Sep., Sko., Sti., *Syph.,* Ther., Thu., Zng.

Pain—Ul. f.

Palate, AFFECTIONS of—Man.

Palms, CRAMP in—Scro.

See also **Psoriasis** PALMARIS.

Palpitation—Adr., Als., Ana., Antf., Arnt.., Avn., Bad., Ca. ar., Can. s., Chl. h., Coc. i., Crt. h., Cup., Dgn., Eps., Fag., Lau., Lo. i., Mag. m., Mor., Oln., Pod.

Palpitation ON WAKING (immediately after falling asleep)—Als.

See also **Heart,** PALPITATION of.

Panaris—Ba. c. (*See also* **Panaritium; Paronychia;** and **Whitlow.**)

Panaritium—Amc., Aps., Ba. c., Buf., Cep., Cis., Hyp., Lyc., Mgt. n., Na. s., Par., Sil. (*See also* **Paronychia;** and **Whitlow.**)

Pancreas, AFFECTIONS of—Iris., Trf. p.

CANCER of—Ca. ar.

DISEASE of—Pan.

DISORDERS of—Pho.

INDURATION of—Cb. a.

Pancreatitis—*Atr.,* Ba. m., *K. i., Mr. sol.*

Pannus—Aps., Ch. m., Mrl.

Panophthalmitis—Phyt.

Paralysis—Abr., *Aco.,* AEs. g., Ags., *Aln.,* Alm., An. oc., Ana., Ag. i., *Ag. n., Arn., Aur., Ba. c.,* Ba.. m., *Bel.,* Brcn., Caj., Calc.,

Ca. cs., Ca. hp., *Cn. i.,* Cap., Crb. o., Cast., Caus., Chn. a.,
Cic. v., *Coc. i.,* Con., Cu. a., *Cup.,* Cur.., Dbn., Dul., Elc.,
For., Glv., Gas., *Gel.,* Glo., *Gph.,* Gua. c., Hlod., Hoa., Hfb.,
Hyo., Hyp., 1gn., K. br., *K. i.,* K. ph., Kar., Lach., Lol., Lyc.,
Men., *Mr. c., Nux,* Oln., Onos., *Opi., Ox. x.,* Oxt., Par., Ptv.,
Pho., Pi. x., Pb., Pb. i., *Rhs.,* Rx. ac., Rut., *Sec.,* Sol, Stn.,
Tan., Tng., Trn., Tep., Tea., Thu., Thyr., Tub., Vrn., Vb. o.,
Zn. p.

Paralysis AGITANS—Ant. t., Au. s., Gel., Hlod., Hyn., Hyo., K. br.,
Lth., Lol., Lyc., Phst., Pb., Trn., Zn. cy., Zn. pi.

ASCENDING —(Con.), (Hfb.), Sfn.

DIPHTHERITIC—Phyt., Pb.

See also **Diphtheritic Paralysis.**

FACIAL—*K. chl.*

See also **Face,** PARALYSIS of.

GENERAL, OF INSANE— K. br., *Pho.*

HANDS AND ARMS, of—Thyr.

LEAD—Sux.

LEFT SIDE, of—Cu. as., Nt. x.

LOCAL—*Phst.*

NERVOUS—Homa.

POST-DIPHTHERITIC—Sec.

PSEUDO-HYPERTROPHIC—Pho.

RHEUMATIC—Lth.

SPASTIC—*Nux,* Sec. (*See also* **Spastic Paralysis;** *and* **Spine,**
. SCLEROSIS, of.)

SPHINCTER VESICAE., of—Chlf.

SPINAL (SPINAL SCLEROSIS—*Lth.,* Phst., Pi. x., Wil. (*See also*
Spine, SCLEROSIS, of.)

VISCERA, of—Fer.

See also **General Paralysis; Hemiplegia; Paraplegia;
Paresis; Pneumogastric Paralysis; Pseudo-hypertrophic
Paralysis; Respiratory Paralysis; &c.**

Parametritis—*Bel., Hep., Mr. sol., Sil.*

Paraphimosis—Col., Dig., Lach., Mgt., Mr. c., Nux, Rhs.

Paraplegia—Anh., (Caul.), Gel., K. trt., Klm., Lth., Man., Ptv., Phst., Pi. x., Pip. m., Rs. v., Sty., Tha., Thyr., Wil.

Paresis, SENILE—Au. i.

 SYPHILITIC—Au. i.

 See also **Cardiac Paresis.**

Paronychia—Dio. (*See also* **Whitlow.**)

Parotid Glands, AFFECTIONS cf—Iris, (Jab.), (Plo.).

 HYPERTROPHY of—Sul. i.

 INDURATION of—Bro.

Parotitis—Am. c., Ba. c., Calc., Cham., Ch. s., Cis., Coc. i., Dio., Dor., Ephr., Gph., Hpz., Hyo., Man., Merc., Mr. bin., Phyt., Sx. p., So. n.

 GANGRENOSA—Athra.

 See also **Mumps.**

Parturition—Ca. fl.

 See also **Labour.**

Pediculosis—Led., Mez., *Na. m.,* Pso., *Sbd., Stp.*

 See also **Phthiriasis.**

Pellagra—Pb. i.

Pelvic Cellulitis—Med.

Haematocele—*Arn., Ham., Sul.*

Pelvis, CONGESTION of—Nx. m.

Pemphigus—Ana., Buf., Clt., Crb. o., Caus., Dul., Jg. c., *Mr. c.* Rn. b., Rn. s., Rap., *Rhs.,* Scro., Syph., Thu.

 NEONATORUM—Mr. p. r.

Penis, CARTILAGINOUS SWELLINGS on—Sbi.

 INFLAMMATION of—Hdy.

 PAINS in—Geu.

 SORES on—Osm.

Pericarditis—Ant. a., Asc. t., Clch., Fnc., Lcs., Phas.

Perichondritis—*Act. r.,* Bel., Cham., *Oln., Pb., Rut.*

Perimetritis—*Bel., Mr. c.*

Perinaeum, PAINS in—Mla.

ULCER on—Paeo.

Periodic Neuralgia—Tox.

 See also **Neuralgia,** PERIODIC.

Periosteum, PAIN in—Rhs.

 SENSITIVE, PAINFUL—Symt.

Periostitis—Au. m., Fe. i., Hec., Man., Na. sa., Pbo., Rut., Stil.

Peripheral Neuritis—Bz. d.

Peritonitis—*Aco., Aps., Ars., Bel., Bry., Calc., Cth.,* Cham., *Chi., Col.,* Con., Crt. h., Eub., Fl. x., K. n., *Lyc.,* Merc., *Mr. c.,* Pyro., Ric., Sbl., So. n., *Sul.,* Til., Ver.

 PLASTIC—*Mr. d.*

 TUBERCULAR—*Pso.*

Perityphlitis—*Ars.,* Crt. h., Ir. t., *Lach.*

Pernicious Anaemia—Pi. x.

 See also **Anaemia.**

Pernicious Fevers— Ver.

Perspiration—*Calc., Fl. x., Smb. n.*

 ABNORMAL—*Mr. sol., Nt. x., Pho.*

 ABSENT—Lach.

 ALTERED—*Cb. a.*

 BLOODY—*Lach., Nx. m.*

 EXCESSIVE—*Chi.,* Eser. *Jab.* Phen.. Pilo. Snc., Su. x.

 HYSTERICAL—*Nx. m.*

 Perspiration, OFFENSIVE—*Pet., Sil., Stp.*

 PROFUSE—*Ph. x.,* Psc.

  See also **Axilla; Feet; Genitals; Hands;** *and* **Sweat.**

Petit Mal—Pho., Zn. cy

Pharyngitis—Am. br., K. chl., Na. i., Sang.

 HERPETIC—Sl. x.

  See also **Atrophic Pharyngitis; Follicular Pharyngitis; Naso-pharyngitis;** *and* **Throat.**

Pharynx, AFFECTIONS of—My. c.

Phimosis—Can. s., *Ham.,* Ja. c., *Mr. Sol.,* Nt. x., Rum., Sbi., Sep., Sil., Sul.

Phlebitis—(Ant. t.), Aps., Crt. h., Mr. cy., *pul.,* Sto. b., Sto. c., Vip.

Phlegmasia Dolens—*Aco.,* Bel., *Bis.,* Bry., Buf., *Ham.,* Hpz., Lach., Lyc., Na. s., *Pul.,* Sul., Urt.

Phlegmon—Dxn., Hpz.

Phlegmonous Inflammation and Ulceration—Athra.

Phlyctenula— Ephr.

Phlyctenular Ophthalmia— Ign.

> *See also* **Eyes;** *and* **Ophthalmia,** SCROFULOUS.
> **Phosphaturia**—Ar. Ip., Ca. p., Guac., Ph. X., Pop. c., Ptl., Sld., Ur. n.

Photophobia—Na. s., Ther., Zin.

Photopsia—Zin.

> *See also* **Headache,** with PHOTOPSIA.

Phthiriasis—Bac., Coc. i., *Sbd.*

See also **Pediculosis.**

Phthisis—Ac. x., Aga., Alo., Ant. a., Arg., Au. ar., Aur., Au. m., Au. m. n., Avi., Bac., Bac. t., Bal., Bl. o., Crd. m., Cet., Chlm., Ccs. c., Con., Cur., Drs., Elp., Erio., Epn., Gad., Ga. x., Gui., Hlx., Icth., K. n., Lchn., Lcs., Nph., Na. cc., Na. p., Na. s., Ol. j., Phel., Pix, Rum., Sbl., Slv., Smb. n., Se. a., Sla., Stn. i., Sti., Su. x., Teu. s., Thyr., Tub., Zn. i.

FLORIDA—Sang., Ther.

HAEMORRHAGICA—Fe. p.

LARYNGEA—Chr. o. (*See also* **Laryngeal** PHTHISIS.)

MUCOSA—Sga.

PITUITOSA—Stn.

PULMONALIS— Pyro.

> *See also* **Consumption; Diarrhoea** of PHTHISIS; **Miller's Phthisis; Stone-cutter's Phthisis; and Tuberculosis.**

Physometra—*Bro.,* Lun., Lyc., *Ph. x.,* Sang., Trn.

Piles—Ant. c.

> *See also* **Haemorrhoids.**

Pimples—Eug., Ephr., K. Chl., Ph. x., Rat.

Pining Boys—Aur.

Pityriasis—*Ars.,* Bac., Ber. a., Caul., *Fl. x., Gph.,* Man., *Mez.,Ter.*
　　Rubra—Eryth., *Na. as.,* Thyr.
　　Versicolor—Cbl. x., sep., Ss. x., Tel.
Placenta, Adherent—Hdr.
　　Praevia—Erig.
　　Retained—Cth.,Pul., Sbi., Sec., Vis.
Plague—Bap.,Buf., Hpz., *Lach., Naj.,* Pest., *Pho.*
Plethora—(Aco.), *Ars.,* Calc.,Fe. i., Ts. fg.
Pleurisy—*Aco.,* Act. s., Ant. a., *Aps., Ars.,*Asc. s., Asc. t., Bel., Bor.,
　　Bry., Can. s.,*Cth.,* Cb. a., Crd. m.,*Chi.,* Chlm., *Fe. m.,* Fe. p.,
　　Gui., *Hep.,* K. ca., K. i., K. n., Lo. i, Mth. b., Phas., Rat.,
　　Rhs., Scil., Sga., Sep., *Sil., Sul.,* Tub., Ziz.
Pleuritic Adhesion—Rn. b.
Pleurodynia—*Aco., Act. r.,* Arn., *Ars., Asc. t., Bry.,Chel.,* Gau.,
　　Gui., *K. ca., Rn., b.,*Rhs.
Pleuro-pneumonia—Cap.
Plica Polonica—Ant. t., Bor., *Lyc.,* Pso., Sars., Ver., *Vin.,* Vi. t.
Pneumogastric Paralysis—Bel.
Pneumonia—A*co.,* Am. m., Ant. a., Ant. i., *Ans., t., Ars., As. i.,*
　　Bel., *Bry.,* Cac., Ca. s., Can. s., Cbl. x., Cep., Chel., Chi. b.,
　　Co. fl., Cup., Elp.,Fe. i., Fe. p., *Hep.,Hyo.,* k. n., k. ph.,
　　Lach., *Lyc.,* Mil., O1. j., *Pho.,* Pod., Rhs., Scil., Sga., *Sul.,*
　　Su. x., Sum., Ver., Ve. v.
　　Acute—*Sang., Tub.*
　　Typhoid—Lchn., Lau., Rhs.
Podagra—Buf.
Poisoned Wounds—Ech. a.
Pollutions—Ac. c., Arg., Idm., Osm.
　　See also **Emissions;** *and* **Seminal Emissions.**
Polypus—Aln., Ber., *Calc.,* Ca. s.,Cb. a., *K. bi.,* K. n.,K. sc.,Lmn.,
　　Med., *Nt. x., Pho.,* Pso., *Sang.,* Sg. n., Teu., *Thu.*
　　Ear, of—Lyc. (*See also* **Ear,** Polypus of.)
　　Eye, of—Lyc.
　　Nose, of—Lyc. (*See also* **Nasal Polypus;** *and* **Nose,** Polypus

of.)

RECTUM, of—K. br.

    See also **Uterus, POLYPUS** of.

Polyuria—Cai., O1. a., Plnt., Pt. m. n.

    See also **Urination, too FREQUENT; Urine, EXCESS** of; *and*
    Urine, INCREASED.

Pork, Effects of—Ac. 1.

Porrigo Capitis—Sum.

    See also **Crusta Lactea;** *and* **Scald-head.**

Post-influenzal Debility—Cyp.

Post-nasal Bleeding—Osm.

Post-Nasal Catarrh—Api. g, Ca. fl., Cri., Hdr., K. bi., Lo. s., Mr.
    bin., Na. as., Na. c., Na. p., Ov. g. p., Pnt., Sg. n., Sin. n.,
    Spi., Sti., Tel.,Thu.,Wye., Yuc.,Zng.

Post-nasal Growths—Osm. (*See also* **Adenoids.**)

Post-Partum Haemorrhage—Can. s., (Cro.), Sec., Trl.

Pot-bellied Children—Snc.

Pott's Disease—Get., Sti.

    See also **Spine.**

Pregnancy—*Aco., Calc., Caus., Pul.*

    AFFECTIONS of—*Coll.,* Cro., *Mr. sol.,* Mur., *Nux,* Sang;.

    ALBUMINURIA of—Gel., Klm.,Thyr.

    BLADDER TROUBLES of—*Pul.*

    BREASTS PAINFUL during—*Con.*

    COMPLAINTS of—Bls., Mos.,Nx. m.

    CONSTIPATION of—Alm.

    CONVULSIONS of—Hfb.

    COUGH of—Vb. o.

    COUGH of, MORNING,—*Bry.*

    DIARRHOEA of—*Ph. x., Pul.*

    DISORDRES of—*Act. r., Bel.,Cth., Cap., Cb. v ., Caul., Cham.,*
    Cyc., Fer., *Ipc.,* K. ca., Sep., Sul.

    DROPSY of—Snc.

    DYSPEPSIA of—Sbd., Sin. a.

HERATBURN of—*Pul.*

IMAGINARY—Caul., Cro., Nux, Thu.,Ver.

NAUSEA of—Lc. v. c., *Mag. c.*, Mag. m., Ph. x.,Pilo.,Stp.

PAINS of, FALSE—*Sec.*

PRURITUS of—Tab.

PYROSIS of—Dio.

SALIVATION of—*Jab.*, Pilo.

SICKNESS of—Bry., Cya., Hep., Lc. x., Onos., Ox. x., *Pet., Pul.,* Snc., Su. x., Sym. r., *Tab.*, Ther. (*See also* VOMITING of; *and* **Vomiting** during PREGNANCY.)

SICKNESS of, MORNING—Iris,Lo. i.

SORE MOUTH of—Sin. a.

Pregnancy, SPURIOUS—Caul., Nux.

TOOTHACHE of—Alm.,Hfb., *Mag.* c., Rap., Tab.

VOMITING of—Alet.,Als., Apm.,Cast., Cer. o.,Gos., *Kre.*, Mr. i. f., Pho., Sep. (*See also* NAUSEA of; SICKNESS of; *and* **Vomiting** during PREGNANCY.)

See also **Jaundice** of PREGNANCY; *and* **Varicosis** during PREGNANCY.

Prepuce, ERUPTION on—Sil.

WARTS on—Ph. x.

Presbyopia—Dbn., Na. c., Onos., Pet.

Priapism—Ank.,Cam., Can. s., Cnb.,Gph., Led., Med., Na. c., Na. hch., OEna., Opu., Pts., Pi. x., **Pip. n.**, Pul., (Rap.), Sel., Sin. n., Yoh., Zn. pi., Zn. v.

Pricking pains—Ar. ds.

Prickly Heat—Led.

Proctalgia—Clch., Ctn., Erig., Ign., K. Ca., K. chl., (Lach.), Lyc Pho., Pb., Sty., Trn., Ve. v.

Proctitis—Alo.,Chm. u., Coll., *Nt. x.,* Pho.,*Pod.*, Sbl.

Progressive Muscular Atrophy—Crb. s., *Pho.*, Phst., *pb.*

Prolapsus Ani—Aral., Ar. m., Ephr., Mgt., Mez., Pb., Plp.

RECTI—Ant. c.

UTERI—Alo.

See also **Anus; Rectum;** *and* **Uterus.**

Prosopalgia—Calc., Chi., Mr. c.,Nt. s. d., Vbs.

    See also **Face,** Neuralgia of; *Neuralgia;* *and* **Toothache.**

    Prostate, Affections of—AEsc., Alo.,Cac., Ephr., Hdrn. a., *K. i.,* Mla.,O1. a., Phyt., Pop. t., Sbl., *Stp.,* Sul. i., Tur.

    Diseases of—Fe. Pi., *Mr. Sol.,* Phas:,Pch.,*Thu.*

    Disorders of—Baro.

    Enlargement of—*Ag. n.,* Ba., c., Dig., *Iod* Prei., *Sbl., Std.*

    Haemorrhage from—Phas.

    Inflammation of—*Pul.* (*See also* **Prostatitis.**)

    Irritation of—Gna., Kre.

    Suppuration of—*Nt. x.*

Prostatitis—Aps., Cn. i., Caus., Chm. u., *Clch.,* Con., Cop., Cub., Cyc., Hpm.; Li. c., Lyc., Mr. d., Pet., Pod., Plg., *Pul.,* Sx. n., Sel., Se. a., Ves.

Prostatorrhoea—Alm., Dph.,Pip. m., Pul., Sel.,Spi., Sul., Tab., Zin.

Prostration—Cchn.,Phst.

    Muscular— Phst.

    See also **Debility.**

Prurigo—Alns., Ank, Hoa., Oop, Rs. v., Rum., Zn. s.

Pruritus—Aln., Ar. dm., Cod., Cop., Dol., Epn., Homa., Lp. a., Mth. pi., Sep., Tab.

    Ani—Pho., Ur. n.

    Mercurialis—Hep.

    Pudendi—Fag., Trn.

    Senilis—Mez.

    Vaginae—Cld., Gph., Gnd.

    Vulvae—Amb., Au. s., Ch. s., Coll., Cvl., Co. c., Frl., Gnd., Hlon., Icth., K. bi., Lil., Ov. g. p., Pi. x., Plat., So. t. ae.

    See also **Pregnancy,** Pruritus of.

Pseudo-hypertrophic Paralysis—Cur.

Psilosis, or Sprue—Frg., Ilx.

Psoas Abscess—Ph. x., Sil., Stp., Symt., Syph.

Psora—Alns., (Bac.), (Pso.), (Sul.), &c.

HEREDITARY—Ped.

Psoriasis—*Ant. t., Ars.,* As. r., Bls., Ber. a., Bor., Cbl. x., Chi., *Chs. x., Cic. v.,* Crl., Cup., Gli., *Gph.,* Iris, K. as.,K. br., K. sc., Lo. i., man., Nph., Nup., *Pet.,* Pho., Pix, Src., Sep., Ste., Stil., Teu., *Thyr.*

PALMARIS—Calc., Crt. h., Med., Sel.

TONGUE, of—Mu. x.

Pterygium—Am. br., Chm. u, Gre., Spi.

Ptomaine poisoning—Pyro.

Ptosis—Caus., Chl. h.,Con., Cur., Ephr., Gel., Gph., Gre., Haem., K. ph., Klm., Med., Mrl., Nx. m, Pi. n., Rhs., Sac. l., Sep., Spa. u., Stn., Syph., Thu., Up., Ver., Zin.

Ptyalism—Dig., Epl.

See also **Salivation**.

Pudenda, OVER-SENSITIVENESS of—Au. m.

Puerperal Convulsions (Eclampsia)— Amb., Ch. s., Chl. h., Chlf., Cia. v., Gel., Hel., Mil., Nx. m., CEna., Opi., Ph. x., Pho., Pilo., Pul., So. n., Thyr., Ve. v.

Puerperal Fever—*Aco.,* Ail., Bry., K. ph., Mil., *Mr.* c., Pul., *Pyro.,* Sbl., Sl. x., Thyr.

Puerperal Fever and Convulsions—Lach.

Puerperal Mania—*Act. r.,* Bel., Hyo., K. ph., Pul., Se. a., Ve. v.

Punctured Wounds— Aps., Aran., Led., Phas.

Pupils, CONTRACTED— Eser.

DILATED— Dbn., So. pc.

Purpura— *Aco., Arn., Ars.,* Cb. v., *Cry. a.,* Chl. h., Crl., *Crt. h., Ham.,* Jg. r., K. chl., Lach., *Mr. sol., Ph. x., Pho., Rs. v.,* Sec., Su. x., Tax.

Purpura, HAEMORRHAGICA—Ter.

Pustules—Hpz., Kre., Pod., So. o.

See also **Malignant Pustule.**

Putrid Fevers—Ech. p., Hpz.

Pyaemia—*Arn., Ars., Ch. s.,* Conc., Crt. h., *Ech a.,* Hpz., *Lach., Mr. sol., Pyro., Rhs.,* Ver.

See also **Blood-poisoning; Septicaemia; &c.**

Pyelitis—*Ars.,* Z. st.

Pylorus, AFFECTIONS of—*Hep.,* Lo. d., Lyc., (Merc.), Ts. p.

    DISEASES of—*Chi., Nux.*

    INDURATION of—Sep.

    PAIN in—Lct. v., Lo. S.

    SUPPURATION of—*Sil.*

    THICKENING of—*Pho.*

Pyrosis—Pr. v., Rob., Sang., Ss. x., Tab.

    PREGNANCY, of—Dio.

    See also **Waterbrash.**

Pyuria—*Bry.*

    See also **Urine.**

Quinine CACHEXIA—Chne., Euc., (Na. m.).

    EFFECTS of—Az.

Quinsy—*Aco., Ba. c.,* Fe. m., Hep., Lach., Lyc., Mr. bin., Pso., Rn. s., Sang., Sg. n., Sep., Trn., Vsp.

    See also **Tonsillitis;** *and* **Tonsils,** INFLAMED.

Rabies—Lach.

Rage—Hyo., (Stp).

    FITS of—Mos.

Railway Spine—Bls.

Ranula—Amb., Am. bz., *Calc.,* Chr. o., Lc. c., *Mr. sol.,* Na. m., Nt. x., Sac. o., Stp., Thl., *Thu.*

Raynaud's Disease—(Bac.), Fe. p., Sec.

Reaction, DEFECTIVE—Amb., Cast., Zin.

Rectum, AFFECTIONS of—*Gph., Hdr.,* Kis., *Nt. x.,* Rut., *Sul.*

    BURNING in—Iris.

    CANCER of—Phyt., Sep., Spi.

    CONSTRUCTION of—Pyr. a.

    CRAMP in—Snc.

    DISEASES of—*Cap.*

    FISSURE of—Sep.

Rectum, INFLAMMATION of—*See* **Proctitis.**

PAIN in—Inu., Pr. p. (*See also* **Proctalgia.**)

PARALYSIS of—Tab.

PROLAPSE of—Ant. c., Ch. s., Clch., Fer., Ign., Mag. p., Rut., So. t. ae.

STRUCTURE of—Syph., Tab., Thio.

> *See also* **Polypus**, RECTAL.

Red-gum—*Ant. c., Aps., Cham., Rhs.*

Reflexes, ABOLISHED—Sfn.

Relapsing Fever—*Bap., Bry., E. pf., Rhs.*

Remittent Fever—*Aco., Ant. c., Ars., Bry., Ch. s., Cin., Crt. h., E. pf., Gel., Ipc.,* Nyc.

Remittent Fever, Infantile—Lpt., Sntn.

Renal Calculi—Ca. ren., Nux, *Ocm.,* Thl.

Renal Colic—Ber., Brc. x., Calc., Dio., Ery. a., E. pu., Ind., Lyc. Med., Nx. m., Ocm., Prei., Ppz., Sars., Se. a., Urt., Zea., st.

Renal Dropsy—Lia.

Respiration, ABNORMAL—*Phyt.*

AFFECTIONS of—*Bro.*

CHEYNE-STOKES—Atp. (*See also* **Cheyne-Stokes Breathing.**)

SLOW—Bz. n.

Respiratory Paralysis—Hfb., (Son. ac.).

> *See also* **Lungs,** PARALYSIS of.

Restlessness—Abs., Cod., Jal., Rut.

Retained Placenta—Cth., Pul., Sbi., Sec., Vis.

Retina, ANAEMIA of—Li. c.

DETACHMENT of—Gel., Nph.

Retinitis—Bz. d., Pho.

ALBUMINURICA— Klm.

Reveries—Sel.

Rhagades—Alm., Calc., Hep., Lyc., Man., Sars.

> *See also* **Anus,** EXCORIATION and CHAPS of; **Chapped Hands;** *and* **Hands,** CHAPPED.

Rheumatic Affections—Bov., Mrl.

Rheumatic Arthritis—Fe. pi. (*See also* **Chronic Rheumatic**

Arthritis; Rheumatic Gout (*below*); *and* **Rheumatoid Arthritis.**)

'**Rheumatic Fever**—Ail., Ign., Spo., *Sul.,* Trm. (*See also* **Rheumatism,** *which includes* **Rheumatic Fever.**)

Rheumatic Gout—*Act. r., Ars., Cap., Caul.,* Fe. pi., *Iod., Sbi.* (*See also* **Chronic Rheumatic Arthritis;** *and* **Rheumatoid Arthritis.**)

Rheumatic Nodes—Agn.

Rheumatic Paralysis— Lth.

Rheumatism—Abr., *Act. r.,* Act. s., Aga., All., Alns., Am. bz., Amm. Ana., Anag., Ank., *Ant. t., Aps.,* Arb., Ar. lp., Arg., Arm., *Arn., Ars.,* As. i., Asc. s., Asc. t., Bad., Bel., Bls., *Bz. x.,* Ber., Bry., Cac., Caj., *Calc.,* Ca. cs., *Ca. p.,* Cam., *Cap.,* Crb. s., Crd. m., Carl., Cas. s., *Caul.,* Caus., Ced., Cham., Chel., Chi., *Ch. s.,* Chr. o., Cnb., Cit., Clem., Coca, Coc. i., *Clch.,* Coll., Col., Clv. d., Cty., Crt. h., Ctn., Cub., Cp. a., Cyc., Dph., Dio., Dir., *Dul.,* Elt., Elc., Euc., E. pf., E. pu., Fag., Fel., Fer., Fe. mg., Fe. m., Fe. p., For., Fnc., Glv., Gas., Gau., Gel., Gin., Glo., Gna., Guac., Gui., Ham., Hlon., Hep., Hyp., Icth., Ict., Ill., *Iod.,* Ird., Iris, Jnc., *K. bi.,* K. cy., K. fc., *K. i.,* K. m., K. n., K. sc., *Klm.,* Kre., Lc. c., Lc. v., Lc. x., Lth., *Led.,* Lpi., Ln. c., Li. c., Li. l., Lrs., *Lyc., Mac.,* Mgt., Mgn. gr., Mlr., Man., Mn. m., Med., *Mr. sol., Mr. v.,* Mr. bin., Mth. b., Mez., Mim., Na. c., Na. 1., Na. p., Na. sa., Nx. m., Nyc., Oln., O1. j., Oxt., Pet., Ph. x., Pho., *Phyt.,* Pin. s., Pip. m., Plat., Ple., Plp., Ptl., *Pul.,* Pl. n., Pyre., Pyr. a., Rn. a., Rn. b., Rhe., *Rho., Rhs.,* Rum., *Rut.,* Sbd., Sac. o., Sl. x., Sxm., Sll., Sang., Snc., Sap., *Sars.,* Scro., Sil., Sko., Sld., Spi., Spo., Stp., *Ste.,* Sti., *Stil.,* Sty., Su. x., Syph., Trx., Tax., Tep., Teu., Til., Ur. x., Urt., Ver., Vic., Vi. o., Vi. t., Wis., Wil., Zin.

ACUTE—*Sul.*

CHRONIC—Sil., *Sul.*

GONORRHOEAL—Dph., Ja. c., *Med.,* Phyt., Pul., Sars., *Sul., Thu.*

HEREDITARY—Sil.

PARALYTIC—Pho.

SYPHILITIC—Phyt.

WANDERING—Ap. a., (K. bi.), Pl. n., (Puls.).

> See also **Muscular Rheumatism; Lumbago; Myalgia;** *and under* **Joints.**

Rheumatoid Arthritis—Fe. pi., Mth. b., Sl. x.

> See also **Chronic Rheumatic Arthritis;** *and* **Rheumatic Gout.**

Rhinitis—Ust.

ATROPHIC—K. bi., Lmn., Sbl.

> See also **Nose,** INFLAMMATION of.

Rhinorrhoea. Cerebro-spinalis—Hd. h.

Rhinoscleroma—Au. m. n.

Rhus Poisoning—An. oc., Ctn., Ech. a., Gph., Gnd., Hph. v., K. sc., Nup., Plnt., (Rhs.), Sang., Vbn.

Rickets—Am. c., *Ars.,* Calc., *Ca. p.,* Fe. m., Hec., Hd. h., K. i., Merc., Nt. x., *Pho.,* Sac. o., Snc., *Sil.,* Ther., Thu.

> See also **Scurvy Rickets.**

Riding in Carriage, EFFECTS of—Coc. i.

Rigg's Disease—(Bac.), Merc., Mr. c.

Rigid Os—Lo. i.

Ringworm—An. oc., Anag., Ant. t., Ar. lp., *Ars., Bac.,* Bap., Ba. m., *Calc.,* Chm. u., Cbs. x., Cup., E. pf., Jg. c., Jg. r., Mez., Ol. j., Phyt., Pso., *Sep., Sul.,* Tel., Vi. t.

> See also **Herpes;** *and* **Tinea.**

Roaring in Horses—Lth.

Rodent Ulcer—Cnd., Fe. pi., Jg. c., Mil., Phyt.

Roseola—*Aco.,* Atp., *Bel.,* Cub.

Rumination—Api. g., Klm:

Rupia—*K. i.,* Thyr.

Sacralgia—Ol. j.

Sacrum, Pain in—*AEsc., Aga.,* Alo., (Ant. t.), *Ber.,* Pnt., Sep., *Tel.*

Saliva, MILKY—Pbo.

    SOUR—Par.

Salivation—Ac. c., All., Arec., Ast. r., Dig., Epl., Eps., Eser., Glv., Hl. o., Hfb., *Iod.,* Ipc., *Iris, Jab.,* K. pm., K. tel., Mgt. n., *Mr. sol., Nt. x.,* Prt., Phyt., Pilo., Pt. m. n., Rhe., Scor., Sin. a., Trf. r., Ver., Vic., Wye.

    INTERMITTENT—Nm. x.

    NOCTURNAL,—Cham., Mth. pu.

    PREGNANCY, of—Jab., Pilo.

Satyriasis—Cn. i., Cth., Fl. x., Hfb., Sx. n., Zn. pi.

Sausages, POISONING from—Ac. x.

Scabies—Ank., Cb. v, Caus., *Pso.,* Rs. v., Sel., *Sul.,* Ter.

    SICCA—Mr. i. f.

    See also **Itch.**

Scald-head—Ars., Chel., (Mlt.), Sum., Ust.

    See also **Crusta Lactea.**

Scalds—Ac. x., Crb. s., Jab.

    See also **Burns.**

Scalp, ECZEMA of—Sel.

    ERUPTION on—*Oln.*

Scalp, PAINFUL—So. t. ae.

    SORENESS of—Sul. i.

Scapula, PAIN in—Chn. a., *Jg. c.*

    PAIN under—Chn. v.

    PAIN under RIGHT—(Chel)

    RHEUMATISM of—Ham.

    See also **Interscapular Pain.**

Scarlatina—*Aco., Ail.,* Am. c., Atp., *Aps.,* Ag. n., *Ars., Ar. t.,* Asi., *Bel., Bry.,* Ca. s., *Cth.,* Cbl. x., Ch. ar., Ch. s., Cin., *Crt. h., Cu. a.,* Dul., *Ech. a.,* Hl. f., Hel., *Hep.,* J g. c., *Lach., Mu. x., Rhs.,* So. n., *Spi.,* Stm., *Ter.,* Ver.

    ANGINOSA—Mnc., Sl. x.

    See also **Anasarca,** AFTER SCARLATINA; *and* **Nephritic Scarlatina.**

Scars—*Fl. x.*, Gas., Hyp., Iod., *Phyt., Sil.*, Thio.

AFFFECTIONS of—Jnc.

INFLAMED—Gph.

School-headache—(Ca. p.), Mag. p., Na. c., (Na. m.), Ph. x., Sbl.

Sciatica—Act. r., Am. m., Ant. a., *Ars.*, As. mt., As. r., Calc., *Cap.*, Crb.o., Crb. s., Crd. m., Carl., Crv., Cham., Cnb., Cof., *Col.*, Dio., Drs., Elt., E. pu., Eub., Gau., Gin., Glo., *Gna.*, Gui., Hdr., Hfb., Hyp., Ign., Ind., Inu., *Iris,* K. bi., *K. ca.*, K. i., K. ph., Lc. c., Lc. v. d., Lach., Lc. x., Lo. s., *Lyc.*, Mag. p., Med., Na. s., Nyc., OEna., O1. j., Pal., Pas., Ph. x., Phyt., Pb., Pod., Plg., Pso., Pl. n., Pyr. a., *Rhs., Rut.*, Sac. 1., Sl. x., Sx. m., Se. a., Sep., So. t. ae., Sld., Stp., Sto. c., Sul., Syph., Tel., Tep., *Ter.*, Thu., Trb., Up., Val., Vis., Xan.

Scirrhus—Lp. a.

See also **Cancer;** *and* **Carcinoma.**

Scleriasis— Elae.

Scleroderma—Elae., Klm., Thyr.

Sclerotitis—Ch. m., Ery. a., Klm., Tan.

Scoliosis—Fe. i.

See also **Spine.**

Scorbutic Affections—Aran.

See also **Scurvy.**

Scorbutus—Ar. m., Cis., K. m.

See also **Scurvy.**

Screaming—*Ant. t., Bor., Bry., Cham., Cic. v.,* K. br., *Pho.*, Ph. chr., *Zin.*

CHILDREN, of—Rhe.

See also **Waking,** SCREAMING on.

Scrofula—AEps., Alns., Alm., Ank., Ar. lp., Asc. t., Aur., Bad., Ba. m., Bro., Calc., Ca. m., Ca. si., Cap., Cb. a., Caus., Chm. u., Cnb., Cis., Coca., Con., Cry., Cur., Dul., Ephr., Fe. i., Fe. m., Fe. s., Get., Gph., Hep., Hpz., K. bi., K. i., Lp. a., Mez., Na. c., Na. p., Pin. s., Pb. i., Sld., Stil., Ts. ff.

Scrofulosis— Ther.

Scrofulous Affections— Ars.

Emaciation—Cet.

Glands—Bac.

Ophthalmia—As. .i., Na. s., O1. j. (*See also* **Ophthalmia,**
SCROFULOUS.)

See also **Eyes,** SCROFULOUS AFFECTIONS of; *and*
INFLAMMATION of; **Joints,** SCROFULOUS; *and* **Laryngitis,**
SCROFULOUS.

Scrotum, Abscess of—Sty.

Scurf—Smb. n.

Scurvy—Agv., All., Aln., Am. m, Aran., Arm., Ar. m., Brs., Cb. v.,
Cry. a., Cet., Cis:, Cit., Coca, Elt., *Ham.*, Jg. r., K. chl., K.
m., K. ph., Lach., *Mr. sol.*, Mu. x., Na. hch., Nm. x., Ph. x.,
Pho., Pso., Rat., Sac. o., Snc., Sin. n., So. t. ae., Stp., Su. x.,
Tep., Uri.

Scurvy Rickets—Aran.

Sea-bathing, Effects of—Ars., Lim.

Sea-sickness—Aml., Apm., Aq. m., Ars., Bor., Cap., Cer. o., *Coc.
i.,* Cuc. p., Eu. co., Glo., Kre., Nct., Nux, *Pet.,* Snc., Stp.,
Tab., Ther.

Seaside, Effects of—Aq. m., Bro.

Sebaceous Cysts—K. br.

Sebaceous Tumours—Aga., Thu.

Seborrhoea—Hdr., *Iod.,* K. br., Lo. i., *Na. m.,* Rap., Sars., Sep.,
Stp., *Vin.*

CAPITIS—Her.

Self-abuse—*Ana., Aps.,* Buf., *Ca. p., Chi., K. br., Na. m., Ph. x., Pi.
x., Stp., Sul.*

See also **Masturbation;** *and* **Onanism.**

Semen, too early Ejaculation of—Tit.

Seminal Emissions—Cim., Cf. t., Gph., Nup., Onos., Ori., Sti., Ur.
n., Vi. o., Vi. t., Voe., Zn. pi., Zn. v., Zng.

NOCTURNAL—Thu.

See also **Nocturnal Emissions.**

Senility—Orc.

PREMATURE— Vip., (Stram.).

Senses, Disordered—Anh.

Sensibility, Loss of—K. br.

Sensitiveness—*Bel., Cham., Ign.*

See also **Hypheraesthesia;** *and* **Hypersensitiveness.**

Sepsis—Pyro.

See also **Antiseptic.**

Septic Diseases—Trn.

Septicaemia—*Ech. a.*

See also **Blood-poisoning.**

Sewer-gas Poisoning—*Bap., Phyt.*

Sexual ATONY, DESIRE LOST—Onos.

EXCESS—Avn., Up.

EXCESS EFFECTS of—Aga., Gel., Symt.

EXCITEMENT—Chn. s., Gin.

IRRITATION—Ori.

MANIA—Cam.

ORGANS, INFLAMMATION of—Cast. .

ORGANS, SPASM, of—Cast.

PERVERSION—Idm., Nux, Plat.

POWER, DIMINISHED—Pal.

WEAKNESS—Ery. a., Ery, m., Gas., Orc., Per.

Shingles—K. m.

See also **Herpes** ZOSTER; **Zona;** *and* **Zoster.**

Shivering—*Aco., Ars., Ast. f., Bap., Cam., Cb. v., Pho.*

Shock—Cof.

Shoulder, AFFECTIONS of—Fer.

PAIN in—Lo. i., Med.

RHEUMATISM of—Sang., Snc., Wil.

RIGHT, PAIN in—Ple., Pl. n., (Sang.), (Urt.).

Shyness—Mli.

Sick-headache—Chlf., Sti.

See also **Headache,** SICK, **Hemicrania; Megrim;**

Migraine.

Side, Pain in—*Act. r.,* Ber., Bry., *Cean., Dio., Ox. x., Pul.*

See also **Stich in Side.**

Sighing—(Ca. p.), *Na. p., Opi.,* Sac. l.

Sight, Affections of—Cin., For. (*See also* **Vision,** Affections of.)

Defective—Bap. c., Elae.

Vanishing of—Cnt. .

Weak—Mep. (*See also* **Eyes,** Sight Weak.)

Sigmoid, Flexure, Cancre of—Spi.

Pain in—Scro.

Sinking Sensation—*Act. r., Ign., Sul.*

Sinuses—Cty., Sil.

Skin, Affections of—AE.ps., All., Buf., Calc., Cim., Elae., Gph., *Hep.,* Her., Hur., Hyd., Icth., (Ign.), Imp., Ind., Jat., K. as., Kam., Lim., Ped., *Pet.,* Prm. o., Pso., Sprn., *Sul.,* Vic.

Darkness of—So. t. ae.

Diseases of—Ana., Lev.

Eruption of—Caus., Ery. m., Eu. a., Lcrt., Led.

Inflammation of, Malignant—Com.

Peeling of—Hl. f.

Rough—Aln.

Sensitive—Rs. d.

Unhealthy—Anag., Mld., *Sel.*

See also **Bronzed Skin,** *and* the various eruptions: **Eczema; Herpes; &c.**

Sleep, Abnormal—*Cnb., Lyc., Nux, Opi.,* So. m.

Disorders of—*Bel.,* Calc., cm. br., *Cb. v.,* Chi., *Gel.,* Homa. *Hyo., Ign.,* Mor., *Pho., Sul.*

Disturbed—Mgt. n.

Dreamful— *Ve. v.*

Dreams, Anxious, in—*Bry.*

Excessive—Lct. v., So. o.

Loss of, Affections from—*Coc. i.*

Overpowering—Nx. m.

RESTLESS—*Rhs.*

SHORT, but REFRESHING —Rn. r.

SUDDEN—Psc.

WHINING in—*Ver.*

    See also **Somnambulism.**

Sleepiness—Coc. i., Dbn., Nx. m., Opi., Scro., So. pc., (Sul.), Thev., Zin.

Sleeplessness—Abs., *Aco., Act. r.,* AEth., Ara. t., Avn., Bls., Bnz., Ca. br., Calc., Cam., Cof., Cchn., Crt. h., Cup., Cyp., Dph., Hyn., Ir. t., K. br., K. ca., K. ph., O1. j., Pas., Phst., Rap., Sap., Scu., Sna. Stn., Sti., Syph., Tea., Ur. n., Val., Zn. o., Zn. p.

EXCESSIVE—Phel.

    See also **Debility,** with SLEEPLESSNESS.

Sloughing—Amm.

Small-pox—An. oc., Athra., *Ant. t.,* Ag. n., *Cbl. x.,* Caus., *Crt. h.,* Cnd., Cu. a., *Ham.,* K. i., K. m., Lach., Mld., *Mr. sol.,* Rhs. Sll., Src., So. n., Vac., Var.

CONFLUENT—Hpz.

HAEMORRHAGIC—Sec.

    See also **Variola.**

Smarting Eruptions—Na. hch.

Smell—DISORDERS of—*Aco., Aur., Bel., Calc., Cbl. x., Dio., Gph. Mag.* m., Sep.

ILLUSIONS of—Ana., Eu. a., *K. bi.,* Lct. v., *Pul., Sang.,* Sul.

LOSS of—*Am. m.,* Chlf., Per. Sang.

PERVERTED—Zn. m.

SENSE of AFFECTED—Der.

SENSE of, too ACUTE—Sep.

Snake-bites—Anag., Cam., Ced., Ech. a., Gne., Lo. p., Lcs., Plnt., Sga.

    . *See also* **Bites** of REPTILES.

Sneezing—Sga.

COUGH, AT END OF—Sga.

FITS of—Sga.

HEAT, with—Sna.

    See also **Colds;** *and* **Coryza.**

Snoring—Opi., Rat., Rhe.

Snow-headache—Glo.

Snuffles—Apo., Smb. n.

Sobbing, Spasmodic—Mag. p.

Somnambulism—*Art. v,* (Cur.), *K. br.,* Klm., Lun., Mgt. n., Na. m.,
    Pho., Sil., Zin.

Somnolence—Coc. i., So. pc., Thev.

    See also **Sleepiness.**

Sore Throat—Ar. dm., Cbn., Chm. m., Chlm., Cis., Dol., Elae., Eu.
    pp., Hl. v., Hur. c., Idm., Lchn., Lo. c., Mnc.

    MALIGNANT—Ch. ar.

        See also **Clergyman's Sore Throat; Syphilitic Sore
        Throat;** *and* **Throat,** SORE.

Spasmodic Twitchings—Cod.

Spasms—Acn., Cam., Cham., Cin., Coc. i., Ccs. c., Cchn., Cup.,
    Fer., Fe. s., Gel., Mli., Mth. b., Nct., Oln., Ox. x., Plat.

    See also **Ciliary** SPASM; **Clonic Spasms; OEsophagus,**
    SPASM of; *and* **Writer's Spasm.**

Spastic Paralysis—Bz. d., Gels., Hyp., (Lch.), Nux, Ple., Sec.

    See also **Paralysis,** SPASTIC; *and* **Spinal Sclerosis.**

Spavin in Horses—Ang., Ca. fl.

Speech, AFFECTIONS of—*Cham., K. br.*

    ARRESTED—Rat.

    DEFECTIVE—Nx. m.

    DIFFICULT—Pip. n., Tep.

    DISORDERED—*Lyc., Nux.*

    EMBARRASSED—Na. m., Tab.

Speech, IMPEDED—Nic.

    LOST—K. cy., OEna.. (*See also* **Aphasia.**)

    THICK—AEs. g., Li. br.

        See also **Stammering;** *and* **Stuttering.**

Spermatic Cord, AFFECTIONS of—Stp.
NEURALGIA of—Ber., Ol. a., Ox. x.
PAIN in—Osm., Oxt., Plg., Se. a.
SWELLING of—Sars.
Spermatorrhoea—Cld., *Ca. p.,* Ca. s., Cm. br., *Cth., Chi., Con.,*
Cyp., Dgn., Dig., Dio., Ery. a.., Erig., Fe. br., *Na. m., Nux,*
Ph. x., Sx. n., Sars., *Sel.,* Sep., *Sil., Stp.,* Sum., Tax., Ter.,
Tur., Zin.
Sphincters, PARALYSIS of—Erg.
RELAXATION of—Oxt.
Spina Bifida—(Bac.), *Bry., Ca. p.,* Pso.
Spinal Cord, DRAWING in—Sch.
PAINS in—Lct. v.
Spinal Exhaustion—Pi. x.
Irritation—*Act. r., Aga., Ag. n.,* Atr., Ch. ar., Ch. s., Chn. s., Coc. i.,
Cup., Dio., Hep., Hyp., *Ign.,* K. ca., Lc. c., Lil., Mth. b., Na.
m., Ol. j., Phst., Phyt., Pi. x., Rn. b., *Sec., Sil.,* Sty. p., *Sul.,*
Trn, *Tel.,* Ther., Zin. (*See also* **Cerebro-spinal Irritation.**)
Irritation (of NUCHA)—Naj.
Paresis—Ird.
Sclerosis—Au. m., Crb. s., Hyn., Phst., Pi. x., Pb., Tm. (*See also*
Paralysis, SPASTIC; *and* **Spastic Paralysis.**)
Weakness—Sul. i., Zn. pi.
Spine, AFFECTIONS of—Ana., Calc., For., Guac., Oln., Par., Zin.
CARIES of—Ph. x., Syph. (*See also* POTT'S CURVATURE)
CONCUSSION of—Hyp.
CONGESTION of—Abs., Onos., Ve. v.
CURVATURE of—(Fe. i.), *Pho.,* Pul., Sul.
DISEASE of—Pb., Rhs.
INJURY to—Nt. x.
NEURALGIA of—Vrn.
PAIN in—Clcn., Hur., Lo. s., Mns., Prf., Tep., Up.
POTT'S CURVATUREof—Get., K. i., (Pho.), *Pyro.,* Sti.
TUMOUR of—Pb.

See also **Myelitis; Railway Spine; Spinal Exhaustion,** &
c.; *and* **Vertebrae,** AFFECTIONS of, & c.

Spleen, AFFECTIONS of—*Aga.*, Aran., Bls., Ber. a., Ber., Ca. cs., Crd.
m., *Cean.*, Chi., Cty., Euc., Eu. a., Hli., K. i., Kis., Lct.v.. Li.
c., Lo. s.. Mlr., Mrl.. Na. s., Prt., Pb., Plg., Plp., Pso., Ptl.
Qer., Rub., Rut., Sac. o., Scil., Sla., Suc.. Su. x., *Urt.*.

CONGESTION of—Az., Ve. v.

COUGH arising from—Scil.

ENLARGEMENT of—Acn., Au. m., Ch. s., Fe. as., Fe. i., Fe. m.,
Mag. m., Mr. bin., Na. m., Pho., Pb. i.

INDURATION of—Agn., Pso.

NEURALGIA of—Zin.

PAIN in—Amb., Am. m., Bap. c., Cai., (Cean.), Chn. v., Dio.,
Dor., For., Gnd., Gn ,Her., Homa., Ilx., Jg. r., Mag. c., Opu.,
Prf., Phyt., Plnt., Prm. o., Rho., Sap., Sul., Vis., Zng.

PAIN, SHOOTING THROUGH FROM FRONT TO BACK—Als.

SHOOTING in—Alm.

SWELLING of—Agn., Ver.

See also **Dropsy,** SPLENIC; **Leucocythaemia** SPLENICA;
Splen algia Splenic Fever; *and* **Splenitis.**

Splenalgia—Arn., (Cean.), Fl. x., Hlon.

See also **Spleen.**

Splenic Fever—Athra.

Splenitis—Cit., Dph.

See also **Spleen.**

Spotted Fever—Am. c., E. pf.

Sprains—Agn., All., Am. c., Am., m., *Arn.*, Carl., Fe. p., Per., Pet.,.
Pho., Pro s., Pso., Rho., *Rhs., Rut.,* Sto. c., Symt.

See also **Ankle,** SPRAIN of; *and* **Strains.**

Sprue—*See* **Psilosis.**

Squint—(Gel.), Pin.s.

See also **Strabismus.**

Staggering—Au. s.

Stammering—Atr., Bov., Buf., Cn. i., Can. S., Caus., Dul., *Hyo.,*

Lyc., Na. c., Na. sa., Nx. m., Ped., Pho., Ph. h., Rut., Sec., Sel., So. n., So. t., Sgu., Spi., *Stm.*

See also **Speech,** ARRESTED, &c.; *and* **Stuttering.**

Staphyloma—Ephr., Ilx.

Starting—*Aga., Cb. v.,Opi., Smb. n., Stm., Sul.*

See also **Waking,** STARTS *and* SCREAMS on.

Stasis—Bls.

Status Epilepticus—OEna.

Steatoma—Stp.

Sterility—Agn., Alet., Ar. lp., Au. m., Ba. m., *Bor.,* Caul., *Con.,* Fil., (For.), Gos., Hlon., *Iod.,* Mil., Na. c., *Na. m.,* Na. p., Pho., Sbl., Su. x., (Ther.), Tur., Wis.

Sternum— Ver.

PAINS in—Am. c., Lc. v., Osm., Paeo., Rn. s., *Rut.,* Sto. c.

PRESSURE on—Mr. ac.

See also **Chest,** PAIN in; *and* **Chest,** STERNUM, PAIN BEHIND.

Stiff-neck—*Aco., Act. r.,* Ana., *Ant. t., Bry.,* Ca. cs., Ca. p., *Chel.,* Chr. o., *Clch., Dul.,* Gn. c., Hl. f., Hyp., Itu, Lchn., Phst., Phyt., Pim., Ple., *Rho.,* Rs. v., Sg. n., Scro., Stp., Vic., Vin., Zn. v.

Stiffness—(Cur.)

Stings—Ac. x., *Arn.,* Crt. h., *Hy. x., Lach., Led., Mos.*

See also **Bee-stings.**

Stitch in Side—Aga.

See also **Side, Pain in.**

Stomacace—Agv., Ard.

See also **Aphthae; Mouth,** ULCERATED *and* **Stomatitis,** ULCERATIVE.

Stomach, AFFECTIONS of—*Ars., Cbl.* x., Con., Cro., *Cnd.,* Dor., Elae., Gn. c., Gui., Hdr., Imp., *K. ca., Kre.,* Lc. c., *Ox. x.,* Rob.

CANCER of—Ac. x., Act. s., Bis., Mag. p., Pt. m., Sec.

CATARRH of—Hy. x., Ill.

COUGH—Lo. s.

CRAMP in—Gph.

DISORDERS of—AEth., *Ant. c.,* Ast. f., *Cb. v.,* Gn. 1., Mag. m., Rhe.

DISTENSION of—Rat.

HAEMORRHAGE from— *See* HAEMATEMESIS.

INFLAMMATION of—*See* **Gastritis.**

NEUROSIS of—Sang.

ULCERATION of—K. ph., Orn., Rat. (*See also* **Gastric Ulcers.)**

Stomatitis—Bap., Ber. a., Bis., Cap., Cb. v., Ir. t., K. chl., Mnc., Merc., Na. m., OEna., Pod., Rn. s., Sl. x., Sul., Ur. n.

ULCERATIVE. —*Ss. x. (See also* **Mouth,** ULCERATED; *and* **Stomacace.)**

See also **Aphthae** *and* **Mouth** INFLAMMATION of.

Stone-cutter's Phthisis—Calc.

Stone in Bladder—Ca. ren.

See also **Bladder,** STONE in.

Stool, BILIOUS—Sg. t.

INEFFECTUAL URGING to—Ger.

See also **Constipation** *and* **Diarrhoea.**

Strabismus—Aln., Alm., Bz. n., Ca. p., Cb. a., Cic. v., Cin., Cu. a., Cyc., Ery. a., Jab., Nux, Oln., Pin. s., Pod., Sap., Scor., Sec., Spi., Stm., Syph., Tab., Zin.

DIVERGENT—Mor., Na. sa.

INWARD, RIGHT—Tan.

RIGHT—Sp. m.

Strains—Ars., Calc., Ca. fl., Lyc., Sil.

See also **Ankle,** SPRAIN of; *and* **Sprains.**

Strangury—Ac. 1., Arm., *Bel., Cam.,* Cth., Epg., E. pu., Jn. v., Lach., Nx. m., Onis., Plg., Pr. s., Sbl., Sbi., Sntn., Sars., Sil., Tax., Ter., Thl.

Stricture—Chm. u., Med., Pb., Pr. s., Rhs., Syph., Ter., Thio.

SPASMODIC—Sec.

URETHRAL—Sul. i. (*See also* **Urethra,** STRICTURE of.)

See also **Rectum,** STRICTURE of.

Struma—Ech. a., Vis.

Strychnine Poisoning—Euc., Oxg.

Stump, IRRITABLE—Symt.

> NEURALGIA in——Am. m.

Stuttering—Cic. v.

> *See also* **Speech,** ARRESTED, &c.; *and* **Stammering.**
> **Stye**—Cyp., Fag., Fe. p., *Hep.,* Lc. f., Pi. x., *Pul.,* Sac. 1.,
> Sga., Sep., So.o., Stn., *Stp.,* Ur. n., Vi. o., Ziz.

Subinvolution. —Na. hch.

> *See also* **Uterus,** SUBINVOLUTION of.

Suffocation,FITS of—Chi.

Sun, EFFECTS of—Cac.,Sel.

> *See also* **Sun—headache;** *and* **Sunstroke.**

Sunburn—Sol.

Sun-headache—Gel., Glo., K. bi., Klm., Stm.

Sunstroke—Aml., Ant. c., *Cac.,* Cam., Cit., Crt. h., Eu. pi., Gel.,
Glo. Hy. x., Hfb., Lyc., Na. m., Opi., Pop. c., Sol., Stm.,
Syph. Ve. v.

> CHRONIC EFFECTS of—Na. c.

Suppressed Eruptions, EFFECTS of—Aps., Bry., (Pso.), (Sul.)

> *See also* **Eruptions,** SUPPRESSED; **Itch,** SUPPRESSED; *and*
> **Suppressions.**

Suppressed Menstruation—As. h.

> *See also* **Menstruation,** SUPPRESSED.

Suppressions—Zin.

> *See also* **Eruptions,** SUPPRESSED; **Feet,** SWEAT of,
> SUPPRESSED; *and* **Itch.** SUPPRESSED.

Suppuration—*Arn.,* Ars., Buf., *Caln.,* Dxn., Fl. x., *Hep., Mr. sol.,*
Mth. b., Mst. s., *Sil.*

> *See also* **Gangrenous** *and* **Fetid Suppurations** *and* **Joints,**
> SUPPURATION of.

Supra-orbital Neuralgia—(Acn.), Mr. c.

> *See also* **Ciliary Neuralgia;** *and* **Neuralgia,** SUPRA-ORBITAL

Surgical Fever— Merc.

See also **Operations,** Effects of; **Traumatic Feve;** *and* **Traumatism.**

Swallowing, Constant—Ar. m.

Constant, while **Talking**—Stp.

Sweat—Am. ac., Bnz., Ca. hp.

    Excessive—Eser. (*See also* **Perspiration,** Excessive.)

    Local—Ple.

    Profuse—*Ph. x.,* Psc.

    Viscid—Phal.

    See also **Perspiration.**

Sycosis—Anan., Ank., *Ant. t.,* Aps:, Ast. r., Au. m. n., Bz. x., Calc., Cast., Cnb., Ephr., K. bi., K. m., Na. s., Pi. x., Sbi., Thu.

    Hahnemanni—Mil., (Nt. x.), Ph. x., (Thu.).

    Menti—Calc.

Sycotic Diathesis—Gph.

    Eruptions—Sto. c.

Syncope—Amg., Prt.

    See also **Fainting.**

Synovitis—Ant. t., Pul.

    See also **Joints,** Synovitis of.

Syphilis—AEps., Ail., Alns., Anag., Anan., Aps., Ag. i., Ag. n., As. i., As. mt., Asa., Asc. t., Au. ar., Au. i., *Aur.,* Au. m., Au. m. n., Bad., Ber. a., Ca. fl., Ca. s., Cltr., Cb. a., Caus., Chm. u., Ch. ar., Chr. o., Cnb., Crl., Cry., Crt. h., Cnd., Cu. s., Ech. a., Eryth., Euc., Eub., Fer., *Fl. x.,* Fnc., *Gph.,* Gui., Hec., Hep., Hpz., Hoa., Hdr., Hyd., Iod., Ja. c., Ja. g., Jg. r., *K. bi.,* K. br., K. chl., K. *i.,* Kre., Lc. c., Lach., Li. c., *Mr. sol.,* Mr. bin., *Mr. c.,* Mr. i. f., *Mez., Nt. x.,* Osm., Pet., Ph. x., Pho., *Phyt.,* Pso., Sang., Sars., Sel., Sti., *Stil.,* Syph., *Thu.,* Thyr., Ul. f., Vi. t.

    Nerves, of— Mr. n.

    See also **Congenital Syphilis; Eyes,** Syphilitic Affections of ; **Headache,** Syphilitic ; **Kerato-iritis Syphilitica; Liver,** Syphilis of; **Syphilitic Deafness,** &c.;

and **Testicles,** Syphilitic Enlargement of.

Syphilitic Deafness—Kre.

Eruptions—Osm., Phyt.

Pains—E. pf.

Sore Throat—Bor., Klm.

Syringo-myelia—*Pho.*

Tabes Mesenterica—Bap., *Calc., Iod., Mr. c.,* Pet., Pb., Pyro., Sac. o.

Tachycardia—Adr.

Tape-worm—Arec., Calc., Ca. cs., Cnb., Cuc. p., Cu. a., Fil., Frg., Grn., Kam., Kou., Plat., Pul., Sbd., Sl. x., Stn.

Tarentula—bites—Lcs.

Tarsal Cysts—Fe. p., Fe. py., K. i.

Tarsal Tumours—Stp., Zin.

Tartar—Sil. m.

    See also **Teeth,** Tartar, on.

Taste, Abnormal—*Lyc.*

    Altered—*AEsc., Ant. t., Ag. n.,* Crv., *Chel.,* Fag., Gne.

    Bad—Rhe.

    Depraved—*Pul.*

    Disordered—Alm., *Arn.,* Bel., Bor., Calc., *Cam., Chi.,* Hdr., *Mag. c., Mag. m., Mr. sol., Mr. c., Na. m., Nt. x., Nux.*

    Illusions of—Pod., *Sul.*

    Loss of—Chlf., *Na. m.,* Per., Pod., *Pul.*

    Perverted—Pod., Zn. m.

Tea, Effects of—Ab. n., *Chi.,* Dio., Lo. i., *Nux, Thu.*

Teeth, Affections of—Eub., *Mr. v., Mez.*

    Caries of—*Calc.,* Hec., Kre., Pip. n., *Sil., Stp.,* Syph., Thu.

    Crumbling—Ph. h.

    Defective—Bac., Fl. x.

    Operations on—Aln.

    Pitted—Bac.

    Tartar on—Ca. ren., Sil. m.

Teething—Gel.

See also **Dentition**; and **Wisdom-Teeth**, EFFECTS of
CUTTING.

Temperature, Lowered—Sap.

Tendo Achillis, AFFECTIONS of—Mu. x.

PAIN in—Ari., My. c., Ttr., Up.

Tendons, CONTRACTED—Caus., Mez.

CREAKING of—K. m.

INFLAMED—Ant. c.

Tenesmus—Ags., Alo., Aph., *Bel., Hep., Ign., Mr. c., Nux,* Pb. chr.,
Pod., Sil., So. t. ae., *Sul.*

Testicles, AFFECTIONS of—Aco., Aur., Ba. m., *Bel., Con.,* Rhs., Stp.

ATROPHY of—Sbl.

INDURATION of—Agn., Bro., Ox. x.

INFLAMMATION of—*Cle., Ham., Spo.*

NEURALGIA of—Na. as., Ol. a.

PAINS in—Osm., Ox. x., Oxt.

RETRACTION of—Ol. a.

SWELLING of—Agn., Ca. p., Var.

SYPHILITIC ENLARGEMET of—Mr. bin.

TUBERCLE of—Bac. t.

TUBERCULOSIS of—Teu. s.

UNDEVELOPED—Aur.

Tetanus—Acn., *Aco.,* Amg., Ang., Atr., Bz. n., *Caln.,* Cam., Can. s.,
Cbn., Crb. h., Crb. s., Cast., Chlf., Cic. m., Cic. v., Crt. h.,
Cur., Glv., Grt., Hel., *Hy. x.,* Hfb., Hyo., Hyp., Ipc., Jas., Jn.
v., K. br., Lau., Led., Mil., Mor., Nct., *OEna.,* Ox. x., Pas.,
Phst., Phyt., Pb., Sntn., Scor., Siu., Son., So. c., So. n., Stm.,
Sty., Sul. h., Tab., Ter., Ther., Thyr., Up., Vrn., Ver., Vb. p.

NEONATORUM—Pas.

See also **Jaws**, CLENCHED; **Lock-jaw; Opisthotonos;** and
Trismus.

Tetany—Aco.

Tetters—Anag., Can., Jg. c., Ph. x.

MOIST and ITCHING—Alm.

Thighs, PAIN in—Ill.

SWEAT on—Rn. g.

Thirst—*Aco., Amm., Ant. t., Arn., Ars., Bel., Bry., Cth., Chi., Crt. h., Dul.,* E. pf., (Na. m.), *Stm., Sul.*

ABSENCE of—*Cyc.,* (Pul.)

Thought, Difficult—So. m.

Thread-worms—*Bap., Cin., Na. p.,* Scir, Sin. a., *Spi., Teuc.*

Throat, AFFECTIONS of—*Aco., AEsc.,* Aln., Alm., Ag. *n.,* Caus., Cen., Gui., *Iod.,* Thev.

ATROPHIC PHARYNGITIS—Sbl.

BURNING in—Pop. c.

CATARRH of—Lc. f., Sum.

CONSTRICTED—Gn. l.

CONSTRICTED, SORE—Lc. x.

CONTRACTION of—Rat.

DEAFNESS—*Hdr., Mr. sol.*

DIPHTHERITIC—Phyt.

Throat, DRYNESS of—Dbn., Onos.

FISH-BONE SENSATION in—Phst.

GRANULAR—Homa., Phyt., Yuc.

HAIR SENSATION in—*K. bi.*

HERPETIC—Phyt.

INFLAMED—*Mr. c.*

MUCUS in—*Na. c., Pho., Pso., Sul.,* Trf. p.

PARALYSIS of—Pop. c.

RISING in—Arnt.

See also **Globus Hystericus;** *and* **Hysteria.**

SORE—Atp., *Aps., Ars.,* Asi., *Ba. c., Bel.,* Bz. x., *Bro., Ca. p., Cth. Cap.,* Chr. o., Epl., Eug., E. pu., Eu. a., Fag., For., Gam., Gn. c., Ger., Gno., Haem., Hli., Hep., Hpt., Homa., *Hdr.,* Hyn., *Ign.,* Ja. g., *K. bi.,* K. ca., K. pm., Lc. c., *Lach.,* Lc. x., Lc. v. f., Lo. s., Lrs., *Lyc.,* Mth. pi., *Mr. v.,* Mr. ac., *Mr. cy.,* Mr. d., *Mr. i. f,* My. c., Naj., Nic., Nym., Onos., Ov.

g. p., Phst., *Phyt.,* Ple., Rx. ac., Rum., Sbd., Sbl., Sl. x., Sg.
n., Snc., Sga., Trf. p., Ts. p., Urt., *Ver.,* Vin., Vis.,Wye., Zin.
See also **Clergyman's Sore Throat; Pharyngitis; Sore
Throat;** *and* **Syphilitic** SORE THROAT.

SORE, CATARRHAL—Sbl.

SORE, VARICOSE—(Ba. m.), (Ham.)

SPASM of—Sum.

ULCERATION of—Elp., ldm., Rum., Syph., Vi. t.

Thrombosis—Antf., Sec.

Tibia, BURNING in—Zin.

PAIN in—Bad., Dul., Mn. o., Nt. s. d., Stp., Sypb., Trb., Ts. p.

Tic Convulsif—Aga., Anan.

Tic Douloureux—Anan., Ccn. s., Der., Gel., K. chl., K. i., Mag. p.
See also **Neuralgia;** *and* **Prosopalgia; &c.**

Ticklishness—Son.

Timidity—Amm., Dt. m.

Tinea Capitis—Bap., Ba. m., Mez., Pso. (*See also* **Ringworm.**)

CILIARIS—Mag. m.

FACIEI—Pso.

VERSICOLOR—(Bac.), (Chs. x.), Mez., (Sep.), (Tel.).

Tinnitus Aurium—Acr. r., Ba. m., Chn. a., Chi., Ch. sal., Ccs. c.,
(Cur.), Fe. pi., K. i., Klm., Kis., Lach., Lct. v., Led., Mag.
c., Pim., Pin. s., Pl. n., Rat., Rho., Sln., Sang., Sg. n., Spi.,
Thio., Ve. n.
See also **Ear,** NOISES in; **Ear,** REPORTS in; **Headache,** WITH
TINNITUS; *and* **Noises** IN THE HEAD.

Tobacco, EFFECTS of—Ab. n., Ch. ar., Ch. m., Gel., Klm., Nct., So.
m. Stp.

HABIT—*Ars., Ca. p., Cam., Chi., Nux, Pho.,* Plnt., *Pb., Spi.*

HEART—Apo., Scu.

INTOLERANCE of—K. bi.

Toe-nails, AFFECTIONS of—Per.

INGROWING—Stp. (*See also* **Ingrowing Toe-nails.**)

Toes, AFFECTIONS of—Rn. s.

Tongue, AFFECTIONS of—Acn., *Aco., AEsc., Ars.,* Au. m. n., *Bel.,*
Caj., *Cb. a.,* Caus., *Dul.,* Glv., *Gel.,* Gre., *Hdr.,* Man., *Mr.*
sol., Mr. v., Mr. c., Mez., Mu. x., Nux, Ox. x., Rhs.

BITING of—Sec., Thu.

BLISTERED—*Na. m.*

BLUE—Gno.

BURNING in—Pod., Snc.

CANCER of—Crt. h., *K. cy.,* Vb. p.

COATED—*Ant. c., Ant. t., Bry.,* (Equ.), *Lyc.,* Oln., *Pul., Sul.*

COATED WHITE—*Na. m.*

CRACKED—*Ar. t., Rms. v.,* So. t. ae., Syph.

CRAMP in—Lyc., Rut.

ERUPTION on—Pip. n.

HEAVY—*Na. m.,* Pip. n.

INDURATION of—Smp.

INFLAMMATION of—*Cth.,* Crt. h. (*See also* **Glossitis.**)

MAPPED—*Mr. v., Rn. s.,* Trx.

NEURALGIA of—K. as., K. i.

NODULES on—*Aur.*

NUMBNESS of—Li. m., Rhe.

OEDEMA of—*Aps.*

PAINFUL—Crv.

PARALYSIS of—Ac. c., Ast. r., Bth., Cap., Caus., Cnn., Guac., Ln.
u., Lo. p., Mrl., Pb., Pyr. a., Tep., Zn. s.

PARCHED—Oln.

PATCHED— Mnc.

PEELING of—*Rn. s.*

PRICKLING on—Lina.

PSORIASIS of—Mu. x.

RINGWORM of—Snc.

ROUGHNESS of—Lina.

SENSIBILITY of, LOST—hch.

SHRIVELLED—Na. Clch.

SORENESS of—Bz. x., Osm., Phel.

SPASM, of—Cbn.

STIFFNESS of—Chm. m., Nic.

Tongue, STRAWBERRY—*Frg.,* Sap.

SWELLING of—Ast. r., Caj., Frg., K. tel., Mns., Mez., Na. hch. OEna., Rut., Vsp., Vip.

THICKENING of—Sul. i.

ULCERATED—*Aps., Ag. n.,* Bap., Bov., *Fl. x.,* Lc. v., *Nt. x.,* OEna. Syph., Thu. .

VESICLES under—Lcrt.,

Tonsillitis—Ba. m., Ca. s., Chn. a., Dul., Fe. m., Gui., Mr. i. f., Rap., Stp., Sul., Ust.

See also **Quinsy; Tonsils,** *and* INFLAMED.

Tonsils, CONCRETIONS in—Pso.

ENLARGED—*Ba. c.,* Bz. x., Bro., *Ca. p.,* Pb. i., Plp.

HYPERTROPHY of CHRONIC—Sul. i.

INFLAMED—Bro. (*See also* **Quinsy; and Tonsillitis.**)

SWOLLEN—Am. m., Gre.

Toothache—Aco.,—A.ct. s., Aga., Agn., Am. c., Amph., Ang., Atp., Aph., Api. g., Aran., Arm., Ast. f., Bis., *Bry.,* Caj., *Calc.,* Ca. cs., Cbl. x., Ced., *Cham.,* Chm. m., Chm. u., Chr. o., Clem., Ccn. s., Cof., Col., Com., Dph., Dig., Dio., Eub., Epn., Fer., Fe. s., Fl. x., Glv., Gel., Glo., Grn., Gui., Gno., Hec., .Hyo., Ign., Ind., Inu., Ipc., Itu., *K. ca., Kre., Mag. c.,* Mag. p., Mag. s., Mgt., Mgt. n., Mn. s., *Mr. sol.,* Mr. i. f., Na. c., Na. hch., Nic., Nx. m,, Onis., Prt., Pet., Phyt., Pip. m., Pip. n., *Plnt.,* Ple., Pr. s., *Pul.,* Rap., Rho., Sbd., Sbi., Snc., Scil., *Sep., Spi., Stp.,* Sul., Tab., Tep., Ther., Thu., Til., Ton., Trb., Val., Ver., Xan., Zn. a.

See also **Eye-teeth, Pains in;** *and* **Pregnancy,** TOOTHACHE of.

Torticollis—Gui.

See also **Wry-neck.**

Touch, Sense of, Disordered—Par.

Trachea, AFFECTIONS of—*Ars., Calc.,* Cb. a., *K. bi., Lach., Nux,*

Rum., *Sil.,* Stn.

CARTILAGES, AFFECTIONS of—(Stil.)

DRYNESS of—*Cb. v.*

IRRITATION of—*Aps., Bro., Sul.*

MUCUS in—*Can. s.*

PAIN in—*Bry., Osm.*

TICKELING in—*Cap., Pho.*

Trachoma—Ch. m., Cu. s., Mrl.

See also under **Eyes; Granular Conjunctivitis;** *and* **Granular Lids.**

Trauma—Cep., Glo., (Su. x.). (*See also* **Traumatism.**)

Traumatic Fever—*Aco., Arn., Ars.,* Cac., *Chi., Lach.,* Merc.

See also **Surgical Fever;** *and* **Traumatism.**

Traumatism—Bls.,Eu. pi.

See also **Operations,** EFFECTS of; *and* **Teeth,** OPERATIONS on.

Travelling, Effects of—Cai., Clcn.

Tremors—*Act. r., Aga., Ant. t., Gel., Ign.,* Lol., *Mr. sol., Stm.*

MERCURIAL—Zn. p.

Trichiasis—Bor., Gph., (Tel.) —

See also **Entropion;** *and under* **Eyes.**

Trichinae—*Ars., Bap.*

Trifacial-nerve Paralysis—Na. m.

Trismus—Acn., AEth., Ag. p., Alm., Bz. n., Crb. o., Chr. o., Cia. v.,. Con., Ln. u., Mor., So. n., So. t., Stm.

Tubercular Diarrhoea—Cto.

Tuberculosis—Avn., *Bac., Bel.,* Bro., *Calc.,* Ch. ar., Fe. i., Hpz., Iof., Lp. a., Led., Mrt., Na. as., Pho., Pyro., Spo., Teu. s., Tub., Ure. See also **Consumption; Laryngitis,** TUBERCULAR; **Phthisis;** *and* **Testicles,** TUBERCULOSIS of.

Tumours—Anan., Aps., Arn., Ast. f., Aur., Au. m. n., *Ba. c.,* Ba. i., Ba. m., Bls., Ber., Bov., *Ca. ar., Calc.,* Ca. s., Chel., Col., Con.,. Cro., Cp. l., Dul., Euc., Epn., Gos., Gph., Hec., K. i., Lach., Lp. a., Lau., Mag. a., Na. sf., Pho., Phyt., Sang., Sil.,

So. t., Stp., Trn., Thio., Thu., Vac.

BREAST, of—Bro., Ca. i. (*See also* **Breast,**TUMOUR of.)

CANCEROUS—Pho.

ERECTILE— Pho.

FATTY—*See* **Fatty Tumours.**

FIBROID—*See* **Fibroma.**

POLYPOID—Pho. (*See also* **Polypus.**)

TARSAL—Stp., Zin.

Turpentine, Effects of—Nx. m.

Twitching—Cam., Cin., Se. j.

    See also **Spasmodic Twitching.**

Tympanites, or **Tympany**—Amb., Asa., *Cb. v.,* Chi., Coc. i., Mor., Opi., Rm. c., So. n., *Ter.*

Typhlitis—Crd; m., Clch., Gam., Gas., Pb., Pyro., Rm. c.

    See also **Appendicitis.**

Typhoid Fever—Abs., *Aga.,* Ail., Ar. t., Bap. c., Bnz., Ber. .a, Cld,. Ca. ar., Calc., Clch., Dor., Dul., Ech. a., Euc., Fe. m., Hel., K. ca., Lo. p., Lyc., Mna., Mos., Nph., Nt. s. d., Nup., Phen., Sec., Sptun., So. n., Sul. h., Sum., Trx., Tri, Ver., Ve. v., Zin., Zn.m.

Typhoid Fever, HAEMORRHAGE in—Aln., Nx. m.

    LACK OF RECUPERATION after —Cast.

    See also **Enteric Fever.**

Typho-malarial Fever—Lcs.

Typhus Fever—*Aga.,* Ail., Alm., Aps., *Ars.,* Asr., Bap., Cld., Cb. v., Cast., *Ch. s.,* Chlf., Chlm., Hdr., Hyn., *Mr. v.,* Mr. bin., Mu. x., Pest., Ph. x., *Pho., Rhs.,* Stm.

Ulceration—Amm., Cb. a., Cry., Cro., Cur., Dor., Hyp., Mst. s. Rn. fl.

Ulcers—Aln., Am. m., Anan., Athra., Ar. lp., Arm., *Ars.,* Asa., *Ast. r.,* Bal., *Bel.,* Bz. x., Bor., Brs., Bro., Ca. si., Ca. s., *Caln.,* Cb. v., Cbl. x., Caus., Cet., Cham., Chlm., Chr. o., Cis.,

Com., Con., *Crt. h.,* Cnd., Cup., Ech. a., Eub., Gli., Get., Gph., Gnd., *Ham.,* Hel., Hl. v., Hpz., Hoa., Hn. m., *Hdr.,* Hfb., Jeq., K. as., *K. bi.,* K. chl., *K. i.,* K. ph., Kre., Lc. c., *Lach.,* Lia., Mgt., *Mr. sol.,* Mr. ac., *Mez.,* Na. m., *Nt. x.,* *Pcao.,* Ph. x., *Pho.,* Phyt., Pb. i., Plg., Pso., Rn. a., Sars., Sec., *Sil.,* So. n., *Sul.,* Su. x., Syph., Syz., Tep., Trac., Xan., Zin.

ILL-CONDITIONED—Anag.

MALIGNANT—Chm. u.

OBSTINATE—Pyro.

VARICOSE—(Crd. m.), Euc., Gas. (Ham.), Pyro.

See also **Rodent Ulcer.**

Umbilicus, ABSCESS of—Pb.

HERNIA of—Pb. .

INFLAMMATION of—Phst., Sac. 1.

OOZING from—Abr.

PAIN in—Ph. x., Prf.

Uraemia—Am. c., Asc. s., Cn. i., *Cbl. x., Cu. a., Opi.,* Phen., Ter., Ure., Urt.

Uraemic Convulsions—Hy. x., Pilo.

Ureter, PAIN in—Scro.

See also **Renal Colic.**

Urethra, CARUNCLE of—Can. s., Euc.

EXCRESCENCES in—Teu.

INFLAMMATION of, CHRONIC—Pet.

IRRITATION of—Onos.

SPASM of—*Nux.*

STRICTURE of—*Clem.,* Euc., Ind., Lo. i., Pet., *Pho., Sil.,* Sul. i.

STRICTURE of , SPASMODIC—*Aco., Dam.*

Urethral Fever—Aco.

Urethritis—Aps., Caus., Cop., Cyc., Dor., K. bi., Li. c., Pip. m., Rm. f.

See also **Gonorrhoea; Gleet;** *and* **Urethra,** INFLAMMATION of, CHRONIC.

Uric Acid, Deposit of—Li. bz.

    Diathesis—Ccs. c., Lys., Thl.

    Excess of—Pip. m.

Uricacidaemia—Pb.

Urinary Affections—Cf. t., Uva.

    Calculi—Lips. (*See also* **Bladder,** Stone in.)

    Difficulties. —Apo. (*See also* **Dysuria;** *and* **Urination, Difficult.**)

    Disorders—Arm., Asp., Caj., Cn. i., Chm. u., Chn. s., Dig., Li. c.

Urination, Delayed—Plnt.

    Difficult—Apo., Dul., Rut. (*See also* **Dysuria.**)

    Difficult, of Childbed—Rhe.

    Frequent, too—*K. ca., Lil., Nux,* Sntn. (*See also* **Polyuria; Urine,** Excess of; *and* **Urine,** Increased)

    Straining—Mag. m.

    Urging to—*Carl.*

Urine, Abnormal—*Aps., Cth., Ign., Lyc.,* Ocm., *Ox. x.*

    Alkaline—K. ac.

    Black—Bz. d.

    Bloody—Pi. x.

    Deposits in—Ard., Spa. u.

    Disorders of—Arb., *Bz. x., Ber., Cap., Caus., Gph.*

    Excess of—Picr., *Scil.* (*See also* **Polyuria; Urination,** Too Frequent; *and* **Urine,** Increased.)

    Fetid—Trp.

    Fishy Odour of—*Ur. n.*

    Incontinence of—Dul., Ery. a., Fer., *Fe. p.,* Hdm. a., *K. br., Kre.,* Lth., *Pul.,* Sbl., *Sep.,* Sil., Trt., Tur., Ur. n., *Vbs.* (*See also* **Enuresis.**)

    Increased—Pin. s., Thri. (*See also* **Polyuria; Urination,** Too Frequent; *and* **Urine,** Excess of.)

    Milky—Cin.

    Offensive—Sto. b.

    Phosphatic—*Ph. x.*

PURULENT—(Ber.)

RED—Rhe.

RETENTION of—Api. g., Equ., E. pu., Hyo., *Opi.*, Ter., Zea. st.

RETENTION of, HYSTERICAL—Zin.

SCANTY—Sld.

Urine, SLIMY—Prei,

STRONG-SMELLING—Bor., Pin. s.

SUPPRESSION of—*Aco.*, Ag. p., *Cam.*, Mds., *Opi.*, Sld., *Ter.*, Zea st., Zng.

Urticaria—Amg., Ank., Atp., Api. g.,. Ar. dm., Bom., Bov., Calc., Ch. s., Chl. h., Cop., Co. c., Crt. h., Cub., Frg., Ga. x., Hli., *Hep.*, K. ca., K. ph., Ln. u., Lips., Med., My. c., Na. p., Phy., Pod., Rhs., Rs. v., Rob. Rum., Sntn., Sko., So. a., So. o., *Sul.*, Ttr., Til., Tri., Urt., Voe.

GIANT—Sntn.

NODOSA—Urt.

TUBEROSA—Bo. lu.

See also **Nettle-rash.**

Uterus, AFFECTIONS of—*Act. r.*, Aln., Ast. r., *Bel.*, *Calc.*, Cur., *Frx.*, *Gel.*, *Ham.*, *Hlon.*, Hdr., *Iod.*, Kre., La. a., *Lil.*, Pal., Prf., Phyt., Sbl., Thl., Vic.

AIR in—*Bro.*

ATONY of—Caul., Lap., Rs. a.

BEARING DOWN in—Gos., *Sep.*, *Til.*, Vb. o.

BLEEDING from—*Sbi.*, *Vin.* (See also HAEMORRHAGE from; *and* **Metrorrhagia.**)

CANCER of—Arg., Caln. (Clt.), Cb. a., Gph., K. ca., Trn., Thl. (*See also* SCIRRHUS of.)

CONGESTION of—*Ve v.*

CRAMPS in—Onos., Pip. n., Vb. o.

DEBILITY of—Als.

DISCHARGE from, OFFENSIVE—Caln.

DISEASES of—*Cham.*

DISPLACEMENTS of—Ab. c., Cbl. x., *Lil.*

FATIGUED—Bls.

HAEMORRHAGE from—Au. m., Aur. m. k., Jn. v., Rs. a., Thl. *(See also* BLEEDING from; *and* **Metrorrhagia.)**

HYPERPLASIA of—Ant. i.

INDURATION of—*Aur.,* Au. m. k., Au. m. n., Mag. m., Plat.

INERTIA of—Opi., Sec.

INFLAMMATION of—Caln., Pul., Til.

INFLAMMATION of, FOLLICULAR—*Hyd.*

MISPLACEMENT of—Hlt., Ov. g. p., Sbl.

NEURALGIA of—Crt. c., Cu. as., Sec., Trn.

PAINS in—Alet., Asc. s., Col., Mag. m., Pl. n.

POLYPUS of—Ca. p., Erod.

PROLAPSE of—Aco., AEsc., Alet., Alo., Ar.lp., Arg., Ca. p., Fe. br., Fe. i., *Frx.,* Hfb., *Mur.,* Nx. m., Nux, Onos., Ov. g. p., Pal. Ph. x., Pod., Pul., Pyr. a., Snc., Sec., Stn., Sul., Su. x., Til.

Uterus, RETROVERTED—OV. g. p. (?)

SCIRRHUS of—Au. m. n. *(See also* CANCER of.)

SODDEN—Na. hch.

SORENESS of—Snc.

SPASM of—Caul.

SUBINVOLUTION of—*Lil.,* Na. hch.

TUMOURS of—Au. m., Frx., Sbl., (Snc.)

ULCERATED—Vsp.

WATER-LOGGED—Na. hch.

See also **Cervix Uteri,** AFFECTIONS of; **Os Uteri,** DILATED; *and* **Rigid Os.**

Uvula, AFFECTIONS of—(Hyo.), Wye.

BURNING in—Ts. p.

ELONGATED—(Hyo.), *Mr. c.,* (Phyt.), Rx. a.c., Sbd.

ENLARGED—Idm., (Phyt.)

PAIN in—Trf. p.

RELAXED—Aln.

SWOLLEN—K. pm.

ULCERATED—Idm.

Vaccination—*Aps., Mr. sol.,* Mez., *Sil.,* Sko., *Sul., Thu.*
EFFECTS of—*Aco.,* Crt. h., Ech. a., Gph., K m., Mld.
Vaccinia—Bel., Pho., *Vac.*
Vaccinosis—Lc. c., *Mld.,* Thu., *Vac.,* (Var.)
Vagina, AIR in—*Bro. (See also* **Physometra.)**
BURNING in—Pop. c.
CYSTS in—Rho.
DISCHARGE from, SEROUS—Lo. i.
HEAT, BURNING *and* ITCHING of—Au. m.
PAIN in—Col.
PROLAPSE of—Nux, Ocm., Stn., (Stp.), Su. x.
PRURITUS of—Hyd.
SPASM of—*Ham., Ign.,* Pb., *Sil. (See also* **Vaginismus.)**
Vaginismus—Aln., Ber., Cac., Hfb., Mag. p., Na. m., Plat., Pb.,
Thu.
See also **Vagina,** SPASM of.
Vaginitis—Cur.
Varicella— Led.
Varices—Calc., Mil., Mu. x., Na. m., Pet., Ph. x.
Varicocele—Crt. h., Ham., Pnt., Rut., Sul., Tab.
Varicose Ulcers—(Crd. m.), Euc., Gas. (Ham.), Pyro.
Varicose Veins—(Amb.), Aps., Crd. m., Caus., Chi., Ch. s., K. as.,
Lc. c., Paeo., Sep.
See also **Veins,** VARICOSE.
Varicosis—Ac. x., Bls., Caln., Crd. b., Crt. h., Fl. x., Lyc., Mgt. s.,
Mr. cy., Pyro., Rn. s., Scir., So. n., Spo., Sto. b., Sto. c., Sul.,
Su x., Vip., Zin.
OF EXTERNAL GENITALS—Zin.
DURING PREGNANCY—Zin.
See also **Arms,** VARICOSIS of.
Variola—Aps., Bap., *Ch. s.,* Pho., Sin. n.
See also **Small-pox.**
Varioloid—Ant. t.
Vegetations—Mr. n.

Veins, DISEASED—*Fl. x.*
　　DISTENDED—Chn. s.
　　FULNESS of—Opi.
　　INFLAMMATION of—*Pul. (See also* **Phlebitis.**)
　　SWOLLEN—Rut.
　　VARICOSE—*Fe. p., Ham., Lach., Pb., Pul.,* Rut. *(See also*
　　　　Varicose Veins; and Varicosis.)
Vertebrae, AFFECTIONS of—Prf.
　　CERVICAL, CRACKING in—Mgt. n.
　　PAIN in—Ov. g. p., So. t. ae.
　　PULSATION in—So. t. ae.
　　TUMOURS of—Trn.
　　　See also **Spine,** AFFECTIONS of, &c.
Vertigo—*Aco.,* AEs. g., Ag. e., Ath., Aur., *Bel.,* Bls., Bzn., *Bor.,* Bro.
　　Bry., Caj., Ca. a.c., *Calc.,* Chi., Chlf., *Coc. i.,* Cf. t., Cnn.,
　　Con., Clv. d., Cul., Cyc., Dt. a., Dgn., Dbn., Eth. n., Ev. a.,
　　Fgs., Fer., *Gel.,* Gre., *K. ca.,* K. n., K. sc, Klm., Lab., Lach.,
　　Li. br., Lo. p., Mgn. gr., Mrl., Mor., Mos., *Na. m., Nux.,*
　　Oln., Oxt., Paeo., Phal., Ph. x., Pin. s., Prm. ve., Qer., Sbd.,
　　Sx. p., Sil., So. a., So. n., Sta., *Sul.,* Tep., Ther., Urt., Ver.,
　　Vsp., Voe., Wis.
　　AURAL—Pilo. *(See also* **Meniere's Disease.**)
　　CADUCA—Na. hch., Wis.
Vesication of Skin—Cth.
Vesicles—Eu. cy.
Veta—*.See* **Mountain Sickness.**
Vicarious MENSTRUATION—Epn.
　　NOSE- BLEED— Lach.
　　　See also **Epistaxis,** MENSTRUAL; *and* **Menstruation,**
　　　VICARIOUS.
Vision, AFFECTIONS of—Crd. b., Ol. j., Sto. c. *(See also* **Sight,**
　　AFFECTIONS of.)
　　COLOURED—Anh.
　　DEFECTIVE—Bap. c., Elae.

DIM—Sg. t., Sprn., Tax.

DISORDERED—Anh., Atr., Aur., Bnz., Cb. a., Cnn., Con., Dig., Dxn., Dbn., Eub., Fe. mg., Grt., Hyn., Hyo., Prf., Prt., Per., Src.

HALLUCINATIONS of—Dgn. *(See also* **Clairvoyance.)**

ILLUSIONS of—Glv., Mor. *(See also* **Clairvoyance.)**

IMPAIRED—Nic.

LOST—Jg. c.

YELLOW—Sntn.

Vitreous, Opacities of—Chlst., Pr. s.

Voice, AFFECTIONS of—*Arn.,* Ber. a., Iod., Prm. ve.

ALTERED—*Ox. x.*

HOARSE—Ar. t., Au. m., Stp. *(See also* **Hoarseness.)**

LOSS of—Arg., *Caus.,* Fe. pi., *Gel., Ign.,* Pho. *(See also* **Aphonia.)**

LOW—Ant. c.

NASAL—Stp.

WEAKNESS of—Coca, Mth. pi.

Vomiting—Acn., Ac. c., AEth., Ag. p., Amm., *Ant. t.,* Ap. a., Apo., *Ars.,* Bis., Brc. x., Ca. m., *Cbl. x.,* Cer. o., *Coc. i.,* Cri. r., Cuc. p., Cu. as., Dxn., Drs., Elt., Eth., E. pu., Eu. i., *Fe. m.,* Fe. p., Gui., Hli., Hmer., Hur. c., *Iod., Ipc.,* Ir. t., *Iris,* Jat., K. ox., Klm., Kre., Lc. x., *Mr. sol., Pet.,* Phal., Rm. f., Sang., Sntn., Sch., Sin. a., Tng., Thev.

BILIOUS—Crt. h.

BLACK—Pix.

CEREBRAL—Apm.

MILK, of—Snc.

MORNING, OF BEER DRINKERS—(Cup.)

PREGNANCY, DURING—*Act. r.,* Ana., Cod., Cvl., Cuc. p., Lo. i. *(See also* **Morning Sickness** of PREGNANCY; **Pregnancy,** SICKNESSof; **Pregnancy,** SICKNESS of, MORNING; *and* **Pregnancy,** VOMITING OF.)

REFLEX—Apm.

WATER, of—Snc.

See also **Abdomen,** OPERATIONS on, VOMITING after; **Carriage Sickness; Sea-sickness;** *and* **Hysterical** VOMITING.

Vulva, ERUPTION on—Cen.

INFLAMMATION of—Cop., Itu.

SORENESS of—Ov. g. p.

Vulva, THROBBING in—Cen.

Vulvitis—Cop., Itu.

Waking, SCREAMING on—*Cham.*

STARTS and SCREAMS on—*Bry.*

WEEPING on—*Cic. v.*

Walking, DELAY in—As. f., *Calc.,* Pin. s., *Sil.*

Wandering Rheumatism—Ap. a., Pl. n.

Warts—Ac. x., An. oc., Ana., Ant. c., Ag. n., Au. m., Au. m. n., Ba. c., Bov., *Calc.,* Ca. o. t., Ct. eq., Cast., Caus., Chel., Chr. o., Cnb., Cp. l., Dul., Eub., Fe: mg., Fe. pi., K. bi., *K. m.,* K. pm., Kis., Lc. c., Lach., Lyc., Mag. s., Med., Na. c., *Na. m.,* Na. s.. Nt. s. d., *Nt. x.,* Pal., Pet. (Phas.), Ph. x., Phyt., Rn. b., Rhs., Rut., Sars., Sep., Stp., *Sul.,* Su. x., *Thu.*

See also **Lupoid Warts;** *and* **Prepuce,** WARTS on.

Water, EFFECTS of—Phst.

Waterbrash—*Bry., Lyc.,* Mag. m., *Nux, Ver.*

PREGNANCY, of—Dio.

See also **Pregnancy,** PYROSIS of; *and* **Pyrosis.**

Weaning, Complaints after—Cyc., Frg.

Wens—*Ba. c.,* Bz. x., *Con.,* Gph., *Hep.,* K. ca., K. i., Lo. i., Nt. x., Ph. x., Phyt., Rhs.

White-leg—Crt. h.

White-swelling—Sul.

Whitlow—All., Am. c., Athra., Asa., Brc. x., Bov., Buf., Calc., *Caln.,* Cep., Chm. u., Dio., Fe. mg., Fl. x., Gno., Hec., *Hep.,*

Iris, K. ph., *Lach.,* Led., Mst. s., *Pho.,* Pul., Sang., Sil., Syph., Thl., Wis.

Whooping-cough—*Aco.,* (Amb.), Am. br., Am. pi., Ana., Ang., Ant. c., *Ant. t., Arn.,* Ars., Bad., *Bel.,* Bry., *Cap.,* Crb. h., Cst. v., Caus., Cep., Cham., Chel., Cin., *Ccs. c., Crl.,* Crt. h., Cu. a., Cup., Cur., *Drs.,* Dul., Fe. p., Gph., Gre., *Hep.,* Hpz., Hy. x., Hyp., *Ipc.,* K. bi., *K. ca.,* K. sc., Kre., Lct. v., Lau., Lo. i., Lyc., Mag. m., Mag. p., Mep., Mos., Mu. x., Nph., Na. m., Nic., *Nt. x., Opi.,* Oxg., Pod., Sbl., Smb. n., Sang., Scil., Sga., Sep., Spo., (Suc.), Thu., Urt., Vac., Ver., Vi. o., Vis., Zin.

Wisdom-teeth, Effects of Cutting—Chei.

Worm Complaints—Cic. v.

Worm Fever—Bel., Chm. m., Ipc.

Worms—Abr., All., Ap. a., *Ars.,* Art. v., *Bap.,* Cld., *Calc.,* Chne., Cic. v., *Cin.,* Euc., *Fe. m.,* Fe. s., Gph., Ind., Iod., Jab., Jat., Lips., Lun., *Lyc.,* Nph., Na. m., *Na. p.,* Nx. m., Nux, Ph. x., Plnt., Pod.,. Ptl., Qua., Rat., Sbd., Sntn., Scil., *Scir.,* Sil., Sin. a., *Spi.,* Spo., Stn., *Sul.,* Sum., Tan., Tel., Ter., *Teu.,* Urt., Zin.

LUMBRICI—*Chn. a.,* Pin. s., Ple., *Sntn.*

See also **Helminthiasis; Tape-worm; Thread-worms;** *and* **Trichinae.**

Worry—Sul.

Wounds—Anag., Aps., *Arn.,* Ars., Bro. x., Bov., *Caln.,* Cro., Erig., Ery. a., E. pf., Ham., Hli., Hel., *Hyp.,* Lach., Led., Pho., Phst., Plnt., Se. a., Symt., Zn. m.

HEALING of, TOO RAPID—Hfb.

PUNCTURED—Phas. (*See also* **Punctured Wounds.**)

See also **Dissection Wounds; Gunshot Wounds;** *and* **Poisoned Wounds.**

Wrist, AFFECTIONS of—Per.

BOILS on—Snc.

PAIN in—Homa., Ple., Rho., Trm.

PARALYSIS of—Hpm.

RHEUMATISM of—Hpm., Vi. o.

Writer's Cramp *or* **Spasm**—Ana., Cya., Eub., Fe. i., Fe. p. h., Gel., Lol., Mag. p., Mr. i. f., Pi. x., Rn. b., Sil., Trl.

Wry-neck (Torticillis)—AEs. g., Atr., Chi. b., Gui., Lchn.

Xerostoma—Ir. t.

Yawning—*Aco., Arn.,* Ca. p., Cast., Chel., Cim., Elt., *Ign.,* Kre., Lct. v., *Lyc.,* Man., *Na. m., Nux,* Rap., *Rhs., Sul.,* Tel.

SPASMODIC—Plat.

Yellow Fever—*Aco., Ars.,* As. h., *Bry.,* Cd. s., Cap., Cb. v., Cep., *Crt. h.,* Cup., Ipc., ,Lpt., Pho., Ver.

Zona— Ag. n., Cis., Com., Gph., K. m.

   See also **Herpes** ZOSTER; *and* **Zoster.**

Zoster—Bor., Iris, K. m.

   See also **Herpes** ZOSTER; *and* ZONA.

Zygoma, Pain in—Sgu.

□□

Part II

Repertory of Causation

REPERTORY OF CAUSATION

NOTE

ALMOST all remedies have relations of some kind to the various accidents and conditions of ordinary life. Their symptoms are made worse or better by heat or cold, rest or motion, by night or by day, or other circumstances or conditions. Many remedies are related to the *effects* of certain conditions. This is not just the same thing as aggra- vation, though allied to it and sometimes identical with it. For instance, *Arnica* removes morbid conditions (apart, of course, from surgical injuries such as broken bones) caused by falls; *Ruta* relieves the effects of bruised bones. It is not correct in either case to describe these as aggravations, and therefore I thought well to arrange such relationships under a separate heading in the *Dictionary.* These. I have now indexed, and repertorised, in the subjoined list.

Although Causation and Aggravation are not the same, they are closely allied. *Rhus* is related to the effects of damp weather, and appears in the list of remedies having this *Causation;* but it also has its symptoms, when not caused by damp, aggravated in a supreme degree by conditions of damp. Therefore the prescriber who uses this list of CAUSES as a rough list of Aggravations also will not go far wrong, and may find no little help from it in some of his cases.

The names of a few remedies have been added which do not

occur in the *Dictionary of Materia Medica*. These, for the most part, I have enclosed in brackets. When a cause is associated with any particular effect, that effect is placed in brackets and precedes the name of the remedy which corresponds to it. For instance, "Washing clothes" causes ill effects to which certain remedies correspond. *Phosphorus* corresponds to headache resulting from washing clothes. In the list of remedies this fact is marked thus: "(headache) Pho." When, in a list of remedies, one of them has a qualifying word or phrase thus prefixed to it, the qualification must be understood to apply to that remedy only, and not to those which follow.

Abdominal Operations—Bis. *(See also* **Operations.**)

Acid Food—Na. m.

Air, Cold—Cam.

_____ Draught of—Cd. s., Lach.

_____ Draught of, cold, when perspiring—Mr. i. f.

_____ Draught of—Cd. s., Lach.

_____ Hot, inhaled from Fire—Cb. v.

Air, Snowy—Con., Sep.

Alcohol—(Ars.), Aur., Bry., Calc., Cd. s., Cb. v., Chi., Crt. h., Dig., Gel., Lach., Led., Lo. i., Nx. m., Nux, Opi., Quer., Rn. b., Sel., Sep., Strp., Sul., Ter., Ver. *(See also* **Beer; Liquors; Wines,** &c.)

Alcoholism—Aga., Ars.

Anger—Alm., Arn., Bry., Cham., Chi., Coc. i., Col., Gel., K. br., Lach., Lyc., Mez., Na. s., Nux, Opi., Pho., Sac. o., Sep., Stp., (red nose) Vin., Zin.

_____ Effects of—(cough) Ant. t., Aur.

_____ Slightest—Rhs.

_____ Slightest Fit of—(trembling and dyspnoa) Rn.b.

_____ Suppressed or Reserved—Aur., Ipec., Stp.

See also **Passion;** *and* **Rage.**

Anxiety—Act. r., Lyc., Smb. n. *(See also* **Care; Mental** Distress, & c.; *and* **Worry.**)

Apprehension—Ag. n.

Arms, Raising—Su. x.

_____ Raising high to lift things—Rhs.

Ascending—Ca. p.

August, Hay-fever of—Cep.

Autumn—(epidemics of spasmodic cough) Cep., (affections in general) K. bi.

Bad Beer—Nx. m.

_____ Eggs—Cb. v.

_____ Fat (rancid)— (Ars.), (Cb.v.).

_____ Fish—Cb. a., Cb. v. Cep.

_____ Food—Cb.v.

_____ Liquors—Cb. v.

_____ Lobster Salad—(Ars.).

_____ News, hearing—Aln., Aps., Art. v., Ca. p., Gel., Paeo., Ph. x., Trn.

_____ Smells—(Bap.), Kre. *(See also* **Noxious Efflvia;** *and* **Sewer gas.**)

_____ Vegetables—Cb. a.

_____ Water, drinking—All, Crt. h.

_____ Wines—Cb. v.

Bath—(suppressed menses) Nx. m.

Bathing, Cold—Mag. p., Phst.

_____ Fresh or Salt Water, in—Rhs.

_____ Sea—Ars., Mag. m.

Bed-sores—Sul., (form soon in typhoid) Val.

Beer—(morning vomiting, Cup.), K. bi., (headache) Rhs., Thu.

_____ Bad—Nx. m.

Bee-stings—Urt.

Bereavement—Plat.

Bites—Hyp., Led.

_____ Dog-bites—Hfb.

_____ Poisonous—Sga.

_____ Snake-bites—Lo. p., Plnt.

Bitter Foods—Na. p.

Blood-letting—Se. a., Scil.

Blood-poisoning—Aga., Lo. p., Pyro. *(See also* **Sepsis.)**

    Blows—Con., Hel., K. m., K. ph., Mag. c., Phst., Pso., Sep.,
     Sul., Symt., Urt.

_____ Head, on—Art. v., Mrl.

Bones, Injuries to—Hec., Rut., Symt.

Boots, Tight—Paeo.

Brain, Concussion of—Su. x.

_____ Overworked—Cu. a.

Bread—Na. m., Zng.

Bruises—(Arn.), Led., Li. c., Paeo., Plnt., Rut., Su. x.

Burns—(or scalds) Caus., K. m., Plnt., Urt.

Business Embarrassments—Act. r., K. br.

_____ Losses—K. br.

Butter—Cb. v.

Cabbage—Pet.

Camp Life—Mlr.

Care—Ars. *(See also* **Anxiety; Mental** Distress, &c.; *and* **Worry.)**

Carriage, Riding in—Lyc., Pet.

Carrying Heavy Weights—Rut.

Catheterism—Mag. p.

Caustic, Lunar—Na. m.

Chafing—Su. x.

Chagrin—Au. m., Bry., Col., Lyc., Ph. x. *(See also* **Vexation.)**

Charcoal Fumes—Opi.

Checked Eruptions, *&c—See* **Suppressed.**

Cheese—Nt. s. d.

Child-bearing—Act. r., Stm.

Chill—Aco., Chi., Klm., Mos., Pul., Spi., Sul., Vis.

_____ Overheated, when—K. sc.

_____ Water, in the—Ars.

Clay, Cold, Working with—Mag. p.

Climbing Mountains—Ars.

Coffee—(abuse of) Grt., Nux, Ox. x., Thu.

Coitus—Aga., Stp.

Cold—Ant. c., Arm., Plg., Rhs.

_____ Air—Cam.

_____ Bathing—Mag. p., Phst.

_____ Catching—Col., Ka. ca., Rho.

_____ Clay, working with—Mag. p.

_____ Damp weather—Lth., Mr. i. f.

_____ Damp, with—Dul., Phyt.

_____ Drinks, effects of, when overheated—Bls.

_____ Dry winds—Aco., Hep.

_____ Exposure to, and damp—Phyt.

_____ Milk, drinking—K. i.

_____ Moist winds—Calc., Cep.

_____ Water, standing in—Mag. p.

_____ Wind—Bry., Cd. s., Mag. p.

_____ Wind, driving in—Sg. n.

Contradiction, Effects of—Aur.

Contusions—Con., (enlarged testicle) Var.

Coryza, Suppressed—Chi.

Cuts—K. m., Plnt., (clean-cut wounds) Stp.

Damp—Cac., Plg.

_____ Cellars—Ter.

_____ Cold weather—(or warm) Gel., Lth., Mr. i. f.

_____ Cold winds and weather, effects of exposure to—Calc.,

Cep.

_____ Cold, with—Dul., Phyt.

_____ Sheets—Rhs.

_____ Warm Weather—Cb. v.

_____ Weather—Gel., Lth., Sin. n., Syph.

_____ Weather, warm or cold—Gel.

Debauchery—Cb. v., Nux, Sel.

Decayed Vegetables, Eating—Cb. a.

Dentition—Cham., Mag. c., Mag. p., Rhe., Stn., Stp.

Deranged Internal Functions—K. m.

Depressing Emotions—Gel.

Diet, Errors in—Dio., Mag. c.

_____ Mixed—Pul.

_____ Poor—Ars.

Disappointed Love—Act. r., Ant. c., Aur., Cac., Ca. p., Hel., Ign., Iod., Lach., Ph. x., Trn., Ver.

Disappointments—Alm., Na. m.

Discharges, Suppressed—Bry., Led., Vi. o. *(See also* **Suppressed** Discharges, &c.)

Dislocations—Pso., Rhe.

Displeasure, Reserved—Aur., Ipc., Stp. *(See also* **Anger.)**

Dissecting Wounds—Pyro.

Distress, Mental—Mag. c.

Disturbance, Emotional—K. br.

Dog-bites—Hfb.

Draught of air—Cd. s., Lach.

_____ Cold, when perspiring—Mr. i. f.

Drenching Rains, Exposure to—Pho.

Drinks, Cold, when overheated—Bls., Na. c.

Drinking Ice-water—Cb.v., Rhs.

_____ Milk, cold—K. i.

Driving in Cold Wind—Sg. n.

Drunkenness—Aga., Ars. *(See also* **Alcohol.)**

Dry, Cold Winds—Aco., Hep.

Early Rising—Mth. pi.

Eating—Cb. a.

_____ Excess in—All., Ant. c., Bry., Dio., Na.m.

_____ Fish, spoiled—Cb. a., Cb. v., Cep.

_____ Fruit—Rho.

_____ Fruit, unripe—Rhe.

_____ Prunes—Rhe.

_____ Veal—K.n.

_____ Vegetables, decayed—Cb. a.

        See also **Bad** Eggs, &c.; **Butter; Cabbage; Cheese; Diet: Fat; Food; Onions; Pastry; Pork; Poultry; Rice; Sausages; Sugar; Sweets.**

Effluvia, Noxious—Crt. h.

Eggs, Bad—Cb. v.

Electric Shock—Mor.

_____ States of atmosphere—Na. c.

Embarrassments, Business—K. br.

Emissions—Stp.

Emotional Disturbance—K. br.

Emotions—(Fer.), Phst., Pso., Stn.

_____ Depressing—Gel.

_____ Pleasurable, effects of—Cof. _(See also_ **Joy,** Sudden.)

_____ Strong—Pho.

_____ Sudden, effects of, especially pleasurable ones—Cof.

_____ **Errors in diet**—Dio.

Eruptions, Checked, Repelled, or Suppressed—Ana., Ant. c., Aps., Bry., Calc., Cam., Caus., Cu. a., Dul., Hep., Ipc., Nx. m., Pet., Pb., Pso., (asthma.) Ptl., (milk crust, nervous paroxysms following) Vi. t., Zin.

Examinations—Ana.

Exanthema, Checked—Hel.

_____ Suppressed—Ver.

Excess—_See_ **Debauchery; Eating; Sexual;** _and_ **Venery.**

Excitement—(Ag. n.), Con., Scu.

_____ Mental—Aga., (headache) Cod., Sac. 1.

_____ Nervous—Arm.

_____ Sexual, indulged in or suppressed—K. ph.

_____ Unusual, as going on a visit—Eps.

  See also **Mental** Excitement, &c.

Exertion—Sel.

_____ Bodily—Alm.

_____ Mental—Nx. m., Pho., Pi. x., Sbd., (tremulousness and
         starting) Vin.

_____ Unusual, as doing a day's shopping—Eps.

Exposure—Klm., Sg. n.

_____ Cold, to—Phyt.

_____ Damp, to—Phyt.

_____ Drenching rains, to—Pho.

Eyes, Injuries to—Symt.

_____ Operations on—Aln.

_____ Over-exertion or Strain of—Onos., Rut., (Sul.).

Failure, Business—Act. r.

Falls—Lc. c., Li. c., Sep., Sti., Stp., Sul., Su. x., Symt., Tel., Ter.,
         Trn.

_____ Height, from—Mil.

Fasting—Dio.

Fat—(Cb. v.), (Ipc.), Na. m., Pul.

_____ Food—Cb. v., Na. m., Na. p., Pul.

_____ Meat—Thu.

_____ Pork—Sep.

_____ Rancid—(Ars.), (Cb. v.).

Fatigue—Act. s., Cai., (headache) Cod., Cof., Fe. pi., Pi. x., Sac. 1.
  (See also **Journeys,** Long; **Over-exertion,** &c.)

Fear—Aco., Ag. n., Cof., Glo., Gph., Lyc., Opi., Pho. *(See also*
  Fright.)

Feeding, Injudicious—Dio., Mag. c.

Indignation—Col. *(See also* **Anger; Passion; Rage.)**

Indulgence, Beer, in—K. bi. *(See also* **Beer.)**

_____ Malt Liquors, in—K. bi.

Injured Honour—Ver.

_____ Pride—Ver.

Injuries—Aco., Bls., Cep., Dul., Glo., Ham., Hep., (Hyp.), Ipc., K. sc., Lach., Lc. v. d., Nux, CEna., (from tight boots) Paeo., Par. Ph. x., Phst., Pso., Rn. b., (gangrene) Sec., Sep., Sil., Stp., (hydrocele) Smb. n.

_____ Bones, to—Hec., Rut., Symt.

_____ Eye, to—Symt.

_____ Head, to—Na. m., (fall) Na. s.

_____ Mechanical—Arn., Fe. p., K. Ph. *(See also* **Wounds.)**

_____ Nerve, to—(Hyp.), (of tooth) Men., Xan.

_____ Periosteum, to—Symt.

_____ Shock, from—Cam., Ver.

_____ Slightest—(spasms) Val.

_____ Spinal, old—Ign.

_____ Spine, lower, to—Calc.

_____ Tetanus, likely to cause—Teu.

Influenza—Scu.

Intemperate Habits—Ag. n. *(See also* **Alcohol; Beer; Debauchery; Drunkenness; Liquors.)**

Internal Functions, Deranged—K. m.

Iodide of Potassium—Aur.

Iodine—Ars.

Jar—Sep.

Jarring—Glo., Snc.

Jealousy—Aps., Hyo., Ign., Lach.

Journeys, Long—Cof.

Joy, Sudden—Opi. *(See also* **Emotions. Pleasurable.)**

Labour, Mental—Pso.

Laughing—(headache) As. mt.

Laundry Work—(Pho.), Sep. *(See also* **Washing.)**

Lead—Opi.

_____ Ulcers maltreated with—Caus.

Lemonade—Sel.

Light, Bright—Glo.

Lifting—Alm., Ca. p., Cb. a., Cb. v., Mil., Pho., (abortion) Sec.

_____ Arms—Su. x.

_____ (Over-lifting)—Agn., (prolapsus uteri) Pod.

Lightning—Crt..h., Mor., (blindness) Pho.

Liquors, Bad—Cb. v.

Lobster Salad, Spoiled—(Ars.).

Lochia, Suppressed—Hyo., Mil., Ve. v., Zin.

Long Journeys—Cof.

Loss of Fluids—Calc., Cb. a., Chi., Na. m., Ph. x., Pho., .Sel., Sil., (Sul.).

Losses in Business—K. br.

Love, Disappointed—Act. r., Ant. c., Aur., Cac., Ca. p., Hel., Ign., Iod., Lach., Ph. x., Trn., Ver.

Lunar Caustic—Na. m.

Malt Liquors, Indulgence in.—K. bi. *(See also* **Beer.)**

Masturbation—Arg., Ag. n., Calc., Chi., Dio., Gel., Lach., Lyc., Na. m., Nux, Plat., Sel., Stn.,Stp.

Mechanical Injuries—Arn., Fe. p., K. ph. *(See also* **Wounds.)**

Melons—Zng.

Menses, Suppressed—Calc., Mil., Se. a., Ve. v., Vis., Xan., Zin.

Mental Application or Excitement—Aga.

_____ Distress—Mag. c. *(See also* **Anxiety;** *and* **Worry.)**

_____ Excitement—Sac. 1. *(See also* **Excitement.)**

_____ Excitement, Excessive—(headache) Cod.

Mental Exertion—Nx. m., Pho., Pi. x., Pso., Sbd., (tremulousnes & and starting) Vin.

_____ Overwork (mental or physical).—Coc. i., Scu.

_____ Shock—Aps.

_____ Strain—Calc.

_____ Strain and worry—Ag. n.

Mercury—Aur., Chi., Hep., Mez., Stp., Thu.

Milk—Mag. c., Na. c., Na. p., Nx. m.

_____ Boiled—(diarrhoea) Sep.

_____ Cold—K. i.

_____ Effects of—Homa.

Milk, Suppressed—Hyo., Mil., Urt., Zin.

Milk-crust, Suppressed—(nervous paroxysms) Vi. t.

Misbehaviour of Others—Clch.

Mixed Diet—Pul.

Moist, Cold Winds—Calc.

Morphia—Ipc., Oxg.

Mountains, Climbing—Ars.

Music—Pho.

Nerves, Injury to—Hyp., (of tooth) Men., Xan.

Nervous Excitement—Arm.

_____ Overstrain, or Physical—Eps.

_____ Shock—Iod.

(See also **Excitement**; *and* **Mental** Excitement, &c.)

Nettle-rash, Suppressed—Urt.

News, Bad—Aln., Aps., Art. v., (unpleasant) Ca. p., Gel., Paeo., Ph. x., Trn.

Night-watching—Caus., Zin., Zn. a.

Nitric Acid—(deafness) Pet.

Noise—Coc. i.

Noxious Effluvia—Crt. h. *(See also* **Bad** Smells; *and* **Sewer-gas.)*

Odours, Strong—Pho.

Onanism—Arg., Ag. n., Chi., Dio., Gel., Lach., Lyc., Na. m., Nux, Plat., Sel., Stn., Stp.

Onions—(Ac. 1.), Thu.

Operations—Aco., (for fistula) Ca. p., (fine shooting pains after) Cep., Ph. x., Stp., Su. x., Zin.

_____ Abdominal—Bis.

_____ Eyes, on—Aln., (photopsia) Sto. c.

_____ Teeth, on—Aln.

Opium—Ver.

Otorrhoea, Suppressed—Zin.

Over-eating—All., Ant. c., Bry., Dio., Nx. m.

Over-exertion—Act. r., Aga., (= agalactia, Caus.), Mil., Ov. g. p., Rhs.

_____ Eyes, of—Onos., Rut., (Sul.).

Over-fatigue—Cof., Sac. 1. *(See also* **Fatigue, Over-exertion,** & c.).

Over-growth—Ca. p.

Over-heated, Becoming—Ant. c., (heat of summer = vomiting) Cb. v., (rheumatism) Spo.

_____ Chill when—K. sc.

_____ Effects of cold drinks when—Bls., Na. c.

_____ Wet, getting, when—Bls.

Over-lifting—Agn., Calc., (head and back, heart disease, Caus.), Gph., Lyc., Ph. x., (prolapsus uteri) Pod., Pr. s., Pso., Rhs., (dyspepsia) Sep.

Over-strain—K. ca., (prolapsus uteri) Pod.

_____ Mental or Bodily—Coc. i., (Cup.), Scu.

_____ Physical or Nervous—Eps., Scu.

Over-study—Ca. p., Na. c., Ph. x.

Over-work—Con., (asthenopia) Cb. v.

_____ Mental or Physical—Coc. i., (Cup), Scu.

Over-worked Brain—Cu. a.

Pain—Cham., (= nervous agitation) Scu.

Passion, Fit of—Ars., Mag. c., Na. m., Plat. *(See also* **Anger;** *and*
          Rage.)

Pastry—Pul.

Periosteum, Injuries to—Symt.

_____ Checked, on a warm summer's day—Fe. p.

Perspiration, Checked—Caj., Clch., Dul.

_____ Cold Draught during—Mr. i. f.

          (See also **Sweat.)**

Physical or Nervous Overstrain—Eps. Scu.

Pleasurable Emotions—Cof.

Poisoned Bites—Sga.

_____ Wounds—Lach.

Poisoning, Blood—Aga., Lo. p., Pyro.

_____ Ptomaine—Pyro.

_____ Sewer Gas—Pyro.

Pork—(Ac. 1.), Pul.

_____ Fat—Sep.

Potassium Iodide—Aur.

Poultry—Cb. v.

Pregnancy—Mag. c.

Pressure—(bed-sores) Paeo.

_____ Tight Boots, of—Paeo.

Pride, Injured—Ver.

Prunes—Rhe.

Ptomaine Poisoning—Pyro.

Punctured Wounds—(Hyp.), Lach., Led., Plnt.

Punishment—Trn.

Quinine—Ars., Cb. a., Ipc., Men., Na. m.

Rage—Aps. *(See* also **Anger;** and **Passion.)**

Rains, Drenching—Pho.

Raising Arms High to Lift Things—Rhs.

Reaching High—Sul.

Repeated Attacks of Gleet or Gonorrhoea—Agn.

Repelled Eruptions—*(See* **Suppressed Eruptions.***)*

Rice—(vomiting) Tel.

Rich Food—*K.* m.

Riding—Ther.

Riding in Carriage—Lyc., Pet. *(See also* **Travelling.***)*

Riding in a Ship—Ars., Pet., Ther.

Rising Early—Mth. pi.

Salt—Cb. v., Na. m., Nt. s. d., Sel.

Salt Food—Cb. v.

Salt Water, Bathing in—Ars., Mag. m., Rhs.

Sausages—(Ars.), Bel.

Scalds or Burns—Caus. *(See also* **Burns.***)*

Scolding—Trn.

Sea-bathing—Ars., Mag. m., Rhs.

Sea-sickness—Coc. i.

Sea-travelling—Ars., Pet., Ther.

Seasons—*See* **August; Autumn; Spring; Summer; Winter.**

Sedentary Habits—Alo.

Self-abuse—Arg., Ag. n., Chi., Dio., Calc., Gel., Lach., Lyc., Na.
   m., Nux, Plat., Sel., Stn., Stp.

Separation from Home—Cap., Ph. x.

Sepsis—Pyro., Trn. *(See also* **Blood-poisoning.***)*

Sewer-gas Poisoning—Pyro.

Sexual Abstinence—Con.

Sexual Abuse—Dig., K. br., Stp.

Sexual Craving—Stp.

Sexual Excess—Agn., (vaginitis or impotence) Arn., Ca. p., Chi.,
   Con., Dig., K.br., Nux, Onos., Ph. x., Pho., Plat., Pb., Smb.
   n., Sec., Symt., Thu., Up.

Sexual Excitement, indulged or suppressed—K. ph.

_____ Intercourse—Aga., Stp.

Sexual Irregularities—Ca. p.

Sexual Musing—(Stp.)

Shame—Opi.

Sheets, Damp—Rhs.

Ship, Riding in a—Ars., Pet., Ther.

Shock—Aco., Hyp., Mag. c., Ph. x., Stm.

_____ Electric—Mor.

_____ Injury, from—Cam., Ver.

_____ Mental—Aps.

_____ Nervous—Iod.

Shopping—Eps.

Skin Affections, Checked—Asa.

Sleep, Loss of—(= agalactia, Caus.), Coc. i.

Smells, Bad—(Bap.), Kre. *(See also* **Noxious Effluvia;** *and* **Sewer-gas.)**

Snake-bites—Lo. p., Plnt.

Sneezing—(= severe pain in r. chest, Bor.)

Snow, Bright—Glo.

Snowy Air—Con., Sep.

Sorrow—Caus. *(See also* **Grief.)**

Spasms—Rhe.

Spinal Injuries, Old—Ign.

Spine, Lower, Injury to—Calc.

Splinters—Sil.

Sprains—(or over-lifting) Agn., K. m., Kre., (bluish swelling of joints) Lach., Pet., Pho., Plg., Pr. s., Pso., Rho., Rs. v., Rut., Sga., Sto. c., Sul., Su. x.

Spring—(colds) Cep., Con., K. bi., Mr. i. f.

Stings—Led. *(See also* **Bee-stings.)**

Stone-cutting—Sil.

Storms, and Thunderstorms—Gel., Mor., Na. c., Na. p., Pho., Pso., Pul., Rho., Syph.

Stormy Weather—Nt. s. d., Pso., Rho.

Strain—Ars., Calc., Cb. a., Cb. v., Na. c., Ov. g. p., Rhs., Snc., Sil. Ter.

_____ Mental—Calc.

_____ and Worry, Mental—Ag. n.

_____ Over-strain, Mental or Bodily—Coc. i., Scu.

Strain, Over-strain, Physical or Nervous—Eps.

Strong Emotions—Pho.

Strong Odours—Pho.

Strychnine—Oxg.

Study—(headache) As. i., Mag. p., Ph. x., Pi. x. *(See also* **Over-study.)**

Sudden Emotion, especially Pleasurable—Cof.

Sudden Joy—Opi.

Sugar—Ag. n., Na. p., Sel.

Sulphur—Thu.

Summer—(diarrhoea) Pod., Sin. n.

Sun—Aco., Ant. c., Aga., Bel., Cac., Cd. s., Coc. i., Crt. h., Gel., Glo., Klm., Lach., Mu. x., (chronic effects) Na. c., Opi., Pr. s., Stm., Stn., Sul., Syph., Ve. v.

Sunstroke—Arg., Cam., Thu.

Suppressed Anger—(effects of) Aur., Ipc., Stp.

_____ Coryza—Chi.

_____ Discharges—Bry., Led., Vi. o.

_____ Eruptions—Ana., Ant. c., Aps., Bry., Calc., Cam., Caus., Cu. a., Dul., Hep., Ipc., Nx. m., Pet., Pb., Pso., (asthma) Ptl., (milk crust, nervous paroxysms following) Vi. t., Zin.

_____ Exanthema—Hel., Ver.

_____ Excitement—K. ph.

_____ Foot-sweat—Arm., Ba. c., For., Merc., O1. a., Sl. x.

_____ Gonorrhoea—Merc., Na. s.

_____ Gonorrhoea, or badly treated—Thu.

_____ Haemorrhoidal flow—Lcs.

_____ Lochia—Hyo., Mil., Ve. n.

_____ Menstruation—Calc., Mil., (from taking bath) Nx. m., Se. a., Ve. v., Vis., Xan., Zin.

_____ Milk—Hyo., Mil., Urt.

_____ Nettle-rash—Urt.

_____ Otorrhoea—Zin.

_____ Sexual Excitement—K. ph.

_____ Sweat—Caj., Calc., Clch., Dul., Fe. p., Na. c.
      Suppressions—Cup., Lo. i., Lo. s., Par., Stm., Sul., Zin.

Surgical Operations—Aco., Bis., (for fistula) Ca. p., (fine shooting pains after) Cep., Ph. x., Stp., Su. x., Zin. *(See also* **Operations.)**

Swallowing—(= pain in r. scapula, Caus.)

Sweat, Suppression of—(feet) Arm., (feet) Ba. c., Caj., Calc., Clch., Dul., (on a warm day) Fe. p., (feet) For., Na. c., (feet) Ol. a., (feet) Sl. x. *(See also* **Perspiration.)**

Sweets—Thu.

Tea—Ab. n., Chi., Coc. i., Dio., Lo. i., Pul., Sel., Strp., Thu.

Teeth, Operations on—Aln. *(See also* **Tooth.)**

_____ Wisdom, Cutting—Chei., Mag. c.

Temperature, Changes of—Na. c., Rn. b.

Thinking—(headache) As. mt., Sbd.

Thunder, Thunderstorms, Storms—Gel., Mor., Na. c., Na. p., Nt. s. d., Pho., Pso., Pul., Rho., Syph.

Tight Boots—Paeo.

Tobacco—Ab. n., (in boys) Ag. n., Ars., Ch. ar., Lo. i., (chewing) Lyc., (amblyopia) Pho., (heart) Scu., (neuralgia) Sep., Spi., Stp., Strp., Thu., Ver.

Tooth, Broken in, injuries to nerves—Men.

_____ Extraction—Ter. *(See also* **Teeth.)**

Travelling—Coc. i. *(See also* **Riding.)**

_____ by Sea—Ars., Pet., Ther.

Typhoid Fever—(remote effects of) Pyro.

Unpleasant News—Ca. p. *(See also* **Bad** News.)

Unrequited Love—Ph. x., Trn. *(See also* **Disappointed Love.)**

Unripe Fruit—Rhe.

Unusual Excitement or Exertion, as going on a visit, or shopping—
        Eps.

Vaccination—(Aps.), K. m., Mld., Mez., Sil., Sko., Thu.

Veal—K. n.

Vegetables, Decayed, Eating—Cb. a.

Venery—Ag. n., (vaginitis in the female, from, impotence in the
        male) Arn., Calc. *(See also* **Sexual Excess.)**

Venesection—Se. a., Scil.

Vexation—Ant. t., Aps., Au. m., (jaundice) Au. m. n., Cam., Ipc.,
        Lach., Lyc., Mag. c., Pet., Plat., Scro., (and anger) Sep. *(See
        also* **Chagrin.)**

Visit, Going on a—Eps.

Voice, Using—Stn.

Wading—Dul. *(See also* **Water,** Chill in the, &c.)

Walking—Sel.

Washing—Dul.

_____ Clothes—(headache) Pho., Ther. *(See also* **Laundry
        Work.)**

_____ Floor—Mr. bin.

Water, Bad, drinking—All., Crt. h.

_____ Chill in the—Ars.

_____ Cold, bathing in—Mag. p., Phst.

Water, Cold, standing in—Mag. p.

_____ Fresh or salt, bathing in—Rhs.

_____ Ice-water, drinking—Cb. v., Rhs.

_____ Sea, bathing in—Ars., Mag. m.

_____ Working in—(Calc.) *(See also* **Wading.)**

Weather, Changes of—Cb. v., Mr. bin., Rn. b.

_____ Cold and damp—Cep., Lth., Mr. i. f.

_____ Damp—Sin. n., Syph.

_____ Damp, warm, or cold—Gel.

_____ Hot—Ant. c., K. bi.

_____ Stormy—Nt. s. d., Pso., Rho. *(See also* **Storms.)**

_____ Warm—Lach.

_____ Warm and damp—Cb. v.

_____ Winter—Sg. n.

Weights, Heavy, carrying—Rut.

Wet, Getting—Ca. p., Clch., Mlr., Mr. bin., Rho., Sep., Vis., Xan.

_____ _____ Feet—Cep., Lo. i., Pul., Xan. .

_____ _____ Head—Bel.

_____ _____ Heated, when—Rhs.

_____ _____ Overheated, when—Bls.

Winds—Klm.

_____ Cold—Bry., Cd. s., Mag. p.

_____ Cold and damp—Cep.

_____ Cold, driving in—Sg. n.

_____ Cold, dry—Aco., Hep.

_____ Walking in—Bel.

Wines—(Ac. 1.), Cof., Lyc., Na. m.

_____ Bad—Cb. v.

Winter Weather—Sg. n.

Wisdom Teeth, Cutting—Chei., Mag. c.

Working with Cold Clay—Mag. p.

_____ Water—(Calc.)

Worms—Cin., Sbd.

Worry—Ign., K. br., Pho. *(See also* **Anxiety; Care;** and **Mental**
Distress, &c.)

Wounds—Arn., Bry., (Caln.), Fe. p., Hyp., K. ph., Led. Pho., Plnt.,
_____ Clean cut—Stp.
_____ Dissecting—Pyro.
_____ Lacerated—(Caln.)
_____ Poisoned—Lach.
_____ Punctured—Lach., Led., Plnt.

Yawning—Cin.

□□

Part III

REPERTORY OF
TEMPERAMENTS

REPERTORY OF
Temperaments, Dispositions, Constitutions, and States

[In this list are given the remedies which have been found, to act most beneficially in certain types of persons, temperaments, sex and age. There are also included complaints and conditions of particular types of persons and constitutions. In the *Dictionary of Materia Medica* these are generally given in the section *Characteristics* under the description "SUITED TO."]

Abdomen, Coldness of, icy, Children with. - Calc.

_____ Enlarged, Children with—(Am.m.), Calc., Sars.

_____ Nervous Attacks when the Aura starts from—Cast.

Abdominal Soreness—Cast.

Accomplishes little, though Busy all the time—Aps.

Acidity, Colic or Spasms with, of Infants—Na.p.

Acute Diseases, Persons weakened by Violent—Ph.x.

Adipsia Disposition to—Pul.

Adults, Males rather than Females—Pb.

Affectionate Disposition—Pul.

After-pains in Women who have borne many children—Cup.

Aged Persons—Ird. (See also **old Age.**)

Agitation, Nervous—Scu.

Air, Open, Aversion to—Cap, Na.c.

_____ Open, Dread of—Cap.

_____ Open, Persons who live in—Cf.t.

Air Passages, Diseases which affect the, in Scrofulous Children—Smb. n.

Alcohol, Constitutions Abused by—Led.

_____ Drunkards, after leaving off—Ca.ar.

Alcoholism, Chronic, Insomnia of—sum.

Alimentary Canal, Irritation of, in Children—Rhe.

Amenorrhoea with Leucorrhoea, Women who have—Xan.

_____ Nervous Women having—Ter.

Anaemia—Ird.

_____ Young Persons subject to—Fer.

Aneamic, Debilitated Subjects of Rheumatic Diathesis—Spi.

_____ (Half- Aneamic, half-Jaundiced) Persons—Pho.

_____ Persons—Calc., Cb.v., Chi., Fer., K. ca., Lyc., Merc., Na. m, Pho., Pi.x., Pul., Sil., Ver.

_____ Women, Pale—Lc.x.

Angina, Varicose, Venis of Pharynx large and blue—Ham.

Angry and Excited, Persons inclined to get—Nux.

_____ on the least occasion—(Cham., Nux.)

Animal Heat Defective, from Defective Oxygenation—Gph.

Animal Heat Diminished, Constitutions with—Alm., Cyc.

Anus, Fiery Red Rash about, in Babies—Med.

Anxiety, Effect of—Smb.n.

_____ Excessive, with all her Complaints—Ca.p.

Apoplectice—Aco., Arn., Ba.c., Bel., Coc. i., Lach., Nux, Op.

Ardent Persons—Nux.

Argentum Nitricum, those who have been treated locally with—Nat.m.

Arthritic, Diathesis—Cham., Led., Sbi.

_____ Pains—Sbi.

Asocarides, Scrofulous Children afflicted with—Spi.

Assimilating Power, Lack of—Sil.

Asthma, Consumptives, of—Mep.

_____ Drunkards of—Mep.

Asthmatic Constitutions—K.n.

Asthmatics, Old—Ill.

Asthmatical and Hysterical Cough, Globus in—Val.

Atmospheric Changes, Skin sensitive to—Rho., Sul.

Autumn, Affections which come on in—Rho.

Aversion, Exercise, to , Mental or Physical—Na.c.

_____ Open Air. to—Cap., Na.c.

Awkward Persons—Aps., Bov.,Cap.

Axilla, Fetid Sweats in, or on Feet and Hands—Nt.x.

Babies, Colic of—Ill.

_____ Nervous—K.ph.

_____ Rash, Fiery Red, about Anus of—Med.

_____ Sour—Su.x.

_____ Urinary Difficulties of—Pts.

_____ Urine Scalding—Med.

Bachelors, Old—Con.

Back and Limbs, Children with pains in, as if beaten—Ph.x.

Backache, Tired, Females who complain of—Hlon.

Bad Temper—Bry.

Bashful People—Coca.

Bathed or Washed, Children who cannot beat to be—Sul.

Big-bellied Children—Sul.

Big Heads, Children with—Calc.,K.i.,Sil.

_____ **Teeth and Small Jaws,** Children with—K.i.

Bile-pigments, Dirty appearance of Knuckles from—Pi.x.

Bilious Attacks, Remittent, Children liable to—Mr.d.

_____ **Temperament**—Aco., Ail., Amb., Ana., Aps., Ars., Bel., Ber., Byr., Cham., Chi., Chio., Col., Cub., Nux, Pet., Pb., Pod., Pul., Sep., Sul.

Temperament, with tendency to constipation—Cub.

_____ **Women**—Plat.

Black-eyed People—Lrs., Nt. x.

Black-haired People—Aur.,Lrs., Mu.x., Nt.x.,Thu.

Bladder, Irritable. of Old Women., —Cop.

Bleeding—Ter. (*See also* **Haemorrhages.**)

_____ Profusely, Wounds—Mil., Pho.

Bloated Persons—Spi.

Blondes—Chel., Col., Cyc., Kre., Pho., Pul., Sel., Sep.

Blood, Head, to the, Women or Girls with tendency to—Jab.

_____ **Irregular Distribution of**—Fer.

_____ **Loss of**—Fe. pi., Ipc.

_____ **Thin, Black, Watery, Copious Flow of**—Sec.

Blotched Skin—Sep.

Blue Eyes—Bel., Bro.,Cap., Lo.i.,Pul.,Spo.

Blueness of Skin—Cb.a.

Bodies, Sickly, Puny, Weak Children with, but with well-
      developed heads—Lyc.

· **Body** has a Filthy Smell, not removed by Washing—Pso.

_____ and Mind, Exhaustion of—Stn.

_____ and Mind, Torpidity of—Cyc.

_____ Sensitiveness of the Surface of the.,—K.i.,Lach.

Boils, Patients liable to—Bel., Lo. p.,Sul.

Bone Affections of Scrofulous Children, when associated with
      Diarrhoea—Sto.c.

Bone contain too little Lime—Calc.

Bowel Complaints of Rickety Children—Med.

Bowels or Stomach, Flatulence in, after meals—Dio.

Boys, Little, Affections of—Abr.

_____ Pining—Aur.

Brain, Affections of, occurring during Cholera Infantum—Nx.m.

Breath, Short—Coca.

Breathlessness and Fatigue, with Flushed Cheeks—Fer.

Broken Skin—Caln.

Broken-down Appearance of Sore Throat—Mr.cy.

_____ **Constitutions**—Chm.u.

Bronchial Affections in Old Persons—Amc.
Bronchitis in Old Persons—Hpz.
Bronchorrhoea in scrofulous Persons—Fe.i.
Brown-haired Persons—Cham.
Brown Skin, Dirty—Sep.
Brunette Temperament—Iod., Nt.x.
Burning Pain from Washing—For.
Business and Professional Men, Worn out—K.ph.
Busy all the time, but accomplishes little—Aps.

Cachectic Appearance, Women of—Sec.
_____ Conditions—Ag.n., Arn., Ars., Calc., Chi., Chm., u.,
        Clem., Iod., Merc., Na.m., Nt.x., Pho., Pi., x., Sec.
Cancer, Thin, Pale, Patients with tendency to—Arg.
Cancers and Glandular Enlargements—Con.
Cancerous History, Patients of—Sars., Scir., Tub.
Capricious and Dainty Children—Sac.o.
Carbo-nitrogenoid Constitutions—Cu.a., Cup.
Caries, Thin, Pale Patients with tendency to—Arg.
Catarrh, Disposed to—Bac., Ba.c., Calc., Cb.v., Caus., Gph.,
        Med., Na.c., Nt.x., Nux., Pso., Pul., Sul., Thu., Tub.
_____ Leucophlegmatic Persons with disposition to—Chi.
_____ Nasal and Pharyngeal, wtih Nervousness, &c—Sum.
_____ Yellow, Tenacious Mucus, with—Sum.
Catarrhal Troubles, Chlorotic People with—Na.m.
Carebral Irritation of Children, from Dentition—Scu.
Chagrin—Ph.x.
Chalky Look, Persons of—Calc.
Chamomile Tea, Hysterical Women who have taken too much—
        Val.
Change of Life, Women never well since—Lach.
Change of Seasons, Affections which come with—Rho., Sul.
_____ **of Weather,** Children who take Cold readily with—Sep.

_____ **of Weather,** Sudden Cases due to—Lpt.

Changed Mentally and Physically by Illness—Lach.

Changes, Damp and Cold, Persons who take Cold from—Dul.

Cheeks, Flushed, in young Persons—Fer.

Cheese, Old, uncooked Fruit, Pastry, &c., Colic from—Dio.

Chest Complaints—K.n.

Chested, Narrow—Calc., Pho.

Childbed—Women in, during Pregnancy, and while Nursing—
          Sep.

Childhood—Opi.

_____ First and Second (children and old persons). Opi.

Children—Ac.x., Cic., Cic. v., Gel., K.br., Merc., Nx.m., Pul.,
          Sbd., Spo., Stm., Teu., Thu., Ver.

_____ Abdomen, large, with—Calc., Sars.

_____ Air Passages, scrofulous Diseases affecting the—
          Smb.n.

_____ Alimentary Canal, Irritation of, in—Rhe.

_____ Ascarides and Lumbrici, afflicted with—Spi.

_____ Big-bellied—Sul.

_____ Big Heads, with—K.i.

_____ Big Teeth, with, and Small Jaws—K.i.

_____ Bilious Attacks, remittent, liable to—Mr.d.

_____ Bowel Complaints of Rickety—Med.

_____ Cerebral Irritation of, from Dentition—Scu.

_____ Chubby—K.bi.

_____ Chubby, Fat—Sga.

_____ Clumsy—Cap.

_____ Cold, who take, readily when the weather changes—
          Sep.

_____ Convulsions of—Pas.

_____ Cough of, after Influenza—Sang.

_____ Cross after sleep, Pushing every one—Lyc.

_____ Cross, outrageously—Hep.

_____ Cross, Whining—Sac.o.

_____ Dainty and Capricious—Sac.o.

_____ Deep-seated Dyscrasia, with—Su.x.

_____ Delicate, Sickly—Pso.

_____ Delicate Skin, with—Bro.

_____ Dentition, during, Puny—Mag.m.

_____ Dentition, during, Rickety—Mag.m.

_____ Disorders of, such as Flatulence and Irritation of the Alimentary Canal—Rhe.

_____ Dropsy, with a tendency to—Sac.o.

_____ Emaciated—K.i.,Sul.

_____ Eruptions about the Eyes, having—Mag.m.

_____ Excitable—Amb., Hy. n., Lyc.

_____ Exhausting Diseases, after—Cb.v.

_____ Faces, with, like Old People—Sars.

_____ Fair—Calc.

_____ Fat—Calc., K.bi.

_____ Fat and Bloated—Sac.o.

_____ Fat, Chubby—Sga.

Children, Flatulence, with, and Irritation of Alimentary Canal—Rhe.

_____ Flushing easily—Calc.

_____ Fontanelles open, with—Calc., Sil.

_____ Glands, Lymphatic, Hard and Enlarged, with—Calc.

_____ Growing Too Fast—Ird., Kre., Ph.x., Pho.

_____ Head Sweats, subject to—Calc.

_____ Insolent—Sac.o.

_____ Intestinal Irritation of—Scu.

_____ Irregular Growth,of—Calc.

_____ Irritable—Ca.br., Lyc.

_____ Jaws, Small, and Big Teeth, with—K.i.

_____ Large Heads, with—Calc., K.i., Sil.

_____ Large-limbed—Sac.o.

_____ Lax fibre, of—Ca.br., Mag.c.

_____ Light Eyebrows, with—Bro.

_____ Light-haired—Bro., Dig.

_____ Little, Diseases of—Cham., Mag.c.

_____ Liver Affections, with—Mag.m.

_____ Lumbrici and Ascarides, Afflicited with—Spi.

_____ Lymphatic—Ca.br.

_____ Lymphatic Glands, with, Hard and Enlarged—Calc.

_____ Marasmus, with—Coca., Pb.

_____ Milk, who cannot take—Ol.j.

_____ Milk who refuse, and get pain in the Stomach if they take it—Mag.c.

_____ Nervous—Amb., Ca. br., Hyn.

_____ Nervous, who have been Frightened—Hyn.

_____ Nervous, Unmanageable when Sick—Lyc.

_____ New-born—Abr., Ipc., Lach.

_____ Nick-nacks, wanting—Sac.o.

_____ Nose-bleed, subject to,—Ter.

_____ Occupy themselves in any way, not caring to—Sac.o.

_____ Odour, having a Disagreeable—Pso.

_____ Old-looking—Kre., Sars.

_____ Old-looking, hard to awaken—Kre.

_____ Pains, with, in Back and Limbs as if beaten—Ph.x.

_____ Pale—Calc.,Mr.d.,Pso.

_____ Peevish—Pso.

_____ Puny—Ird.

_____ Puny, during Dentition—Mag.m.

_____ Puny, Rickety, having eruptions about eyes—Mag. m.

_____ Puny, Sickly—Lyc., Mag.c.

_____ Restless, Hot, Kick off clothes at night—Sul.

_____ Rickety, Bowel Complaints of—Med.

Children, Rickety, during Dentition—Mag.m.

_____ Ride, who cannot, in Jolting Conveyances—K.i.

_____ Scarlatina, recovering from—Pts.

_____ Scrofulous—Am.c., Ba.m., Cur., Dig., Merc., Mr.d.

_____ Scrofulous, Afflicted with Ascarides and Lumbrici—Spi.

_____ Scrofulous, Bone Affections of, when associated with Diarrhoea—Sto.c.

_____ Scrofulous, Diseases of, which affect the Air Passages—Smb.n.

_____ Scrofulous, liable to Remittent Bilious Attacks—Mr.d.

_____ Scrofulous, with Worm Diseases during Dentition—Sil.

_____ Sickly, Delicate—Pso.

_____ Sleeplessness, and tendency to Spasms, with—Sum.

_____ Slender and Slim—Ph.x.

_____ Slow in Movement—Calc.

_____ Spasms, with tendency to—Sum.

_____ Strumous—Hep.

_____ Substantial Food, caring nothing for—Sca.o.

_____ Sutures Open, with—Calc., Sil.

_____ Sweats, with, Irregular and Partial—Calc.

_____ Swelling of Cervical and other Glands, with—Mr.d.

_____ Tall, Slender—Ph.x.

_____ Teething, when—AEth., Mag.p., Na.m.

_____ Tongue Coated moist white, with—Ant.,c.

_____ Touched, who cannot bear to be—Ant.c.,K.i.

_____ Unhealthy-looking, having a Disagreeable Odour—Pso.

_____ Unmanageable when Sick—Lyc.

_____ Urination and Defecation, inclined to frequency of—K.i.

_____ Washed or Bathed, who cannot bear to be—Sul.

_____ Weak, with well-developed Heads—Lyc.

_____ Weak-limbed—Ird.

_____ White Complexions, with—Dig.

_____ White Skins, with—Bro., Sep.

_____ Withered Old Men, like—Ag.n.

_____ Worms, having—Sul.,Ter.*See also* **Infants**

Chilliness, Disposition to—Pul.

Chilly Persons always Shrinking from Cold—Asr.

_____ Persons who always feel—Led.

Chlorosis with Erethism—Fer.

Chlorotic Conditions—Cyc.

‾‾‾‾‾‾ **Girls**—Alet.

Chlorotics—Alm., Bel., Calc., Cb.v., Cham., Coc. i., con.,Fer., Gph., Hlon., H.ca., Lach., Lyc., Na.m., Nt. x., Pho., plat., Pul., Sep., Sul.

Chlorotics, Catarrhal Troubles, with—Na.m.

Cholera Infantum, Affections of the Brain occurring during— Nx.m.

Choleraic Affections in Old Age—Aeth.

Choleric Persons—Aco., Bry., Cham., Cof., Col., Ign., Lach., Lyc., Nux, Pho., Plat., Stp., Ver.

‾‾‾‾‾‾ **Persons with Dark Hair**—Nux.

‾‾‾‾‾‾ **Women with Freckles and Red Hair**—Lach.

Choreic Affections, Nervous Hysterical Patients subject to—Trn.

‾‾‾‾‾‾ **Affections when Whole Body or Right Arm and Left Leg are involved**—Trn.

Chronic Ailments of Sedentary Persons—Alm.

‾‾‾‾‾‾ **Ailments of Women**—Sbi.

‾‾‾‾‾‾ **Diseases** and Enfeebled Patients—Gn.q.

‾‾‾‾‾‾ **Diseases,** Persons suffering from, who take Cold easily—Nt.x.

‾‾‾‾‾‾ **Sufferers from Diarrhoea**—Calc., Fer., Kre., Mag. m., Mu.x., Ph.x., Pho., Sil., Ver.

Chubby Children—K.bi.

‾‾‾‾‾‾ **Fat Children**—Sga.

Circulation, Excitement of the —Val.

Clear Complexion—Stn.i.

Climacteric Flushings—Sum.

‾‾‾‾‾‾ **Period,** Sufferings at the—Act.r., Ca.ar., Dig., Mur., Su.x.

Climatic Changes, sudden, Cases due to—Lpt.

Climaxis, Fat Women approaching the—Ca.ar.

Climbing—*See* **Mountaineers**.

Clothes, Children Kick off, at night—Sul.

Clumsy, Children—Cap.

Coffee, Persons addicted to—Nux.

Cold Abdomen, Children with—Calc.

_____ Air, Sore Throats that are ≤ from—Sbd.

_____ Children Who readily take, when the weather changes—
          Sep.

_____ and Deficient in Vital Reaction, People who are—Ver.

_____ Disposition to take—Aco., Ana., Ba.c., Bcl., Calc., Cb.
          v., Caus, Cham., Dul., Gph., K.ca., Merc., Na.c.,
          Na.m., Nt.x., Nx.m., Nux, Pho., Pul., Sep., Sil., Sul.

_____ Extremities, Sallow People with—Lyc.

_____ Getting, in cold weather—Bor.

_____ Indoors or Out, Persons always—Gph.

_____ Persons who always feel—Led.

_____ Persons who take, in cold damp weather—Dul.

_____ Persons who take, easily, disposed to Diarrhoea—Nt.x.

_____ Scrofulous Subjects sensitive to—Cis.

_____ Weather, Bronchial Affections in Old People during—
          Amc.

Colic or Spasms, with Acidity, in Infants—Na.p.

Colic or Cramps from excessive Venery—Col.

_____ Error in Diet, from—Dio.

_____ Excess in Eating, after—Dio.

_____ Old Cheese, from, in Persons of Weak Digestion—Dio.

_____ Uncooked Fruit, after—Dio.

_____ Babies, of—Ill.

_____ Tea-drinkers, of—Dio.

Complexion, Clear—Stn.i.

_____ Dark. Bry., Cof., Iod., Kre., Lrs., Lyc., Nt.x., Pi.x., Sul.,
          Thu., Vi.o.

_____ Fair—Lo.i., Lcs., Sbd.

_____ Fair, Girls with—Vi.o.

_____ Jaundiced—Pb.

_____ Light—Bel., Hep., Sel., Sil., Sul.

_____ Livid—Kre.

_____ Olive-brown—Aur.

_____ Pale—*See* **Pale Children,** & c.

_____ Sallow—Lyc.

_____ Swarthy—Chi., Nt.x.

_____ White, Children with—Dig.

Comprehension, Slow, when Sick—Lyc.

Condiments, Persons addicted to—Nux.

Congestion, Pulmonary, Subjects liable to—Lips.

Congestions, Portal System, of—Sul.

Congestions, Sanguine Temperaments inclined to—Sep.

Constipation, Extreme, in Girls—Fer.

_____ Literary men liable to—Nic.

_____ Lymphatic Persons disposed to, or to Morning Diarrhoea—Sul.

_____ Persons of Bilious Temperament, with tendency to—Cub.

Constitutions, Alcohol, Abused by—Led.

_____ Animal Heat Diminished, with—Alm., Cyc., Gph.

_____ Asthmatic—K.n.

_____ Bilious—Chi., Pb. (*see also* **Bilious Temperament.**)

_____ Broken-down—Chm.u.

_____ Carbo-nitrogenoid—Cu.a., Cup.

_____ Debilitated—Ars., Calc., Cb.v., Chi., Iod., K.ca., Na.m., Nux, Ph.x., Pho., Pul., Sep., Slp., Spi.

_____ Delicate—Nx. m.

_____ Delicate, with Pure White Skin—Sep.

_____ Dry—Chi., Lyc., Nux, Pb.

_____ Feeble—*See* **Feeble Persons,** &c.

_____ Gouty—Ca. p., Sti.

_____ Hydrogenoid, possessing an increased capacity to contain water—Arn., Na.s., Nt.x., Nx.m., Thu.

Constitutions, Lax Fibre, with—Hep.

_____ Leucophlegmatic—Agn., Am.c., Ars., Bel., Calc., Cast., Chi., Cyc., Fe. p., Kre., Na.c., Pul., Sep., Ust.

_____ Lymphatic—Dig., Hep.

_____ Nervo-sanguine or Sanguine—Ver.

_____ Nervous—Aco., Act. r., Ail., Amb., Am.c., Ana., Aps., Arn., Ars., Asa., Bel., Bor., Bry., Cham., Chi., Coc.i., Cof., Gel., Glo., Hyo., Ign., Lo.p., Mag.m., Nux, Pho., Pso., Pul., Sec., Sep., Sil., Stp. (*See Also* **Nervous** Affections, &c.)

_____ Nervous, disposed to Haemorrhoids—Sul.

_____ Neuralgic—Sti., Val.

_____ Phthisical—Bac., Fe.i., Pho., St., Tub.

_____ Psoric—Alm., Bac., Hep., Sul., Pso., Tub.

_____ Scorbutic—Jg.c.

_____ Scrofulous—Aps., Ars., Asa., Aur., Ba.c., Bro., Ca.ar., Calc., Ca.p., Cb.a., Caus., Chm. u., Con., Fe.i., Gel., Gph., Hep., Iod., Jg.c., Lyc., Merc., Mr.bin., Na.m., Pso., Rhs., Sc.a., Sep., Sil., Spi., Spo., Sul. (*See also* **Scrofulous** Children. &c.)

_____ Slow, Torpid—Am.m., Caus., Clem., Coc. i., Dul. Hep., K.bi., Kre., Pul.

_____ Weakly—Alm., Am.c., Ars., Calc., Cb.v., Caus., Chi., Cis., Fer., Fl.x., Hel., Iod., Ka.c., Lach., Lyc., Na. m., Nux, Ph.x., Rhs., Sep., Sil., Stn., Sul., Ver., Zin. (*See also* **Weakly** Persons.)

Consumptives, Asthma of—Mep.

Convulsions of Children—Pas.

Cool, Dry Skin—Nx. m., Vi.o.

_____ **Dry Skin,** Persons with, who do not easily perspire—Nx.m.

Corpulent People—Bl.o.

Cough, Influenza, after, of children—Sang.

_____ Severe, after Whooping-caugh—Sang.

_____ Sleeplessness due to, or to Nervousness—Sti.

Coughs, Nervous—Crl.

Cramps or Colic from excessive Venery—Col.

_____ Fruit, from—Col.

_____ Lead Poisoning, from—Col.

_____ Nervous Women with, awfter server illness—Cast.

Critical Period of Life, and Pubescence—Sep.

Cross, Children, after Sleep, pushing every one away—Lyc.

_____ **Children,** Outrageously—Hep.

_____ **Whining Children**—Sca.o.

Dainty and Capricious Children—Sac.o.

Damp, Cold Changes, Persons who take Cold from—Dul.

Damp, Syphilitic Subjects who are sensitive to—Phyt.

Dark Complexion—Bry., Cof., Iod., Kre., Lrs., Lyc., Nt. x., Pi.x.,
        Sul., Thu., Vi.o.

_____ **Eyes**—Aur., Gph., Iod., Lach., Mu.x., Nt.x.

_____ **Hair**—Aco., Arn., Bro., Bry., Caus., Con., Gph. Ign.,
        Iod., K.ca., Mu.x., Nt.x., Nux, Pho. Plat., Sang., Sep.

_____ **Hair,** Choleric Persons with—Nux.

_____ **Hair, Hysterical Subjects with**—Vb.o.

_____ **Haired Persons of Lithic or Sycotic Diathesis**—Sars.

Debauchees, Thin, Irritable, Venous—Nux.

Debilitated—Ars., Calc., Cb. v., Chi., Iod., K. ca., Na.m., Nux,
        Ph.x., Pho., Pul., Sep., Slp.

_____ **Anaemic Subjects of Rheumatic Diathesis**—Spi.

Debility—Cb. a., Cb.v., Cyc., Hep., Lach.

_____ Great, following Flushes of Heat—Dig.

_____ Nervous, after Influenza—Cyp., Scu. _See also_
        Depression; Exhaustion; Weakness.

Decaying, Patients Whose Teeth are always—Lo.p.

Deception, Persons disposed to—Nux.

Decrepit Old Persons—Sec.

Deep Ulcers, Thin Patients with—Arg.

Defecation and Urination, Children inclined to Frequency of—
K.i.

Defective Nutrition—Ol. j., Phe. l., Sil.

Deficient in Silica, Patients who are—Lo.p.

_____ in **Vital Reaction**—Cb.v., Pso., Ver.

_____ **and Weak Nutrition,** Feeble, Irritable Persons who
have—Phel.

Delicate—Act.r., Am.c., Cb.v., Chi., Fer., Kre., Hlon., K.i., Led.,
Lyc., Sec., Sep.

_____ **Children.** Sickly—Pso.

_____ **Constitutions**—Nx.m.

_____ **Constitutions with Pure White Skin**—Sep.

_____ **Eyelashes**—Pho.

_____ **Girls,** fearfully constipated with Low Spirits—Fer.

_____ **Organisation,** Women of—Xan.

_____ **Skin**—Bro., Caus.

_____ **Women**—Eu.pi.

Dentition—Act.r., Bor., Pas., Scu., Sil., Ter.

_____ Cerebral Irritation of Children from—Scu.

_____ Complaints during—Cof.

_____ Puny Children, during—Mag.m.

_____ Rickety Children, during—Mag.m.

_____ Scrofulous Children, who have Worm Diseases,
during—Sil.

Dentition, Suckling and Children during—Rhe.

**Depression of Nervous and Vital Powers after Long
Sickness**—Scu.

_____ of Vital Powers—Cb.v.

Despair of Perfect Recovery—Pso.

Despondent and Without Hope, Phthisical Patients who are—
Stn.

Destructive Tendency, Persons of—Trn.

Diarrhoea—Chi., Sil., Sto.c.

_____ Chronic, sufferers from—Calc., Fer., Kre., Mag.m.,

Mu.x., Ph.x., Pho., Sil., Ver.

_____ Early Stages of—Rhe.

_____ Morning, or Constipation, Lymphatic Persons with—Sul.

_____ Persons disposed to, who take Cold easily—Nt. x.

_____ Profuse, Watery of Old People—Gam.

Diathesis, Gouty—Cham., Led., Sbi.

_____ Lithic Acid—Lyc.

_____ Lithic or Sycotic, Dark-haired Persons of—Sars.

_____ Psoric—Aln., Bac., Hep., Pso., Tub.

_____ Rheumatic—Act.r., Bry., K.bi., Led., Phyt., Rhs., Spi.,
          Sti.

_____ Scrofulous—*See* **Scrofulous.**

_____ Scrofulous or Mercurial—Fe.i.

Diet, Error in, Persons liable to Colic from—Dio.

Digestive Powers, Feeble—Dio., Nic.

_____ Feeble, in Elderly People—Pr.v.

Dirty Appearance about Knuckles (from Bile Pigments)—Pi.x.

Dirty-brown Bloated Skin, Puffed Flabby Persons with—Sep.

**Dirty, Filthy People with Greasy Skin and Long Matted
        Hair**—Sul.

**Dirty-looking Persons who are always Speculating on
        Religious or Philosophical Subjects**—Sul.

**Dirty People in whom the Body has a Filthy Smell which no
        amount of Washing can remove**—Pso.

Disagreeable Odour, Children, Unhealthy-looking, having a—
        Pso.

_____ **Odour,** Patients who Emit—Pso.

Diseases, Putrid, Persons with—Ars., Kre.

Disinclination for Labour, Blonde Leucophlegmatic Subjects
        having—Cyc.

Disposition, Affectionate—Pul.

_____ Gay—Ver.

_____ Gentle—Pul.

_____ Hasty—Lo.p.

_____ Haughty, when Sick—Lyc.

_____ Irritable—Kre.

_____ Malicious—Nux.

Disposition, Melancholic—Asr., Lach., Mac., Mur., Nux, Pul., Ver.

_____ Mild—Aln., Coc.i., Ign., Ph.x., Pul., Sep., Vi.o.

_____ Sad—Kre., Lach.

_____ Spiteful, Malicious—Nux.

_____ Tenacious and Irascible—Nux.

_____ Voluptuous—Ced.

_____ Yielding—Pul.

Disturbances, Menstrual, Women with—Ag.n.

Draughts, Effects of whilst Perspiring, in Scrofulous and Syphilitic Patients—Mr.i.f.

Dread Open Air, Patients who—Cap.

Dream about Water, Persons who—Ve.v.

Dried-up-looking Women—Ag.n.

_____ **Nervous Persons**—Amb.

Drinkers—Opi.

Drinking, Men addicted to—Sep.

Dropsical Affections, Disposition to—Chi.

_____ **Persons**—Na.m.

_____ **or Semi-Dropsical,** Lower Part of Body, Upper Wasted—Lyc.

Dropsy, Children with a tendency to—Sac.o.

Drugged Subjects—Nux., Thu.

Drunkards—Cd.s., Lach.

_____ After leaving off Alcohol—Ca.ar.

_____ Asthma of—Mep.

_____ Old—Ill.

Dry Constitution—Chi., Lyc., Nux, Pb.

_____ **Habit,** Vigorous Persons of—Nux.

_____ **Skin, and Cool**—Nx. m.,Vi.o.

_____ **Skin, Profuse Saliva, Diarrhoea Night-Sweats**—Sil.

Dulness of Head—Ag.n.

———— of Intellect—Mac.

Dwarfish—Ba.c.

Dyscrasia, Deep-seated; Child is weak, with no other symptoms—Su.x.

———— Deep-seated, Weakness which seems to come from— Su.x.

Dysmenorrhoea of Nervous Women—Ter.

Dyspepsia of Old People—Nx.m.

Earliest Months of the Year, Complaints which come on in— Mez.

Earthy, Yellow, Wrinkled Skin—Spi. (*See also* **Wrinkled;** and **Yellow.**)

Eat, unable, yet has constant sinking—Grt.

Eating, Excess in, Persons subject to Colic after—Dio.

———— Fruit Uncooked, Persons liable to Colic after—Dio.

Eating Old Cheese or Pastry, Person liable to Colic after—Dio.

———— Pork, Persons who suffer from—Pul.

Elderly Persons—Aga., Alm., Amb., Ant.c., Aps., Bap., Ba. c., Ca.p., Cb.a., Cb.v., Cham., Chi., Cic., Clch., Con., Fl.x., Gph., Hdr., Iod., K.ca., Kre., Lyc., Mil., Na.m., Na.s., Nt.x., Nx.m., Opi., Sbd., Sec., Su.x.

Emaciated—Alet., Am.c., Ba.c., Fl.x., Mag.p., Na.m.

———— **Children**—K.i., Sul.

———— Robust and Fleshy Persons who suddenly become— Smb.n.

Emotions, Mental, Sufferings from—Smb.n.

———— Moral, Persons weakened by a long succession of— Ph.x.

———— Excitable Persons , anxious for—Sep.

Emphysematous Persons—Ipc.

Enfeebled Patients, and Chronic Diseases.Gn.q.

_____   Special Senses, Persons with—Cyc.

Engorged Venous System—Cb.v.

Enlargements, Glandular—Clem., Con.

Entertaining Persons—Bel.

Epigastrium, Faintness at, in Forenoon—Sul.

_____   Persons who refer all their Sufferings to the—Sul.

Epilepsy—Pas.

Epistaxis, Subjects of—Abr.

_____   **or other Loss of Blood,** Persons with a history of—
Fe.pi., Ipc.

Epithelium, Sqamous, Syphilitic Affections of Muicous Surfaces
covered with—Mr.i.f.

Erethism, Chlorosis with—Fer.

Eruptions about the Eyes, Children having—Mag.m.

_____   Suppressed—Pso., Sul.

Excess in Eating, Colic after—Dio.

Excesses, Persons suffering from—Ph.x.

_____   Sexual, Cramps and Colic from—Col.

_____   Sexual, Persons exhausted by—Sep.

Excitable—Cham., Con., Gel., Hyo., Ign., Nux.

_____   **Children**—Amb., Lyc.

_____   **Children,** Highly—Hyn.

_____   **Persons,** Exceedingly, and Anxious for Emotions—Sep.

_____   **Persons,** with Weakness—Lun.

_____   **Temperament** (especially Females)—Ced., Ign.

_____   **Temperaments,** Nervous Affections occuring in—Val.

Excited, Women of rigid fibre who are easily, (also opposite
Temperament)—Con.

Excitement, Mental and Nervous, Disorders from—Cyp.

_____   Reflex, Nervous—Cyp.

_____   Sexual, disposed to—Sep.

Exercise, Mental or Physical Aversion to—Na.c.

Exertion, Great Mental, Dark-haired Persons who make—Coca,
Nux. Pi.x.

_____ Least, Red Face from—Fer.

Exhausted by Disease—Ird.

Exhausting Diseases, Children after—Cb.v.

Exhaustion, Mind and Body, of—Stn.

_____ Nervous—Stn.

Extremities, Cold, Sallow People with—Lyc.

Eyebrows, Light, Children with—Bro.

Eyelashes, Delicate—Pho.

_____ Long—Stn.,

Eyes, Black—Lrs., Nt.x.

_____ Blue—Bel., Bro.,Cap., Lo.i., Pul., Spo.

_____ Dark—Aur., Gph., Iod.,Lach., Mu.,x., Nt.x.

_____ Eruptions about, in Puny, Rickety Children—Mag.m.

_____ Hollow, Thin Patients with—Arg.

_____ Light—Lcs.

Face, Children with, like old people—Sars.

_____ Pale—Pul., Sil.

_____ Red (also in Hectic)—Ol.j.

_____ Red, from Least Exertion—Fer.

Faintness in Epigastrium in Forenoon, Patients with—Sul.

Fair Children—Calc.

_____ **Complexion**—Lo.i., Lcs., Sbd.

_____ **Complexion,** Girls with—Vi.o.

_____ **Hair,** Hysterical Subjects with—Vb.o.

_____ **Haired People**—Cup., K.bi., Spo.

_____ **People**—Bro., Ipc.

_____ **Skin**—Pho.

Fasting, Persons who have Bowel Complaints from—Dio.

Fat Children—Calc., K.bi.

_____ **Children,** Bloated—Sac.o.

_____ **Children,** Chubby—Sga.

_____ **Persons**—Am.m., Ant. c., Bac., Ca.ar., Calc., Coca,

Cro., Fer., K.bi., K.ca., Lyc., Pho., Sul.

_____ **Persons** of Lax Fibre—Sga.

_____ Tendency to be—K.ca., Pho.

_____ **Women** approaching the Climaxis—Ca.ar.

See also **Obesity.**

Fatigue, Great, and Breathlessness in Girls with Flushed Cheeks—Fer.

Fatigue, Over-fatigue, Insomnia due to—Chl.h.

Fatigued, Females easily, by any work—Hlon.

Fear, Terror and Timidity—Spo.

Fearful Persons—Coc.i.

Feeble Digestive Powers—Dio., Nic.

_____ **Digestive Powers** in Elderly People—Pr.v.

_____ **Muscular Development,** Intellect keen—Lyc.

_____ **Old Men**—Con.

_____ **Persons,** with Deficient and Weak Nutrition—Gn.q., Phel.

_____ **Women**—Agn., Sec.

Feet, Soles of, Hot—Sul.

Females especially of Nervous Temperament—Ced., Sc.a., Xan.

_____ Nervously run down—Hlon.

_____ Suited more to, than Males—Nt.o.

_____ Tall, Slender, Thin, having retained a good deal of Sprightliness and Moral Power (Teste)—Sga.

Fetid Sweat on Hands, Feet, or in Axilla—Nt.x.

Fibre, Firm, Fleshy—Bry.

_____ Lax, Children of—Ca.br., Mag.c.

_____ Lax, Fat Person, of—Sga.

_____ Lax, Muscular Women of—Sec.

_____ Lax, Persons of—Cap., Hep., Mag.c., Mr.bin.

_____ Lax, Stout Persons of—Ipc.

_____ Lax, Women of—Spo.

_____ Relaxed—Fe.i., Nt.x.

_____ Rigid—Caus., Con., Nt.x. Nux, Plat., Sep.

_____ Rigid, Women of—Con.

_____ Tense—Nux.

Filthy People with Greasy Skin and Long Matted Hair—Sul.

_____ **Smell Which no amount of Washing can Remove**—
Pso.

Firm, Fleshy Fibre—Bry.

Fitful Mood, Persons of—Ver.

Flabby—K.ca., Trl.

_____ **Muscles**—Aga., Calc., Hep., K.ca., Sil., Spo., Ver. (See
also **Muscles.**)

_____ **Persons with Yellow or Dirty-brown Blotched Skin**—
Sep.

_____ **Skin,** and Ill-nourished—Mr.d.

_____ **Vessels** and Lax Fibre, Women of—Sec.

Flatulence, Children who suffer from, and Irritation of the
Alimentary Canal—Rhe.

_____ Meals, after, in Stomach or Bowels—Dio.

Fleshy Fibre—Bry.

_____ **People**—All., Mag.p.

_____ Persons inclined to be—Lo.i.

Fleshy Persons, Lymphatic Temperament of—Thu.

_____ Robust Persons who suddenly become Emaciated—
Smb.n.

_____ Women inclined to be—Pul.

Flooding after every Labour, Women who have—Trl.

Fluids, Loss of, Strong People Weakened by—Ph.x.

Florid Women—Glo.

Flushed Cheeks, Young Persons with, Fatigue, and
Breathlessness—Fer.

Flushes of Heat all over Body, followed by Perspiration—Sul.

_____ **of Heat, followed by Great Debility**—Dig.

Flushing, Easily—K.i.

_____ **Easily in Children**—Calc.

Flushings, Climacteric—Sum.

Fontanelles, Open—Calc., Sil.

Food, Substantial, Children caring nothing for—Sac.o.

Foxy Persons—Trn.

Freckled People—Sul.

Freckles and Red Hair, Choleric Women with—Lach.

Frivolous Persons—Aps.

Fruit, Cramps from—Col.

_____ Eating, Persons affected by—Bor.

_____ Uncooked, Pastry, Old Cheese, &c., Colic caused by—
Dio.

Full-blooded Persons—Ve.v.

_____ Persons with great Irritability, Restlessness, and
Hastiness—Sul.

Gay Disposition—Ver.

Gentle Disposition—Pul.

Girls or Women, with tendency to Blood to Head—Jab.

_____ Chlorotic—Alet.

_____ Delicate, fearfully constipated, with Low Spirits—Fer.

_____ Or Women , with Dry Skin—Jab.

_____ Flushed Cheeks, Fatigue, and Breathlessness, with—
Fer.

_____ Home-sick—Ca.p., Cap.

_____ Impressive, Mild, of Fair Complexion—Vi.o.

_____ Little, and Women, of Nervous Temperament—Se.a.

_____ or Women with scanty Menses—Con., Jab.(See also
Menses.)

_____ Mild, impressionable, fair—Vi.o.

_____ Puberty, at—Aur.

_____ School—Ca.p.

_____ Tall, Thin, Nervous—Vi.o.

Glands, Affections of Persons having—Gph.

_____ Cervical and other, Children having swelling of—Mr.d.

_____ Lympahatic, Hard and Enlarged, in Children—Calc.

Glands, Persons subject to diseases of the—Pso.

Glandular Enlargements and Cancers, Subjects of—Con.

_____ Swellings and Indurations—Clem.

Globus in all Asthmatical and Hysterical Coughs—Val.

Gouty Complaints—Ter.

_____ Constitutions—Ca.p., Sti.

_____ Diathesis—Cham., Led., Sbi.

Greasy Skin and long matted hair, dirty, filthy people with—Sul.

Grief, Persons affected by—Smb.n.

Growth, Children of Irregular—Calc.

_____ Children of too Fast—Ird., Ph.x.

_____ Young People of too Rapid—Kre., Pho., Ph.x.

Growing too Fat—Pho.

Habits, Sedentary—Aco., Alm., Am.c., Ana., Asr., Calc., Coc.i.,
Con., Na.am., Nux, Pet., Sep., Sil., Sul., Ter.

Haemorrahages from Gums, Nose, Rectum, in robust, sanguine
persons—Rut.

_____ Passive, copious flow of thin, black, watery blood—Sec.

Haemorrhagic Patients—Pho.

Haemorrhoidal Troubles—Cap., Plat.

Haemorrhoids, Nervous Constitutions disposed to—Sul.

_____ Tendency to, with Venous Constitution—Nux.

Hair, Black—Aur., Lrs., Mu.x., Nt.x., Thu.

_____ Brown—Cham.

_____ Dark—Aco., Arn., Bro., Bry., Caus., Con., Gph., Ign.,
Iod., K.ca., Mu.x., Nt.x., Nux, Pho., Plat., Sang.,
Sep.

_____ Dark, Choleric persons with—Nux.

_____ Dark, Hysterical Subjects with—Vb.o.

_____ Dark, in Persons of Lithic or Sycotic Diathesis—Sars.

_____ Dark, Persons with, of rigid fibre, mild, easy

disposition—Sep.

_____ Dark, Women with—Plat.

_____ Dark, Women esp., with, disposed to stoop—Pho.

_____ Fair—Cup., K.bi., Spo.

_____ Fair, Hysterical Subjects with—Vb.o.

_____ Light—Aga., Aur., Bel., Bor., Bro., Cap., Cham., Clem., Coc.i., Con., Dig., Hep., Hyo., K.bi., Lo.i., Merc., Mez., Na.c., Opi., Pet., Pul., Sbd., Spi., Spo., Su.x., Thu., Ver.

_____ Long matted, filthy people with Greasy Skin and—Sul.

_____ Red—Pho., Sep., Sul.

_____ Red, and Freckles, Choleric Women with—Lach.

_____ Sandy—Pul.

_____ Soft—Pho.

Hair, Stiff, Straight—Nx.m.

Hands, Affections of Palms of—Ana.

_____ Fetid Sweat on—Nt.x.

_____ Hot Palms—Sul.

_____ Hot and Sweaty—Sul.

_____ Sweaty—Sul.

_____ Warts on Palms of—Ana.

Hastiness, Irritability, and Restlessness in Full-blooded Persons—Sul.

Hasty Disposition—Lo.p.

Haughty Disposition when Sick—Lyc.

Head, Blood to the, in Women or Girls—Jab.

_____ Dulness of—Ag.n.

_____ Large, in Children—Calc., K.i., Sil.

_____ Sweats in Children—Calc.

Headaches, Mental Causes, from—Ag.n.

_____ Nervous Literary Men suffering from—Nic.

_____ Nervous Women, of—Ter.

Heart, Nervous Palpitation of the—Val.

_____ **or Liver Affections,** Hydrothorax depending on—Mr.s.

_____ Palpitation of, from least Motion—Dig.

Heat, Animal Defective, from Defective Oxygenation—Gph.

_____ Animal, Diminished, Constitutions with—Alm., Cyc.

_____ Flushes of followed by great Debility—Dig.

_____ Flushes of followed by Perspiration—Sul.

_____ Persons overcome by—Gui.

Heels, Rheumatic Inflammation of—Sbi.

Hepatic Troubles, Predisposed to—Lyc., Pod.

Hepatic and Lung Troubles, Lean Persons predisposed to—Lyc.

Herpetic Constitutions—Lyc.

High-living, those used to—All.

Hollow Eyes, Thin Patients with—Arg.

Home-sick Girls—Ca.p., Cap.

Hopeless and Despondent Phthisical Patients—Stn.

Hopelessness, Despair of Perfect Recovery—Pso.

Horses' Urine, Odour of Urine like—Nt.x.

Hot Countries, Tetanus of—Pas.

_____ **Hands,** sweaty—Sul.

_____ **Palms**—Sul.

_____ **Soles**—Sul.

_____ **Vertex**—Sul.

Hurry, People who do everything in a—Su.x.

Hydrocele of New-born Children—Abr.

Hydrogenoid Constitution—Arn., Na.s., Nt.x., Nx.m., Thu.

Hydrothorax depending on liver or Heart Affections—Mr.s.

Hypochondriacs—Alo., Coc., i., Lcs., Pb., Val.

_____ Subject to Skin Diseases—Lyc.

Hysteria and **Neuralgia,** subjects who suffer from—Val.

Hysterical—Act. r., Ana., Asa., Calc., Cast., Cham., Coc.i., Con., Gel., Hyo., Ign., Mag. m., Mos., Na.m., Nux. Nx. m., Plat., Pul., Sep., Stn., Sul., Trn., Vb.o.

_____ Complaints complicated with Uterine Diseases— Mag.m.

_____ Cough, Globus in—Val.

_____ Men—Cro., Mos.

_____ Nervous, Irritable Subjects in whom the Intellectual
Faculties predominate—Val.

_____ Nervous Patients subject to Choreic Affections—Trn.

_____ Nervous Persons—Ag.n.

_____ Subjects, slender—Vb.o.

_____ Subjects with dark hair—Vb.o.

_____ Subjects with fair hair—Vb.o.

_____ Temperament—Gel.

_____ Women and Men—Mos.

_____ Women who have taken too much Chamomile tea—Val.

Illness, changed mentally and physically by—Lach.

_____ Severe, Women with weakness after—Cast.

Imbecility—Arg.

Impatient Persons—Nux.

Impressionable Girls, Fair—Vi.o.

Indigestion, Melancholic People troubled with—Nux.

_____ Women suffering long from—Mag.m.

Indolent Persons—Am.m.

Indulgence, Sexual, excessive—Smb.n.

Indurations and Swellings of Glandular System—Clem.

Infancy, Complaints during—Cof.

Infants, Acids, redundant, suffering from—Na.p.

_____ Colic with Acidity, in—Na.p.

_____ Fed to Excess with milk and sugar—Na.p.

_____ Fontanelles open, with—Calc.,Sil.

_____ Spasms with Acidity, in—Na.p.

_____ Tongues coated moist, white—Ant.c.

Inflammation, Rheumatic , of heels—Sbi.

Influenza , Cough after, in Children—Sang.

_____ Nervous Weakness following—Cyp., Scu.

Insensitive to well-chosen Remedies—Opi.

_____ To well-chosen Remedies, after too much Medicine—
Teu.

Insolent Children—Sac.o.

Insomnia, Chronic, Alcoholism of—Sum.

_____ Overfatigue, due to—Chl.h.

See also **Sleep;** and **Sleeplessness**

Intellect, Dulness of—Mac.

_____ Keen, feeble muscular development—Lyc.

Intestinal Irritation of Children—Scu.

Intestines as if falling down, Sensation of, in Pregnant or
Parturient Women—Pod.

Intoxicated easily with Stimulants—Con.

Irascible Persons—Nux, Pb.

_____ Temperament and Tenacious Disposition—Nux.

Irregular Distributions of Blood—Fer.

_____ Growth of Children—Calc.

_____ Partial Sweats of Children—Calc.

Irresolute Temperament—Mez.

Irritable Bladder of Old Women—Cop.

_____ Children.Ca.br., Lyc.

_____ Nervous. Hysterical, Intellectual Subjects—Val.

_____ Persons—Aco., Ag. n., Ars., Bry., Cham., Coc.i., Col.,
Dul., Gel., Hyo., Ign., K.ph., Kre., Lips., Lyc., Mac.,
Nux.Phel., Pho., Plat., Sec., Sil., Stp., Val.

_____ Persons who are always—Nux.

_____ Persons, Nervous, with Dry Skin, profuse Saliva,
Diarrhoea, Night Sweats—Sil.

_____ Thin, Venous Debauchees—Nux.

_____ Women of Nervous Temperament—Sec.

Irritability—Bry., Sul.

_____ Bodily, Want of, and mucles lax—Opi.

_____ Restlessness and Hastiness in Full-blooded Persons—
Sul.

Irritation, Alimentary Canal, of, and Flatulence, in Disorders of

Children—Rhe.

_____ Cerebral, of Children, from Dentition—Scu.

_____ Intestinal, of Children—Scu.

Jaundiced Complexion—Pb.

_____ Half-Anaemic, Half-Jaundiced Persons of Waxy, Translucent Skin—Pho.

Jaws small, and Teeth big, Children with—K.i.

Jealous—Aps., Lach.

Jolting Conveyances, Children who cannot ride in—K.i.

Jovial—Bel.

Keen Intellect, with feeble muscular development—Lyc.

Kick-off Clothes at night, Restless, Hot Children who—Sul.

Knuckles, dirty appearance about, from Bile Pigments—Pi.x.

Labour, Disinclination for—Cyc.

_____ Flooding after every—Lach., Trl.

Labours, Tedious,when Patients becomes Nervous and Excitable—Pas.

Lack of Animal Heat—Alm., Cyc., Gph.

Lack of Reaction—Cb. v.

Lactic Acid, Diseases caused by excess of—Na. p.

Ladies, Old Maiden—Bro., Calc., Con.

Languor, Paresis easily produced, lax connective tissue—Sep.

Large Blue Veins of Pharynx; Varicose Angina—Ham.

_____ Head, in Children—Calc., Sil.

_____ Limbed Children—Sac.o.

Laughter, easily moved to—Pul.

Lax Connective Tissue, Languor, easily produced Paresis— K.ca., Sep.

_____ Fibre—Cap., Mr.bin.

_____ Fibre, Children of—Ca.br., Mag.c.

_____ Fibre, Constitutions with—Hep.

_____ Fibre, Fat Persons of—Sga.

_____ Fibre, Persons of—Cap., Fe.i., Hep., Mag. c., Mr.bin., Nt.x.

_____ Fibre, Stout Persons of—Ipc.

_____ Fibre, Women of—Sec., Spo.

_____ Muscles—Bor., Cap., Merc., Sil., Thu.(*See also* **Muscles.**)

_____ Muscles, and want of bodily irritability—Opi.

_____ Pale, Lean Persons—Ac.x.

_____ Skin—Bor., Merc.

_____ Temperament—Cld.

Laziness, Tendency to—Cyc., Lach.

Lazy Persons—Cap.

Lead Poisoning, Cramps from—Col.

Lean Persons—Ac.x., Amb., Ars., Chi., Cof., Gph., Iod., Kre., Lach., Lyc., Merc., Na.m., Nt.x., Pet., Pho., Pb., Sec., Sil., Stn., Sul., Ver.

_____ Lax, Pale Persons—Ac.x.

_____ Persons, predisposed to Lung and Hepatic conditions— Lyc.

_____ Stoop-shouldered Persons who walk and sit stoped— Sul.

Leucophlegmatic—Agn., Am.c., Ars., Bel., Calc., Cast., Chi., Cyc., Fe.p., Kre., Na.c., Pul., Sep., Ust.

_____ Persons with disposition to Catarrh—Chi.

Leucorrhoea with Amenorrhoea—Xan.

_____ Subjects of, with Disinclination for Labour—Cyc.

Life, Change of, Women never well since—Lach.

_____ Critical period of, and Pubescence—Sep.

_____ Extremes of (Children and Old People)—Ver.

_____ Sedentary, Persons who lead a—Nux.

Lifting too Much—Mil.

Light complexion—Bel., Hep., Sel., Sil., Sul.

_____ Complexion, fine skin, pale face—Sil.

_____ Eyebrows, Children with—Bro.

_____ Eyes—Lcs.

Light Hair—Aga., Aur., Bel., Bor., Bro., Cap., Cham., Clem.,
Coc.i., Con., Dig., Hep., Hyo., K.bi.,Lo.i., Merc.,
Mez., Na.c., Opi., Pet., Pul., Sbd., Spi., Spo., Su.x.,
Thu., Var.

Light-haired Children—Bro., Dig.

Light skin—Pet.

Limbs, Pains in the, and Back of Children, as if beaten—Ph.x.

_____ Tired feeling extending into—Hlon.

Lip, Pallor of—Fer.

Liquors, Spirituous, Addicted to—Lach., Nux, Opi.

Literary Men liable to Constipation—Nic.

Literary Men and others suffering from Nervous Headaches—
Nic.

Literary Sedentary Men, sick and chilly—Asr.

Lithic-acid Diathesis—Lyc.

_____ Diathesis, or Sycotic, Dark-haired Persons of—Sars.

Little Boys, Affections of—Abr.

_____ **Children,** Diseases of—Cham., Mag.c.

_____ **Girls** of Nervous Temperament—Se.a.

Lively—Aco., Bel.

_____ Perception—Ign., Pho.

Liver Affections, Children with—Mag.m.

_____ Affections, Hydrothorax depending on, or on Heart
Affections.Mr.s.

Livid Complexion—Kre.

Long Sickness, Weakened by—Fil., Scu.

Loose and Open, Everything seems—Sec.

Loss of Blood—Fe.pi.

Loss of Fluids, Persons of originally strong constitution
weakened by—Ph.x.

Loss of Voice, Tendency to—Hlt.

Love Persons who easily fall in—Ign.

_____ Persons who have been crossed in—Ca.p.

Low Spirits, Anaemic Girls with—Fer.

Low State of Vital Powers—Cb.v.

Lumbrici and Ascarides, Scrofulous Children afflicted with—
　　　　Spi.

Lung Troubles, Predisposed to—Bac., K.bi., Lo.i., Lyc., Pho.,
　　　　Sang., Sil., Tub.

Lung and **Hepatic Conditions,** Lean Persons disposed to—Lyc.

Lymphatic Children—Ca.br.

_____ Glands, in Children, hard and enlarged—Calc.

_____ Persons with Constipation or Morning Diarrhoea—Sul.

_____ Temperament—Alo., Bel., Ca. ar., Caus., Dig., Hep.,
　　　　Lach., Mur., Phel. Sul.

_____ Temperament, very fleshy persons of—Thu.

_____ Temperament, Nervous—Fil., Sep., Vi.o.

_____ Temperament, unhealthy skin, dark complexion, &c.,
　　　　Persons of—Thu.

Magnetised, Nervous Weak Persons who like to be—Pho.

Maiden Ladies, Old—Bov., Calc., Con.

Malarial Cases—Bl.o.

Malarious Fever—Fe.i.

Males—Mr.c. _See also_ **Men.**

_____ Adults, rather than Females—Mr.c., Pb.

_____ Suited less to, than to Females—Nt.o.

Malicious, Spiteful Disposition—Nux.

Marasmus, Children with—Coca, Pb.

Medicine, too much, Over-sensitive Condition produced by, and
　　　　Remedies fail to act—Teu.

Melancholic Disposition—Asr., Lach., Mac., Mur., Nux, Pul.,
　　　　Ver.

_____ or Sanguine Lymphatic Temperament—Mur.

Melancholy People troubled with Indigestion—Nux.

Memory, Weak, Persons of—Lyc.

Men—Act.s., Mag.p., Mr.c., Nt.o., Pb.

_____ Acts more on than on females—Mr. c., Pb.

_____ Drinking, addicted to—Sep.

_____ Hysterical—Cro., Mos.

_____ Literary, Sedentary, who are sick and chilly—Asr.

_____ Old and Feeble—Con. (*See also* **Old Age, &c.**)

Menses coming on some days after the proper time—Pul.

_____ Scanty, in Women or Girls—Con., Jab.

_____ too Frequent and too Profuse—Calc., Plat.

Menstrual Disturbances, Women liable to—Ag.n.

Mental Causes, Headaches from—Ag.n.

_____ Emotions, Sufferings from—Smb.n.

_____ Exertion, great, Dark-haired Persons who make—Nux.

_____ Over-excitement, Nervous Disorders from—Cyp.

_____ or Physical Exercise, Aversion to—Na.c.

Mental or Physcial Shock, Weakness from—K.ph.

_____ Strain, Persons who are wearing out under—Coca.

Mentally and Bodily Overtaxed Persons—Coca,Pi.x.

_____ and Physically Changed by Illness—Lach.

Mercurial or Scrofulous Diathesis—Fe.i.

_____ Patients—Aur.

_____ Syphilitic Affections—Lach.

Mercurialisation, after—Pod.

Mercury, People who have taken much—Asa., Lach., Mr.bin.

Mild Disposition—Alm., Coc.i., Ign., Ph.x., Pul., Sep., Vi.o.

_____ Easy Disposition, Persons of, with rigid fibre and dark hair—Sep.

_____ Impressive Girls of fair complexion—Vi.o.

Milk, Children who cannot take—Ol. j.

_____ Children who refuse, and get pain in their stomach if they take it—Mag.c.

_____ Infants fed to excess with, and sugar—Na.p.

Mind and Body, Exhaustion of—Stn.

_____ and Body, Torpidity of—Cyc.

Miscarriage, Tendency to—Sbi.

Mischievous Persons—Pul., Trn.

Mistrustful, When sick—Lyc.

Monomania, Religious, Disposed to—Pb., Sul.

Moral Emotions, Debility after a long succession of—Ph.x.

Morning Diarrhoea, or Constipation, Lymphatic Persons with— Sul.

Mothers—*See* **Nursing; Pot-bellied; Pregnancy; Pregnant; Women,** After-pains , &c.

Motion, Palpitation from Least—Dig.

_____ Symptoms set up by—Fer.

Mountaineers—(Ars.), Ver.

_____ Movement, children slow in—Calc.

Mucous Membranes, Affections of—Gph.

_____ Membranes, Pallor of—Fer.

_____ Surfaces covered with Squamous Epithelium, Syphilitic Affections of—Mr.i.f.

Mucus, Yellow, Tenacious, Catarrh with discharge of—Sum.

Muscles, Flabby—Aga., Calc., Hep., K.ca., Sil., Spo., Ver.

_____ Lax—Bor., Cap., Merc., Sil., Thu.

_____ Lax, with want of Bodily Irritability—Opi.

_____ Soft—Hep.

Muscular Development feeble, Intellect keen—Lyc.

_____ Fibre, lax, Women of—Sec., Spo.

_____ System relaxed—Sbd.

_____ System weakened—Sbd.

_____ Weakness—Mac.

Narrow-chested Patients—Calc., Pho.

Nasal and Pharyngeal Catarrch, with Nervousness, &c—Sum.

Natures, Sensitive—Mos., Pho.(*See also* **Sensitive.**)

_____ Spoiled—Mos.

Negroes—Sul.

Nervo-sanguine or Sanguine Temperament, Young People and Women of—Ver.

Nervous—Aco., Act. r., Ail., Amb., Am.c., Ana., Aps., Arn., Ars., Asa., Asr., Bel., Bor., Bry., Cham., Chi., Coc.i., Cof., Dig., Gel., Glo., Hyo., Ign., Lo.p., Mag.m., Nux, Pho., Pso., Pul., Sec., Sep., Sil., Stp., Sul., Val.

_____ Affections, especially in subjects of Sycosis—Lun.

_____ Affections occurring Excitable Temperaments—Val.

_____ Agitation—Scu.

_____ Attacks when the Aura starts from Abdomen—Cast.

_____ Babies—K.Ph.

_____ Bilious Temperament—Amb.

_____ Children—Amb., Ca.br., Hyn.

_____ Children who have been frightened—Hyn.

_____ Children, unmanageable when sick—Lyc.

_____ Constitutions disposed to Haemorrhoids—Sul.

_____ Coughs—Crl.

_____ Debility after Influenza—Scu.

_____ Disorders from Mental Over-excitement—Cyp.

_____ Dried-up looking—Amb.

_____ Excitable, when the Patient becomes, with tedious labours—Pas.

_____ Excitement, reflex—Cyp.

_____ Exhaustion—Stn.

_____ Girls, tall, thin—Vio.

_____ Headache, Literary Men suffering from—Nic.

_____ Hysterical Patients subject to Choreic Affections—Trn.

_____ Hysterical Persons—Ag.n.

_____ Irritable, Hysterical subjects in whom the Intellectual Faculties predominate—Val.

_____ Irritable Persons with Dry Skin, profuse Saliva,

        Diarrhoea, Night Sweats—Sil.

_____ Palpitation of the Heart—Val.

_____ Persons, who dread a storm—Rho.

_____ Temperament—Crl., Gel., Ign., Sep.

_____ Temperament (esp.females)—Ced., Sc.a., Xan.

_____ Temperament, Persons of, quick motioned—Sul.

_____ Temperament, Women and Little Girls of—Se.a.

_____ and Vital Powers, depression of, after long sickness—
        Scu.

Nervous, Weak Persons who like to be magnetised—Pho.

_____ Weakness follwing, Influenza—Cyp., Scu.

_____ Women—Cast., K.br., Sec., Se. a., Xan.

_____ Women, Amenorrhoea, subject to—Ter.

_____ Women, Dysmenorrhoea, subject to—Ter.

_____ Women, Headache, subject to—Ter.

_____ Women with Pains, Cramps, &c., after severe illness—Cast.

Nervously run-down Females—Hlon.

Nervousness or Cough, Sleeplessness due to—Sti.

_____ with Nasal and Pharyngeal Catarrh—Sum.

Neuralgia, Subjects who suffer from—Sti., Val.

Neuritis, Traumatic—Cep.

Newborn Children—Abr., Ipc., Lach.

Nick-nacks, Little Children wanting—Sac.o.

Nose, Haemorrhages from, Gums, Rectum—Rut.

_____ Picking—Sum.

Nose-bleed of Children—Ter.

Nurses, Diseases of —Cham.

Nursing Mothers, worn out, distracted by nervous babies—K.ph.

_____ Women —Rhe., Sep.

Nutrition, Defective—Ol.j., Sil.

_____ Weak and deficient—Phel.

Obesity—Cap.

_____ People inclined to—K.br., Sga.(*See also* **Fat.**)

Occupy themselves in any way, Children not caring to—Sac.o.

Odour, Disagreeable, Patients emit—Pso.

_____ Urine of, like Horses' Urine—Nt.x.

Old Age—Aur., Ird.

_____ Age, Bronchial Affections of—Amc., Hpz.

_____ Age, Bronchitis of—Hpz.

_____ Age, Choleraic Affections in—Aeth.

_____ Age, Complaints of—Fl.x., Ter.

_____ Age, Premature—Fl.x., Stum.

_____ Age, Weakness of—Nx.m.

_____ Asthmatics—Ill.

_____ Bachelors—Con.

_____ Cases of Syphilis—Mr.bin.

_____ Decrepit Persons—Sec.

_____ Drunkards—Ill.

_____ Maiden Ladies—Bro., Calc., Con.

_____ Maids, Premature—Fl.x.

_____ Men, feeble—Con.

Old People—Ac.x., Alo., Amb., Cb.a., Cb.v., Cic. v., Coca, Con., Lach., Na.m., Sbd., Sga., Sul. Su.x., Teu., Ver.

_____ People, Bronchial Affections in—Amc., Hpz.

_____ People, Children with faces like—Sars.

_____ People, Dyspepsia of—Nx.m.

_____ People and Children (first and second childhood)—Opi.

_____ People, great weakness, with—Nt.x.

_____ People, Profuse Watery Diarrhoea, esp. of—Gam.

_____ Withered Man, child like an—Ag.n.

_____ Women—Kre., Lyc.

_____ Women especially—Su.x.

Old-looking Children—Kre, Sars.

Old-looking Children, hard to awaken—Kre.

Old Maiden Ladies—Bro., Calc., Con.

Olive-brown Complexioned People—Aur.

Open-air, Aversion to—Cap., Na.c.

_____ Dread of—Cap.

_____ Persons who live in—Cf.t.

Organisation, Women of Delicate—Xan.

Oriflces, Affections of—Gph.

Outrageously Cross Children—Hep.

Over-dosed with Mercury—Asa., Lach., Mr.bin.

Over-drain of the System—K.ph.

Over-excitement, Mental, Nervous disorders from—Cyp.

Over-fatigue, Insomnia due to—Chl.h.

Over-lifting—Mil.

Over-sensitive Condition which too much Medicine has
            produced—Teu. (*See also* **Drugged Subjects.**)

Over-sensitive Persons, Physically and Mentally—Sil.

Over-strain of the System—K.Ph.

Over-taxed Persons, Mentally and Bodily—Coca, Pi.x.

Oxygenation Defective, from Deficient Animal Heat—Gph.

Paines, Children with, in Back and Limbs—Ph.x.

_____ Women of, at Climacteric—Su.x. (*See also*
            Climacteric.)

_____ Cramps, &c., in Nervous Women—Cast.

Pale Children—Calc., Mr.d.,Pso.

_____ Face—Pul., Sil.

_____ Face Fine Skin, Light Complexion, Weakly Persons
            with—Sil.

_____ Lax, Lean Persons—Ac.x.

_____ Persons—Ac. x., K.i., K.ph., Led., Spi.

_____ Skin—Arg.

_____ Thin Patients with tendency to Caries—Arg.

Pale Women—Eu. pi., Lc.x., Sec.

Pallor, Lips, of—Fer.

_____ Mucous Membranes, of—Fer.

Palms of Hands, Affections of—Ana.

_____ Hot—Sul.

_____ Warts on—Ana.

Palpitation from Least Motion—Dig.

_____ Nervous, of the Heart—Val.

Paralyses, Functional, of all descriptions—Gel.

_____ Professional—Gel.

Paresis, Easily Produced, Lax Connective Tissue, Languor—Sep.

Particular Persons, very—Nux.

Parturient Women with Sensation as if Intestines were Falling Down—Pod.

Peevish Children—Pso.

Peevishness—Sul.

Pepper, Persons Addicted to—Nux.

Perception, Quick—Ign., Pho.

_____ Slow—Oln.

Period of Life, Critical, and Pubescence—Sep.

Persons, Professional, Paralyses of—Gel.

Perspiration, following flushes of Heat, all over the body—Sul.

Perspire Easily, Persons who do not—Nx.m.

_____ Profusely, Patients who—Lo.p.

Perspiring, Effects of Draughts while—Mr.i.f.

Pharyngeal and Nasal Catarrh, with Nervousness, &c—Sum.

Pharynx, Veins of, Large and Blue; Varicose Angina—Ham.

Philosophical or Religious Subjects, Dirty-looking Persons always Speculating on—Sul.

Phlebitis—Ham.

Phlegmatic—Alo.,Asa., Cld., Cyc., Dul., Lach., Mez., Pul., Sga.,Src.

_____ Habit, Women of—Alo.

Phthisical Patients—Bac., Pho., Thu.

_____ Patients who are despondent and without hope—Stn.

Phthisis in Third Stage—Fe.i.

Physical Shock, or Mental, Weakness from—K.ph.

_____ Strain, Persons who are Wearing out under—Coca.

Physically and Mentally Changed by Illness—Lach.

Pining Boys—Aur.

Plethora, Venous—Cb. a., Cb.v.

Plethoric—Aco., Arn., Ars., Aur., Bel., Bry., Chi., Fer., Sel.,
Hyo., Nt.x., Pho., Pul., Sec., Stm.

_____ Persons, Ailments of—Stm.

_____ Subjects—Coca, K.i., Lips., Sec., Sul., Ve.v.

Plethroric Subjects, with great Soreness—Hyp.

_____ Women—Glo.

_____ Women Suffering from Inflammation of the Heels—Sbi.

Pleuritic Diseases—Ziz.

Pneumonia—Fe.i.

Prok, Ill Effects caused by Eating—Pul.

Portal System, Persons Subject to Congestions of—Sul.

Pot-bellied Mothers, Yellow Saddle across Nose, Faint from
least Motion—Sep.

Pregnancy, Women during in Childbed, and while Nursing—Sep.

Pregnant Women—Aet., Anac., Cham., Nx.m., Pul., Rhe., Sep.

_____ or Parturient Women with Sensation as if Intestiness
were Falling Down—Pod.

Premature Old Age—Fl. x., Stm.

Professional and Business Men, Worn-out—K.ph.

_____ Persons, Paralyses of—Gel.

Prolapsus Uteri, Affected with—Bel., Hlon., Nux., Pod., Sep.

Psoric Constitutions—Alm., Bac., Hep., Pso., Sul., Tub.

Puberty, Girls at—Aur.

Pubescence, and the Critical Period of Life—Sep.

Public Speakers—Stn.

**Puffed, Flabby Persons with Yellow or Dirty-brown Blotched
Skin**—Sep.

Pulmonary Affections with Liver Involvement—Sang.

_____ **Congestion,** Subjects liable to—Lips.

_____ **Puny** Children—Ird.

_____ Children, Dentition during—Mag.m.

_____ **Sickly** Children—Lyc., Mag. c.
Putrid Diseases, Persons with—Ars., Kre.

Quick Perception—Ign.
_____ in Perception and in Executing—Ign.
_____ Persons—Pho.
Quick-motioned Persons of Nervous Temperament—Sul.
Quick-tempered Persons—Sul.
Quinine, Cases previously Maltreated with—Az., Na. m. (See also **CAUSATION.**)

"Ragged Philosophers."—Sul.
Rainy Weather, Cases ≤ in—Bl.o.
Rapid Progress of Disease—Stn.i.
Rapidity in Executing—Ign. (*See also* **Quick.**)
Rapidly, Children and Young Persons who have Grwon too—Ird., Kre., Ph.x., Pho.
Rash, Fiery Red, about Anus of Babies—Med.
Reaction, Vital, People who are deficient in—Cb.v., Pso., Ver.
Readily-affected Persons, Nervous, Sanguine—Glo.
Recovering from Scarlatina, Children—Pts.
Recovery, Persons who Despair of Perfect—Pso.
Red Face (also in hectic)—Ol.j.
_____ Face from least Exertion—Fer.
_____ Fiery Rash about Anus of Babies—Med.
_____ Hair—Pho., Sep., Sul.
_____ Hair and Freackles, Choleric Women with—Lach.
_____ Sediment in Urine—Lyc.
Relaxed Fibre—Fe.i., Nt.x.
_____ Habit, Women of—Alo.
_____ Muscular System—Sbd. (*See also* **Muscles**; and **Muscular.**)

_____ Tissues—K.ca.

Religious Monomania, Disposed to—Pb.

_____ or Philosophical Subjects, Dirty-looking Persons who are always Speculating on—Sul.

Remedies Fail to Act, when after too much Medicine—Teu.

_____ Well-chosen, Persons Insensitive to—Opi.

Remittent Bilious Attacks, Children liable to—Mr.d.

Renal or Vesical Symptoms prominent—Ber.

Restless Children, Hot, Kick off Clothes at Night—Sul.

_____ Persons—Ars., Dul., Sul.

_____ Persons who are easily Startled—Pso.

Restlessness, Excessive, ≥ by moving about—Mac.

_____ and Hastiness in Full-blooded Persons, with great Irritability—Sul.

Rheumatic Diathesis—Act. r., Bry., K.bi., Led., Rhs., Sti., Ter.

_____ Diathesis Aneamic, Debilitated Subjects of—Spi.

_____ Inflammations of Heels—Sbi.

_____ Subjects sensitive to Damp Weather—Phyt., Sti.

Rheumatism, Chronic—Ter.

Rickety Children, Bowel Complaints of—Med.

_____ Children during Dentition—Mag.m.

_____ Puny Children, having Eruptions about Eyes—Mag.m.

Ride in Jolting Conveyances, Children who cannot—K.i.

Riding Persons Intolerant of—Bor.

Rigid Fibre—Caus., Con., Nux, Nt.x., Plat., Sep.

_____ Fibre, Dark Hair, Mild Disposition—Sep.

_____ Fibre, Women of—Con.

_____ *See also* **Fibre.**

Robust Persons—Ail., Rut.

_____ Persons, Fleshy, who suddenly become Emaciated—Smb.n.

Romantic Young Persons—Ant.c., Ign.

Rosy Skins—Sep.

Run-down, Nervously, Females—Hlon.

Sad Disposition—Kre.

Sadness, Tendency to—Lach.

Saliva, Profuse, Nervous, Irritable Persons with Dry Skins and—
Sil.

Sallow People with Cold Extremities—Lyc.

_____ **People** of Slow Comprehension—Lyc.

_____ **Skin**—Fl.x.

Sandy Hair—Pul.

Sanguine—Aco., Arn., Aur., Cof., Fer., Glo., Hyo., Ign.

Sanguine or Nervo-sanguine Temperament, Women of—Ver.

_____ or Sanguine Lymphatic Temperament—Mur.

_____ Temperament—Aco., Arn., Aur., Cof., Fer., Glo., Hyo.,
Ign., Led.,Mur., Pho., Rut.

_____ Temperament Inclined to Congestions—Sep.

_____ Women—Plat.

Scanty Menses in Women or Girls—Con., Jab.

Scarlatina, Children Recovering from—Pts.

Scarred Tissue, Specific Relation to—Sil., Thio.

School-girls—Ca.p.

Scorbutic Conditions—Jg.c.

Scrawny Women—Ag.n., Amb., Sec.

Scrofulous—Aps., Ars., Asa., Aur., Ba.c., Bro., Ca. ar., Calc., Ca. p.,
Cb.a., Caus., Chm.u., Con., Dul., Fe.i., Gel., Gph.,
Hep., Iod., Jg. c., Lyc., Merc., Mr.bin., Mr.i.f., Na.m.,
Pso., Rhs., Sc.a., Sep., Sil., Spi., Spo., Sul.

_____ Children—Am.c., Ba.m., Cur., Dig., Merc., Mr.d.

_____ Children Afflicted with Ascarides and Lumbrici—Spi.

_____ Children, Bone Affections of, when Associated with
Diarrhoea—Sto.c.

_____ Children, Diseases which Affect the Air-passages of—
Smb.n.

_____ Children who have Worm Diseases during Dentition—
Sil.

_____ Diathesis in Persons Subject to Various Congestions,

esp. of Portal System—Sul.

_____ or Mercurial Diathesis—Fe.i.

_____ Persons, Bronchorrhoea in—Fe.i.

_____ Subjects Sensitive to Cold Air—Cis.

Seasons, Change of, Affections which come on in—Rho., Sul.

(*See also* **Autumn; Earliest; Spring; Storm; Thunder; Weather.**)

Sedentary Habits, Persons of—Aco., Alm., Ana., Calc., Coc.i., Con., Na.m., Nux, Pet., Sep., Sil., Sul., Ter.

_____ Literary Men, Sick and Chilly—Asr.

_____ Persons, Chronic Ailments of—Alm.

_____ Women—Am.c.

Semi-dropsical, Lower Part of Body, Upper wasted—Lyc.

Senses Enfeebled or Suspended—Cyc.

Sensitive—Ail., Asa., As., Bor., Gel., Glo., Ign., K.Ph., Mos., Nux., Pho.

_____ Persons, Physically and Mentally—Sil.

_____ Scrofulous Persons, to Cold Air—Cis.

_____ Sexual Organs, Exceedingly—Plat.

_____ Syphilitic Subjects, to Damp Weather—Phyt.

_____ Touch, to Affected Parts very—Gui., Hep.

_____ Women—Eu.pi., Glo., Ign.

Sensitiveness Diffused—K.i.

_____ Great, produced by too much medicine—Teu.

_____ Great, of ulcers to slightest contact—Hep.

_____ Of the surface of the body—K.i., Lach.

_____ Sexual Excesses Fe., pi., Ph. x.

_____ Excesses, Persons Exhausted by—Sep.

_____ Excitement, Persons that are disposed to—Sep.

_____ Indulgence, Excessive—Smb.n.

_____ Organs exceedingly Sensitive—Plat.

Shock, Mental or Physical, Weakness from—K.ph.

Short-breathed People—Coca.

Sick, Haughty when—Lyc.

_____ Violent when—Bel.

_____ Weak Children, Unmanageable when—Lyc.

Sickly, Delicate Children—Pso.

Sickness, Long, Depression of Nervous and Vital Powers after—
         Scu.

Silica, Patients who are Deficient in—Lo.p.

Sinking, Constant, but cannot Eat—Grt.

Singers—Stn.

_____ Helped to Hold the Voice—Mth.pi.

Skin, Affections of—Gph.

_____ Affections, Dirty People prone to—Sul.

_____ Atmospheric Changes, Excessively Sensitive to—Sul.

_____ Blotched—Sep.

_____ Blueness of—Cb.a.

_____ Broken—Caln.

_____ Cook, Dry—Nx.m., Vi.o.

_____ Dark—Ign., Iod.

_____ Delicate—Bro., Caus.

Skin, Delicate, Children with—Bro.

_____ Dirty Brown or Yellow, Flabby Persons with—Sep.

_____ Dry and Cool—Nx.m., Vio.

_____ Dry, Profuse Saliva, Diarrhoea, Night-sweats—Sil.

_____ Dry, Women or Girls with—Jab.

_____ Earthy, Yellow, Wrinkled—Spi.

_____ Fair—Pho.

_____ Fine, Pale Face, Light Complexion—Sil.

_____ Flabby and Ill-nourished—Mr.d.

_____ Greasy, and Long Matted Hair—Sul.

_____ Diseases, Hypochondriacs subject to—Lyc.

_____ Lax—Bor., Merc.

_____ Light—Pet.

_____ Pale—Arg.

_____ Rosy—Sep.

_____ Sallow—Fl.x.

_____ Tawny—Iod.

_____ Those subject to Diseases of the—Pso.

_____ Translucent—Pho.

_____ Unhealthy, of Persons of Lymphatic Temperament—Thu.

_____ Waxy—Pho.

_____ White—Bro., Sep.

_____ White, Children with—Bro.

_____ White, Pure, with Delicate Constitutions—Sep.

_____ Wrinkled—Bor.

_____ Wrinkled, Yellow, Earthy—Spi.

_____ Yellow—Iod., Spi.

_____ Yellow, or Dirty brown, Blotched, Puffed, Flabby Persons with—Sep.

Sleep, Children Cross after, Pushing every one away—Lyc.

_____ Patient Lying long in Bed before he can—Pul.

Sleeplessness due to Nervousness or to Cough—Sti.

_____ Nervousness and Tendency to Spasms, esp. in Children—Sum. *See also* **Insomnia.**

Slender—Alm., Bry., Calc., Pet., Pho., Vi.o.

_____ Tall Children—Ph.x., Pho.

_____ Tall Females—Sga.

_____ Tall, Hysterical Subjects—Vb.o.

_____ Tall Persons—Pho., Vi.o.

Slight Persons—Kre.

Slim, Slender Children—Ph.x.

Slow to Act—Hep.

_____ Comprehension, Sallow People of—Lyc.

_____ in Movement, Children—Calc.

Slwo Perception—Oln.

_____ Torpid Constitution—Am.m., Caus., Clem., Coc.i., Dul., Hep., K.bi., Kre., Pul.

Sluggish—Am.m., Coc.c., K.bi.

Smell, Filthy of Body, not removed by Washing—Pso. (See also

Odour.)

Smelling-bottle, Women always having Recourse to—Am.c.

Soft Hair—Pho.

_____ Muscles—Hep. (*See also* **Muscles.**)

_____ Tissues—K.ca.

Soles, Hot—Sul.

Soreness, Abdominal—Cast.

_____ Great, in the Plethoric—Hyp.

Sore Throat, Chronic, of Public Speakers—Mr.cy.

_____ **Throats** that are < from Cold Air—Sbd.(*See also* **Throats,** Sore.)

Sour Babies—Su.x.

_____ Smell, Persons of—Mag.c.

Spare—Alm., Chel.

_____ Habit, Women of—Xan.

(*See also* **Thin.**)

Spasmodic Complaints complicated with Uterine Diseases— Mag.m.

Spasms or Colic, with Acidity, of Infants—Na.p.

_____ Tendency to, with Nervousness and Sleeplessness, esp.in Children—Sum.

Speak, it Hurts the Patient to—Mr.cy.

Speakers, Public—Stn.

_____ Public, Chronic Sore Throat of—Mr.cy.

Speculating on Religious and Philosophical subjects, Persons who are always—Sul.

Spiteful, Malicious Disposition—Nux.

Spoiled Natures—Mos.

Sprains—Mil.

Sprightliness and Moral Power, thin Females having retained a good deal of—Sga.

Spring, Affections which come on in—Rho.

Spirituous Liquors, Addicted to—Lach., Nux, Opi.

Standing, Persons to whom it is the most Uncomfortable

Position—Sul.

Startled Easily, Restless Persons who are—Pso.

Sterile—Am.c., Bor., Cth., Merc., Pho., Phy.

Stimulants, Persons easily Intoxicated with—Con.

Stomach or Bowels, Flatulence in, after Meals, causing Colic—
    Dio.

Stonecutters' Ailments—Sil.

Stoop, Inclination to, in Young Persons—Pho.

Styooping Persons—Cof.

Stoop-shouldered—Pho., Sul.

_____ Lean Persons who walk and Sit Stooped—Sul.

Storm, Nervous Persons who Dread a—Rho.

Stout Persons—Ail., Mag.p.

_____ Persons of Lax Fibre—Ipc.

_____ Women—Am.c.

Straight, Stiff Hair—Nx.m.

Strain, Mental or Physical, Persons who are Wearing out under—
    Coca., Pi.x.

_____ of the System, too great—K.ph.

Strong Persons—Mag.p.

_____ Persons weakened by Loss of Fluids—Ph.x.

Strumous Persons—Thu.

Studiously Inclined—Nux.

Submissive—Pul.

Substantial Food, Children caring nothing for—Sac.o.

Sucklings and Children during Dentition—Rhe.

Sudden Cases due to Climatic Changes—Lpt.

Sugar and Milk, Infants Fed to Excess with—Na.p.

Summer Weather, Persons who are < in—Lach.

Sun, Persons who cannot stand the—Lach.

Sunken Countenance, Women of—Sec.

Suppressed Eruptions, Diseases caused by—Sul.

_____ Eruptions, those who have had—Pso.

Suppuration, great Tendency to—Hep.

Surface of the Body, Sensitiveness of—K.i., Lach.

Suspended Senses, or Enfeebled—Cyc.

Sutures Open, Children with—Calc., Sil.

Swarthy Complexion—Chi., Nt.x.

Sweating, Easy—K.ca.

Sweat, Fetid, on Feet, Hands, or in Axilla—Nt.x.

_____ Hands, on—Sul.

_____ Head, on, Children with—Calc.

_____ Irregular and Partial., Children with—Calc.

Swelling of Cervical and other Glands in Children—Mr.d.

_____ and Induration of Glands—Clem.

Sycosis—Med., Mld., Nit.ac., Thu., Vac.

Sycotic or Lithic Diathesis, Dark-haired Persons of—Sars.

_____ **Persons**—Thu.

_____ **Subjects** esp., Nervous Affections of—Lun.

Syphilis, Old cases of—Mr.bin.

_____ Subjects of Hereditary or Acquired—Plo.

Syphilitic Mercurial Affections—Lach.

Syphilitic Subjects—Asa., Aur., Cnb., Fl.x., K.bi., K.i., Merc., Mr.i.f. Mt., Nt.x., Syph., Thu.

_____ Subjects who are Sensitive to Damp Weather—Phyt.

_____ Taint—Clem., Syph.

Tall—Arg.n., Cof., Kre., Pho., Ust.

_____ Children, Slender and slim—Ph.x.

_____ Girls, thin, nervous—Vi.o.

_____ Slender, hysterical subjects—Vb.o.

_____ Slender persons—Pho., Vi.o.

_____ Slender, thin, sprightly females—Sga.

Tawny Skin—Iod.

Tea-drinkers, Colic of—Dio.

Tears, Easily moved to—Pul.

Tedious Labours, Patient nervous and excitable—Pas.

Teeth Big and Jaws Small, Children with—K.i.

_____ Patients whose Teeth are always decaying—Lo.p.

Teething Children—Aeth., Mag.p., Na.m.

Temper, Bad—Bry.

Temperament, Bilious—Aco., Ail., Amb., Ana., Aps., Ars., Bel.,
        Ber., Bry., Cham., Chi., Chio., Col., Cub., Mr.d.,
        Nux, Pet., Plat., Pb., Pod., Pul., Sep., Sul.

_____ Brunette—Iod., Nt.x.

_____ Choleric—Cof., Col.

_____ Excitable—Amb., Ced., Cham., Con., Gel., Hyo., Hyn.,
        Ign., Nux, Sep., Val.

_____ Excitable (esp. females)—Ced., Ign.

_____ Excitable, nervous affections occurring in—Val.

_____ Excited easily (also opposite Temperament.)—Con.

_____ Hasty—Lo. po., Sul.

_____ Hysterical—_See_ **Hysterical.**

_____ Impatient—Nux.

_____ Impressionable—Vi.o.

_____ Indolent—Am.m.

_____ Irascible—Nux.

_____ Irresolute—Mez.

_____ Irritable—_See_ **Irritable.**

_____ Lax—Cld. (_See also_ **Lax Connective Tissue, &c.**)

_____ Leuco-phlegmatic—Agn., Am.c., Ars., Bel., Calc.,
        Cast., Chi., Cyc., Fe. p., Kre., Na.c., Pul., Sep., Ust.

_____ Lymphatic—Alo., Bel., Ca.ar., Caus., Dig., Hep., Lach.,
        Mur. Phel., Sul.

Temperament, Lymphatic, Children of—Ca.br.

_____ Lymphatic, in very Fleshy Persons—Thu.

_____ Lymphatic, with Dark Complexion, Unhealthy Skin,
        &c—Thu.

_____ Lymphatico-nervous—Fil., Sep., Vi.o.

_____ Melancholic—Asr., Lach., Mac., Mur., Nux, Pul., Ver.

_____ Melancholic or Sanguine Lymphatic—Mur.

_____ Mild—*See* **Mild Disposition.**

_____ Mischievous—Pul., Trn.

_____ Mistrustful when Sick—Lyc.

_____ Nervous—*See* **Nervous.**

_____ Nervous (esp. females)—Ced., Se.a.

_____ Nervous, Women and little Girls of—Se.a.

_____ Nervous, Persons of, quick-motioned—Sul.

_____ Phlegmatic—Alo., Asa., Cld., Chi., Cyc., Dul., Lach., Mez., Pul., Sga., Src.

_____ Restless—Ars., Dul., Mac., Pso., Sul.

_____ Sanguine—*See* **Sanguine.**

_____ Sanguine, inclined to congestions—Sep.

_____ Sanguine or Nervo-sanguine, Women of—Ver.

_____ Sensitive—See **Sensitive.**

_____ Slow, Torpid—Am.m., Caus., Clem., Coc.,i., Dul., Hep., K.bi., Kre., Pul. (*See also* **Slow** to Act, &c.)

_____ Women of Nervous—Se.a.,Xan.

_____ Women and Little Grils of Nervous—Se.a.

Tenacious, Irascible Disposition—Nux.

Tense Fibre—Nux. (*See also* **Fibre.**)

Terror, Fear, and Timidity—Spo.

Tetanus of Hot Countries—Pas.

Thin—Alm., Aps., Ag. n., Chel., Chi., Lach., Nux, Pho., Spi., Ust.

_____ Black Watery Blood, copious flow of, Passive Haemorrhages—Sec.

_____ Females having retained a good deal of Sprightliness and Moral Power—Sga.

_____ Girls, Tall, Nervous—Vi.o.

_____ Irritable, Venous Debauchees,—Nux.

_____ Pale Patients with tendency to Caries—Arg.

_____ Patients with deep Ulcers—Arg.

_____ Patients with Hollow Eyes—Arg.

_____ Women—Amb., Plat., Sec., Sga., Xan.

Throats, Sore, Chronic, of Public Speakers—Mr.cy.

_____ Sore, Old Chronic, that are ≤ from Cold Air—Sbd.

_____ Sore, with Rawness in Spots, and Broken-down
Appearance—Mr.cy.

Thunder, Persons who are particularly Afraid of—Rho.

Timid Persons—Coca,coc.i.

Timidity, Fear, and Terror—Spo.

Tired Feeling extending into Limbs—Hlon.

Tissue, Connective, Active with new Growth, &c—Sil.

_____ Connective, lax, with Languor ans easily-produced
Paresis—Sep.

_____ Relaxed—K.ca.

_____ Scarred, specific relation to—Sil., Thio.

_____ Soft—K.ca.

Tongues Coated Moist White, Infants and Children with—Ant.c.

Torpid, Slow Constitutions—Am.m., Caus., Clem., Coc.i., Dul.,
Hep., K.bi., Kre., Pul. (See also **Slow** to Act, &c.)

Torpidity of Mind and Body—Cyc.

Touch, Affected Parts very Sensitive to—Gui., Hep.

Touched, Children who cannot bear to be—Ant. c., K.i.

Translucent Skin—Pho.

Traumatic Neuritis—Cep.

Trembling, Internal—Caul., Su.x.

Tremor, Quivering—Gel.

Tubercle, Tendency to—Arg.

Tuberculous Persons—Ca.ar., Na.m., Tub., Vi.o.

Ulcers, Deep, Thin Patients with—Arg.

_____ Sensitiveness, Great, to Slightest Contact of—Hep.

Unclean Persons—Cap.

Undernourished States—Lyc.

Unhealthy-looking Children having a Disagreeable Odour—
Pso.

Unhealthy Skin of Persons of Lymphatic Temperament—Thu.

Urinary Difficulties of Babies—Pts.

_____ Difficulties in Women—Mth.pi.

Urination and Defecation, Frequency of, Children inclined to—
K.i.

Urine, Limpid, Profuse Flow of—Val.

_____ Red Sediment in—Lyc.

_____ Scalding, Babies with—Med.

_____ Strong Odour of, like Horses'—Nt.x.

_____ Transparent, with Red Sediment—Lyc.

Uterine Disorders, Women who Suffer from—Act.r., Caul., Coc.
i., Hlon., Mag.m.

_____ Diseases Complicated with Hysterical or Spasmodic
Complaints—Mag.m.

Uterus, Women with Prolapse of—Bel., Hlon., Nux, Pod., Sep.

Vaccination, Ailments from—Thu.
See also CAUSATION.

Varicose Angina, Veins of Pharynx large and blue—Ham.

_____ Veins, Young Persons with—Fe.p., Ham.

Various Congestions, esp. of Portal System, Persons subject to
scrofulous diathesis—Sul.

Veins—*See* **Phlebitis;** *and* **Varicose.**

Venery, excessive, those liable to cramps and colic from—Col.

Venous Constitution with tendency to Haemorrhoids—Nux.

_____ Constitutions—Cb.a.

_____ Plethora—Cb.a., Cb.v.

_____ System Engorged—Cb.v.

_____ Thin, Irritable Debauchees—Nux.

Vertex, Hot—Sul.

Vesical or Renal Symptoms, Prominent—Ber.

Vessels, Flabby, no action, in Women of lax fibre—Sec.

Vigorous Persons of Dry Habit—Nux.

Violent, Acute Diseases, Persons weakened by—Ph.x.

Violent when Sick—Bel.

Vital and Nervous Powers, Depression of, after long sickness—
Scu.

_____ Powers, low state of—Cb.v.

_____ Reaction, People who are deficient in—Cb.v., Pso., Ver.

Voice, helps Singers to hold the—Mth.pi.

_____ Tendency to loss of—Hlt.

Voluptuous Disposition—Ced.

Wakefulness—Val.

Warts on the Palms—Ana.

Washed or Bathed, Children who cannot bear to be—Sul.

Washing, Burning Pain from—For.

_____ Cold, renewed Burning Pain from—For.

Wasted, Upper part of Body, lower semi-dropsical—Lyc.

Water, Persons who Dream about—Ve.v.

Waxy Skin—Pho.

Weak Children, Unmanageable when Sick—Lyc.

_____ **Children** with well-developed Heads—Lyc.

_____ Digestion—Dio., Nic.

_____ Digestion of elderly People—Pr.v.

_____ Limbed Children—Ird.

_____ Memory, Persons of—Lyc.

_____ Nervous Persons who like to be magnetised—Pho.

_____ People—Alet., Coca., Spi.

Weakened by Long Sickness—Fil.

_____ Muscular System—Sbd. (_See also_ **Muscular.**)

_____ Persons—Lach.

Weakened by Violent, Acute Diseases—Ph.x.

Weakly—Alm., Am., c., Ars., Calc., Cb.v., Caus., Chi., Fer., Fl.x.,
Hel., Iod., Ka.c., Lach., Lyc., Na.m., Nux, Ph.x.,
Rhs., Sep., Sil., Stn., Sul., Ver., Zin.

_____ Persons, excitability, with—Lun.

_____ Persons, fine skin, pale face, light complexion,with—
        Sil.

Weakness which seems to come from Deep-seated Dyscrasia—
        Su.x.

_____ Great, old people with—Nt.x.

_____ Muscular—Mac.

_____ Nervous, following Influenza—Cyp.

_____ Old age of—Nx.m.

_____ Out of proportion to the Disease—Su.x.

_____ Shock, mental or physical, from—K.ph.

_____ Women with, after severe illness—Cast.

Wearing-out, Mental or physical strain, under—Coca.

Weather Changes, Children who take Cold readily when the—
        Sep.

_____ Cold, Bronchial Affections in Old People during—
        Am.c.

_____ Cold, Wet, getting cold in—Bor.

_____ Damp, syphilitic subjects who are sensitve to—Phyt.

_____ Rainy, Cases ≤ in—Bl.o.

_____ Summer, persons who are ≤ in—Lach.

Whining and Cross Children—Sac.o.

White Complexions, Children with—Dig.

_____ Moist, Coated Tongues, Infants with—Ant.c.

_____ Pure Skin and Delicate Constitutions—Sep.

_____ Skin—Bro., Sep.

Whooping-cough, severe Cough *after*—Sang.

Widows—Aps.

Wine, Persons addicted to—Nux.

Women—Cro., Ipc., Merc., Nx.m., Pul.

_____ Affections of—Chi.

_____ After-pains of Women who have borne many
        Children—Cup.

_____ Amenorrhoea, Nervous Women subject to—Ter.

_____ Anaemic—Lc.x.

	Bilious—Plat.
	Bladders, irritable, old Women with—Cop.
	Blood to the Head, with tendency to—Jab.
	Cachectic appearance of—Sec.
	Chamomile tea, Hysterical Women who have taken too much—Val.
	Change of Life, never well since—Lach.
	Childbed, in—Sep.
	Choleric, with Freckles and Red Hair—Lach.
	Chronic ailments of—Sbi.
Women,	Climaxis, approaching the—Ca.ar.
	Dark Hair, with—Plat.
	Dark Hair, with disposed to stoop—Pho.
	Delicate—Eu.pi.
	Delicate organisation, of—Xan.
	Diseases of—Mag.m.
	Dried-up looking—Ag.n.
	Dry Skin, with—Jab.
	Dysmenorrhoea of nervous—Ter.
	Excited, easily—Ign.,
	Excited, easily, also of opposite temperament—Con.
	Excited, not easily—Con.
	Fat, approaching the climaxis—Ca.ar.
	Feeble—Ag.n.,Sec.
	Fleshy, inclined to be—Pul.
	Flooding after every labour—Trl.
	Florid—Glo.
	Freckles and Red Hair, with, choleric—Lach.
	Headache of nervous—Ter.
	Heels, Inflammation of the, plethoric, suffering from—Sbi.
	Hysterical—Mag.m., Mos.
	Hysterical, who have taken too much Chamomile Tea—Val.

_____ Indigestion, suffering long from—Mag.m.

_____ Irritable Bladders, Old Women with—Cop.

_____ Irritable, nervous temperament of—Sec.

_____ Lax muscular fibre, of—Sec., Spo.

_____ Many Children, who have borne, after-pains of.Cup.

_____ Menses scanty, with—Con., Jab.

_____ Menstrual Disturbances, with—Ag.n.

_____ Nervous—Cast., K.br., Sec., Se.a., Xan.

_____ Nervous, Amenorrhoea, subject to—Ter.

_____ Nervous, with Cramps, &c., after severe Illness—Cast.

_____ Nervous, Dysmenorrhoea, subject to—Ter.

_____ Nervous, Headache, Subject to—ter.

_____ Nervously run-down—Hlon.

_____ Nursing—Rhe., Sep.

_____ Nursing, worn out by Nervous Babies—K.ph.

_____ Old—Con., Kre., Lyc., Su.x.(See also Old Age, &c.)

_____ Old, irritable Bladders, with—Cop.

_____ Old, Prematurely, Unmarried—Fl.x.

_____ Old Unmarried—Bro., Calc., Con.

_____ Pale—Eu.pi., Lc. x., Sec (See also Pale Face, &c.)

_____ Phlegmatic habit, of—Alo.

_____ Plethoric—Glo.

Women, Plethoric, suffering from Inflammation of the Heels—
Sbi.

_____ Pregnancy, during in Childbed, and While Nursing—
Sep.

_____ Pregnant—Alet., Ana., Nx.m., Cham., Rhe., Pal. Sep.

_____ Pregnant, or Parturient, with Sensation as if Intestines
were falling down—Pod.

_____ Relaxed habit, of—Alo.

_____ Rigid fibre, of—Con.

_____ Sanguine—Plat.

_____ Sanguine or Nervo-sanguine Temperament, of—Ver.

_____ Scrawny—Ag.n., Amb., Sec.

_____ Sedentary—Am.c.

_____ Sensitive—Eu.pi., Glo., Ign.

_____ Smelling Bottle, having constant recourse to—Am.c.

_____ Spare habit, of—Xan.

_____ Sterile—Am.c., Bor., Cth., Merc., Pho., Phy.

_____ Stout—Am.c.

_____ Sunken Countenance, of—Sec.

_____ Tall and Slender—Sga.

_____ Thin—Amb., Plat., Sec., Sga., Xan.

_____ Thin, having retained a good deal of Sprightliness and Moral Power—Sga.

_____ Urinary difficulties in—Mth.pi.

_____ Uterine Disorders, with—Act.r., Caul., Coc.i., Hlon., Mag.m.

_____ Weakness in, after severe illness—Cast.

_____ Widow—Aps.

_____ Worn-out—K.ph., Mag.m.

Work—*See* **Labour;** *and* **Laziness.**

Worm Diseases, Scrofulous Children with, during dentition—Sil.

Worms, Children having—Sul., Ter.

Worn-out Business and Professional Men—K.ph.

_____ Nursing Mothers distracted by Nervous Babies—K.ph.

_____ Persons—Pi.x.

_____ Women—Mag.c., Mag.m., Mag.p.

Wounds which Bleed Profusely—Mil., Pho.

Wrinkled Skin—Bor., Spi.

_____ Skin, Yellow, earthy—Spi. (**See also Yellow** Skin.)

Yawning, Complaints which are concomitant to—Cin.

Yellow Saddle across Nose, Pot-bellied Mothers with—Sep.

_____ Skin—Iod., Spi.

_____ Skin, or dirty brown, blotched, Puffed, Flabby persons with—Sep.

_____ Tenacious Mucus, Catarrh with discharge of—Sum.

Yielding Disposition—Pul.

Young—Aco., Apo., Aur., Bel., Ca.p., Gel., Ign., Mag.p., Mil.,
Pul., Stm., Ver.

_____ and fat—Ant.c., Calc.

_____ Persons, Ailments of—Stm.

_____ Both Sexes, of—Sep.

_____ Growing too rapidly—Ird., Kre., Ph.x. Pho.,

_____ Lively—Aco.

_____ Retarded in Growth—Ba.c.

_____ Stoop, with Inclination to—Pho.

_____ Varicose Veins in—Fe. p., Ham.

_____ Romantic—Ign.

Zealous Persons—Nux.

□□

Part IV
Clinical Relationships

SECTION 8

Clinical Relationships

NOTE

THIS section of the Repertory gives in tabular form the chief
clinical relations of all remedies of the Materia Medica so far
as they have been noted.They are included under the following
headings : "Complementary Remedies," "Remedy Follows
Well," "Remedy is Followed Well by," "Compatible
Remedies," "Incompatible Remedies," "Remedy Antidotes,"
"Remedy is Antidoted by." There is also added the duration of
action of remedies so far as these have been noted.

The term "compatible" is a generic term, and includes all
the remedies ofthe first three columns—i.e., the "complementary" remedies, those which the remedy "follows well," and
those which it is "followed well by"—but the column
"Compatible Remedies" has been included because some
remedies have been noted as compatible with others, without
further qualification.

Many remedies have not yet had their clinical relationships
noted. But I have not excluded them on this account; and
spaces are thus provided for the insertion of their related remedies when found later on in practice.

REMEDY	Complementary Remedies	Remedy Follows Well	Remedy is Followed Well by	Compatible Remedies
Abies c.				
Abies n.				
Abrotanum			Aco. and Bry. (pleurisy), Hep. (boils)	
Absinthium				
Acalypha i.				
Aceticum ac.				
Aconitium.	See Aco.			
Aconitum.				
Aconitum c.				
Aconitum f.				
Aconitum l.				
Aconitum n.	Arn. (bruises injury to eye) cof. (fever, sleeplessness, intolerance of pain), Sul.	Often indicated after Arn., Cof., Sul., Ver.	Arn., Ars., Bel., Bry., Cac., Cth., Coc. i., Hep., Ipc., K. br., Merc., Pul., Rhs., Sep., Sil., Spo., sul. (also for abuse of Aco.), Sul.	

Incompatible Remedies	Remedy Antidotes	Remedy is Antidoted by	Duration of Action	REMEDY
				abies c.
				Abies n.
				Abrotanum
	Ba. m. (some times)			Absinthium
				Acalypha i.
Arn., Ac. x. < the effects of Bel., Lach., Merc. Disagrees when given after Bor., Caus Nux, Ran., b., Sars.	Aco., Anaesthetics, Ar,. t, Asr., Cof., Eub., Hep., Ign., Opi., Pb. (colic); sausage poisoning, Sep., Stm., Tab.	Potencies by Aco. and Tab. for depressing agonising feeling; Mag.c. Large doses by Calc. (water), Mag. (fluid). For gastric, plumonary, and febrile symptoms. Na m. and afterwards Sep.	14-40 d.	Aceticum ac.
				Aconitium
				Aconitum.
				Aconitum c.
				Aconitum f.
				Aconitum l.
	Arn., Asp. (sometimes), Ast. f., Bel., Bry., Cac., Oth., Cham., Chel., Cinm., Cit., Cof., Cro., Dol., Glo., Gph., Klm. (Kre.), Lyc., Mrl., Mez., Morphia (secondary effects of) Nux, Pet., Sep., Sol., spo., Sty. (?), sul.., Ther. (sensitiveness to noise), Ver., Vb. o. (epididymitis)	Ac. x., Alcoh., Bel., Ber., Cham., Cit., Cof., Nux, Par., Sul., Ver., Wine.	1 hour top several weeks	Aconitum n.

REMEDY	Complementary Remedies	Remedy Follows Well	Remedy is Followed Well by	Compatible Remedies
Actaea r.				
Actaea s.		Nux.		
Adonis V.				
Adrenalin				
Aesculus g.				
Aesculus h.		Coll., Nux, Sul.		
Aethiops ant.				
Aethusa	Calc.			
Agaricus emet.				
Agaricus m.		Bel., Calc., Merc., Opi., Pul., Rhs., Sil.	Bel. Calc., Cup., Merc., Opi., Pul., Rhs., Sil., Trn., (typhoid with "rolling of the head").	
Agaricus ph.				
Agave am.				
Agnus c.			Ars., Bry., Ign., Lyc., Pul., Sel., Sul.	
Agraphis n.				
Agrostemma g.				
Ailanthus g				
Aletris f.				
Allium cepa	Pho., Pul., Sars., Thu.		Calc. and Sil. in polypus.	

Incompatible Remedies	Remedy Antidotes	Remedy is Antidoted by	Duration of Action	REMEDY
	Tansy poisioning	Aco. (the sleeplessness); Bap. (≥ the headache and nausea); Lcs. (?)		**Actaea r.**
				Actaea s.
				Adonis V.
				Adrenalin
				Aesculus g.
		Nux (pile symptoms)		**Aesculus h.**
				Aethiops ant.
	Opium, Pb, (?).	Vegetable acids	20-30 d.	**Aethusa**
				Agaricus emet.
		Brandy, Calc. (≥ icy coldness), Cam., Charcoal), Cof., Fat or Oil ≥ stomach. Pul., Rhs., (nightly backache), Wine.	40 d.	**Agaricus m.**
				Agaricus ph.
				Agave am.
		Cam., Na. m. (headache), strong solutions of table salt.	8-14 d.	**Agnus c.**
				Agraphis n.
				Agrostemma g.
		Alcohol, Nux, Rhs.		**Ailanthus g**
All., Alo., Scil.	Cld.	Arn. (toothache) cham. (abdominal pains) Cf. t. (onion breath), Nux (coryza recurring in August), Thu. (offensive breath and diarrhoea after eating onions), Ver. (colic with despondency).	1 d.	**Allium cepa**

REMEDY	Complementary Remedies	Remedy Follows Well	Remedy is Followed Well by	Compatible Remedies
Allium s.	Ars.			
Alnus				
Aloe				
Alstonia c.				
alumen				
Alumina	Bry., Fer.	Arg., Bry., Lach., Sul		
Ambra g.			Lyc., Pul., Sep., Sul.	
Ambrosia a.				
Ammoniacum				
Ammonium ac.				
Ammonium benz.				
Ammonium bro.				
Ammonium carb.			Bell., Calc., Lyc., Pho., Pul., Rhs., Sep., Sul.	
Ammonium mur.				
Ammonium mur.			Ant. c., Cof., Hot-bath, Merc., Nux, Pho., Pul., Rhus.	
Ammonium ph.				
Ammonium pi.				
Ampelopsis				
Amphisbaena				

Incompatible Remedies	Remedy Antidotes	Remedy is Antidoted by	Duration of Action	REMEDY
Alo., Cep. Scil.		Lyc.		Allium
				Alnus
All., Cep.	Paeo	Aln. (vomiting blood), Cam. > for a while, Lyc. and Nux > the ear-ache, Mustard Sul.	30–40	Aloe
				Alstonia c.
	Lead poisioning, calomel and other mercurials, Alo. (vomiting blood)	Cham. (cramps in abdomen), Ipc. (nausea and vomiting), Nux, Sul.		Alumen
	Bry., Cham., Lach., Lead.	Bry., Cam., Cham., Ipc., Pul	40–60 d.	Alumina
	Nux, Stp. (esp. the vuluptuous itching of scrotum.	Cam., cof., Nux, Pul., Stp.	40 d.	Ambra g.
				Ambrosia a.
	Chl. h.	Arn., Bry.		Ammoniacum
	As. h. (sometimes)			Ammonium ac.
				Ammonium benz.
				Ammonium bro.
Lach.	Bro., Cen., Charcoal fumes, Plo., Rhs., and stings of insects.	Vegetable acids., Arn., Cam., Fixed Oils, Hep., Lach.	40 d.	Ammonium carb.
	In sugasr water, Colch. poisioning	Vegetable acids, Ag. n. and Vinegar		Ammonium caus.
		Bitter almonds, Cam., Cof., Hep., Nux.	20–30 d.	Ammonium mur.
				Ammonium ph.
				Ammonium ph.
				Ampelopsis
				Amphisbaena

REMEDY	Complementary Remedies	Remedy Follows Well	Remedy is Followed Well by	Compatible Remedies
Amygdalae am. aq.				
Amylenum n.				
Anacardium oc.				
Anacardium or.		Lyc., Plat., Pul.	Lyc., Plat., Pul	
Anagallis arv.				
Anantherum				
Angophora				
Angustura v.			Bel., Ign., Lycop., Sep.	
Anhalonium lew.				
Anilinum				
Anthemis n.				
Anthoxanthum				
Anthracinum		Ars. (burning and ulceration), Ph. x.	Au. m. n. (periosteal swelling of lower jaw), Sil. (cellulitis).	
Anthrokokali				
Antifebrinum				
Antimonium a.				
Antimonium c.	Scil.	Ipc., Pul.	Calc., Lach., Merc., Pul., Sep., Sul.	
Antimonium i.				

Incompatible Remedies	Remedy Antidotes	Remedy is Antidoted by	Duration of Action	REMEDY
		Cofee (strong) opi (convulsions), Water (cold) poured overhead.		**Amygdalae am. aq.**
	Chlf. (failure of respiration), Sty. (convulsions).	Cac. (cardiac constriction).		**Amylenum n.**
		Iodine (locally) Rhs.		**Anacardium oc.**
	Rhs. if there are gastric symptoms going from r. to l.	Clem., Cof., Ctn., Jg. c., Rn. b., Rhs.	30–40 d.	**Anacardium or.**
				Anagallis arv.
Wines and spirits		Aromatic liquors		**Anantherum**
		Ipc.		**Angophora**
	Merc.	Bry. (belly-ache after milk), Chel. (sharp, cutting pain from just beneath r. scapula to chest), Cof. (not Cam.)	20–30 d.	**Angustura v.**
				Anhalonium lew.
				Anilinium
		Chi. is useful after abuse of chamomile tea when hemorrhage from uterus results.		**Anthemis n.**
				Anthoxanthum
		Aps., Ars., Cam., Cbl. x., Cb. v., Kre., Lach., Pul. Rhs., Sil., Sl. x.		**Anthracinum**
				Anthrokokali
				Antifebrinum
				Antimonium a.
	Pb., Pl. n., Sep., Stings of insects	Calc., Hep., Merc.	40 d.	**Antimonium c.**
				Antimonium i.

REMEDY	Complementary Remedies	Remedy Follows Well	Remedy is Followed Well by	Compatible Remedies
Antimonium m.				
Antimonium s. a.				
Antimonium t.		Pul. (nausea in chest, gonorrhoeal suppressions), Sil. in dyspnoea from foreign substances in larynx, Ter. (symptoms from damp cellars), Var.	Ba. c., Cam., Cin., Ipc., Pul., Sep., Sul., Ter.	Pho. in hydrocephaloid, worn-out constitutions, laryngitis, pneumonia
Antipyrinum				
Aphis c. g.				
Apis	Na. m. (the "chronic" of apis).	Bry (when cephalic cry appears), Hel. (when torpor sets in), Hep., Iod., Lyc., Merc., Sul.	Ars. (hydrothorax), Gph. (tetter on ear-lobe), Iod. (swollen knee), K. bi. (scrofulous ophthalmia), Lyc,. (staphyloma), Pho. (diphtheria), Pul., Stm. (mania), Sul. (hydrothorax, pleurisy, hydrocephalus).	
Apium g.				
Apocynum an.				
Apocynum can.				
Apomorphinum				
Aqua m.				
Aquilegia V				
Aralia r.				
Aranea d.				
Aranearum t.				
Aranea s.				
Arbutus a.				
Arctium l.				
Areca				

Incompatible Remedies	Remedy Antidotes	Remedy is Antidoted by	Duration of Action	REMEDY
				Antimonium m.
				Antimonium s.a.
	Ba. c., Bry., (dyspepsia), Cam., Caus. (dyspepsia), Ctn., Iod., (relieves the vertigo of Mil.), Sep., Vac., Var.	Asa., Chi., Coc, i., Con. (pustules on genitals), Ipc., Lau., Merc., Opi. (Opium in large doses is the best antidote in poisoning), Pul., Rhs., Sep.		Antimonium t.
				Antipyrinum
				Aphis c. g.
Pho., Rhs., (in eruptive diseases).	Athra., Asp., Cth. (the cystitis) Chi., Dig., Iod., Na. p. (Urticaria), Vac., Vsp.	Cth., Ipc., Lach., Lc.x., Led., Na.m. Massive doses, poisionings and stings are aitidoted by Na. m. (the crude salt, solutions, and potencies); Sweet-oil (which contains salt); Onions; Ammonia; Urtica; powdered Ipec. applied locally		Apis
				Apium g.
				Apocynum an.
				Apocynum can.
				Apomorphinum
				Aqua m.
				Aquilegia V
				Aralia r.
	Chi., Merc., Quinine	amoking tobacco		Aranea d.
				Aranearum t.
				Aranea s.
				Arbutus a.
				Arctium l.
				Areca

REMEDY	Complementary Remedies	Remedy Follows Well	Remedy is Followed Well by	Compatible Remedies
Argentum cy.				
Argentum iod				
Argentum met.		Al., Plat.	Calc., Pul., Sep.	
Argentum n.		Bry., Caus. (urethral affections), Spi. (dyspepsia), Spo. (goitre), Ver. (flatus)	Calc., Hfb., K. ca., Lyc. (flatus), Merc., Pul., Sep., Sil.	
Aristolochia mil.				
Aristolochia ser.				
Armoracia s.				
Arnica	Aco., Ipc., Ver.	Aco., Aps., Ipc., Ver.	Aco., Ars. (action aided by Ars. in dysentery and varicose veins), Bel., Bry., Cac., Calc., Cham., Chi., Con., Hep., Iod., Ipc., Nux, Pho., Pul., Rhs., Sul., Su. x.	
Arsenicum a.	All., Cb. v., Na. s., Pho., Thu.	Aco., Aga., arn., Bel., Cham., Chi., Ipc., Lach., Ver.	Aps., Aran., Bel., Cac., Cham., Chel., Chi., Cic., Fer., Fl. x., Hep., Iod., Ipc., K. bi., Lyc., Merc., Nux ; Rhs. follows well in skin affections, esp. in cases treated allopathically with large doses of arsenic; Sul., Ver.	

Incompatible Remedies	Remedy Antidotes	Remedy is Antidoted by	Duration of Action	REMEDY
				Argentum cy.
				Argentum iod
		Merc., Pul., (an occasional does of Pul. favour action of Ag. n. in ophthalmia)	30 d	**Argentum met.**
Cof. (it increases the nervous headache), Vsp.	Amm., K. i. (fulness and indigestion after each dose), Op., effects of tobacco	Ars., Iod., Merc., Milk., Na. m. (chemical and dynamic). Antidotes to Ag. n. and Nt. x. are Calc., Pul., Sep.; next in importance, Lyc., Pho., Rhs., Sil., Sul.	30 d.	**Argentum n.**
				Aristolochia mil.
				Aristolochia ser.
				Armoracia s.
Injurious in bites of dogs or rabid or angry animals. Wine < unpleasant effect of Arn.	Amc., Am. c., Caln., Cep. (toothache) Chi., Ch. s., Cic. v., Fer., Ham., Ign., Ipc., Phst., Sga.	*If potencies :* Aco., Ars., Cam., Chi., Cic. v., Fer., Ign., Ipc., Sga. *If massive doses :* Cam., Ipc., Coffee (headache)	6-10 d.	**Arnica**
	Athra, Ag. n., Arn., Ca. a., Cb. v., Chi., Ch. s. Elp., Fer., Gph., Hep., Hyp. (weakness or sickness on moving), Iod., Ipc., K. bi., Lach., Leo., Mag. c. Mag. m., Mlr. No. II., Merc., Na. m. (bad effects of sea-bathing), Nux, Pho,. Pb. Smb.n., Sty., Tab., Thri., Ver.	*Chemical antidotes :* Animal charcoal, Hydrated peroxide of iron, Limewater, Magnesia. *Dynamic antidotes:* Opium; it may be administered by clyster if not retained on stomach; Brandy and stimulants if there is depression and collapse ; Sweat spirit of nitre in large quantities of water if urine is suppressed. *If poisonous doses :* Milk, Albumen,	Antidoted by. If poisonous doses (continued) : Demulcent drinks, followed by emitics of Mustard, Sulphate of Zinc, or Sulphate of Copper (Tartat emitic is too irritating); Castor oil is the best purgative *(If potencies:* Cam., Cb. v., Chi., Ch. s., Eub., Fer., Gph., Hep., Iod., Ipc., Lach., Merc., Nx. m., Nux, Smb. n., Sul., Tab., Ver. 60-90 d.	**Arsenicum a.**

REMEDY	Complementary Remedies	Remedy Follows Well	Remedy is Followed Well by	Compatible Remedies
Arsenicum br.				
Arsenicum hy.				
Arsenicum i.	Pho	Con. in sensitive lump in breast, and Sul. in phthisis pulmonalis		
Arsenicum m.		In pterygium after failure of Nux and Spi.		
Arsenicum s. f.				
Arsenicum s. r.				
Artemisia V.	Art. v. acts better when given with wine than with water	Aco., Bel., Bry., Cin., Hel., Iod.	Caus.	Stm., Pul., and Aur. (in alternation).
Arum dracon.		Ant. t. and Clch. in laryngismus.		
Arum dracun.				
Arum it.				
Arum m.				
Arum t.		Caus., Hep., Nt. x., Sng.	Eub.	
Arundo m.				
Asafoetida			Chi., Merc., Pul.	
Asarum e.			Bis., Caus., Pul.,, Sil.	
Asclepias s.				
Asclepias t.				

Incompatible Remedies	Remedy Antidotes	Remedy is Antidoted by	Duration of Action	REMEDY
				Arsenicum br.
		Am. ac. (breathing), drinks containing sulphuretted hydrogen, Nux (fever), sinapisms (breathing)		Arsenicum hy.
	Relieves the diarrhoea of Mil.	Bry. > pain and pyrosis		Arsenicum i.
		Bel. (sore throat), Na. c. (syphilitic symptoms).		Arsenicum m.
				Arsenicum s. f.
				Arsenicum s. r.
				Artemisia Y.
Cld.				Arum dracon.
Cld.				Arum dracun.
Cld.				Arum it.
Cld.		Butter, Milk, Sweet oil, Mil. (?). Gum > pungent effect on mouth.		Arum m.
Cld.		Ac. x., Bel., Buttermilk, Lc. x., Pul.	1–2 d.	Arum t.
				Arundo m.
	Alcohol, Ant. t., Caus., Ln. u. (?), Merc. Pul.	Cam., Caus., Chi., Merc., Pul., Val.	20-40 d.	Asafoetida
	Cit	Ac. x., Cam., vegetable acids and vinegar	8–14 d.	Asarum e.
				Asclepias s.
				Asclepias t.

REMEDY	Complementary Remedies	Remedy Follows Well	Remedy is Followed Well by	Compatible Remedies
Asimina t.				
Asparagus				
Astacus fl.				
Asterias r.		Bel., Calc., ,Cb. a., Con., Sil., Sul.		
Astragalus m.				
Athamantha				
Atropinum				
Aurum ar.				
Aurum br.				
Aurum i.				
Aurum met.			Aco., Bel., Calc., Chi., Lyc., Merc., Nt. x., Pul., Rhs., Sep., Sul.	
Aurum mur.				Sulphur springs
Aurum mur. k.				
Aurum m. n.				
Aurum sul.				
Avena s.				
Azadiracta i.				
Bacillinum	Ca. p. goes with this remedy very well. So do Hdr., Lach. asnd K. ca			
Bacillinum t.				
Badiaga	Iod., Merc., Sul..		Lach.	
Balsamum p.				
Baptisia c. a.				
Baptisia t.				

Incompatible Remedies	Remedy Antidotes	Remedy is Antidoted by	Duration of Action	REMEDY
				Asimina t.
	Cof.	Aco (prostration, feeble pulse, pain in shoulder), Aps.		Asparagus
				Astacus fl.
Cof. Nux. (Ipc. > after Nux <).		Pb., Zin.		Asterias r.
				Astragalus m.
				Athamantha
Antagonised by Gel.	Chl. h., Gel., Mor., Muscarine, Opium, Plo	Bel., Opi., Phst		Atropinum
				Aurum ar.
				Aurum br.
				Aurum i.
	Chronic effects of alcohol, K. i., Merc., Spi.	Bel., Cam., Chi., Coc. i., Cof., Cup., Merc., Pul., So. n., Spi.	50–60 d.	Aurum met.
		Bel., Cnb., Merc.		Aurum mur.
				Aurum mur. k.
Alcohol. Cof.				Aurum m. n.
				Aurum sul.
				Avena s.
				Azadiracta i.
				Bacillinum
				Bacillinum
				Badiaga
				Balsamum p.
				Baptisia c. a.
				Baptisia t.

REMEDY	Complementary Remedies	Remedy Follows Well	Remedy is Followed Well by	Compatible Remedies
Barosma				
Baryta c.	Dul.	Ars., Scil., Sul.	Ant. t., (Calc.), Con., Pho., Pul., Rhs., Sep., Sil., Sul	Before and after Sul.
Baryta i.				
Baryta m.		Ars. in extravasations of blood		
Belladonna	Calc.	Ars., Cham., cup., Hep., Lach., Merc., Nt. x., Pho	Aco., Ars., Cac., Calc., Cb. v., Cham., Chi., Con., Dul., Hep., Hyo., Lach, Merc., Mos., Mu. x., Nux., Pul., Rhs., Sga., Sep., Sil., Stm., Sul., Val., Ver.	
Bellis perennis	Van			Van
Benzinum				
Benzinum d.				
Benzinum nit.				
Benzoicum ac.		In gout after Clch., after abuse of Cop. in suppression of gonorrhoea, in enuresis after failure of K. n.		
Benzoin				
Berberis a.				
Berberis V.	An occasional dose of Lyc. helped action of Ber.	Bry., K. bi., Rhs., Sul.		
Bismuthum		Evo. (headache).	Bel., Calc., Pul., Sep.	

Incompatible Remedies	Remedy Antidotes	Remedy is Antidoted by	Duration of Action	R E M E D Y
				Barosma
Calc.		Ant. t., Bel., Cam., Dul., Merc., Zin.	40 d.	**Baryta c.**
				Baryta i.
		Absinthe (the vomiting).		**Baryta m.**
Dul., Vinegar, < by Ac. x.	Aco., Atp., As. mt. (some times), Ar. t., Art., Aur., Au.m., Bar. c., Ber., Ced., Chi., Clch., Cop., Cro. Cup., Fer., Grt., Hep., Hyo., Iod., Jab., K. m., Klm., Lach., Mag. p., Mrl., Merc., Mor., Nt., o. (?), Nux., Opi., Osm. (laryngeal cararrh), Pal. (headache), Phyt., Plat., Pb., Rhs., Rum., Sars.,. Sga., Sol., Stm., Val.,; Oil of turpentine; Sausage poisoning	If effects of large doses, Vegetable acids, infusion of galls, or green tea, Cof., Hyo. If effects of small doses, Aco., Cam., Cof., Hep., Hyo., Opi.,Pul., Sbd. (salivation), Vinum.	1–7 d.	**Belladonna**
				Bellis perennis
				Benzinum
		Sty		**Benzinum d.**
				Benzinum nit.
Wine, which < pains in k i d n e y s , drawing in knees, &c.				**Benzoicum ac.**
				Benzoin
				Berberis a.
	Aco.	Bel., Cham.		**Berberis V.**
		Calc., Cap., Cof., Nux.	20–50 d.	**Bismuthum**

REMEDY	Complementary Remedies	Remedy Follows Well	Remedy is Followed Well by	Compatible Remedies
Blatta am.				
Blatta or.				
Boletus lar.				
Boletus lur.				
Boletus sat.				
Bombyx pro.				
Boracicum ac.				
Borax.			Calc., Nux.,	
Bothrops lan.				
Bovista		It has cured where Rhs. seemed indicated and failed.	Alm., Calc., Rhs., Sep.	
Brachyglottis r.				
Brassica n.				
Bromium		Iod., Pho., Spo.	Ag. n., K. ca.	Ag. n. (generally after Bro.), K. ca. (emphysema).
Brucea ant.				
Brucinum				
Bryonia.	alum., Rhs. Alumina is the "cronic" of Bry.; and Kali c. and Nat. m. hold a similar but less pronounced relation to it.	Aco., Amm., Nux, Opi., Rhs., Sul.	Alum., Ars., Bel., Cac., Cb. v., Drs., Hyos., Kali. c., Mu. x., Nux, Pho., Pul., Rhs., Sbd., Sep., Sil., Sul.	
Bufo	Salamandra in spilepsy and brain softening.			

Incompatible Remedies	Remedy Antidotes	Remedy is Antidoted by	Duration of Action	REMEDY
				Blatta am.
				Blatta or.
				Boletus lar.
				Boletus lur.
				Boletus sat.
				Bombyx pro.
				Boracicum ac.
Ac. x., Vinegar, Wine	Cham.	Cham., Cof.	30 d.	Borax
				Bothrops lan.
Cof.	Effects of Tar applied locally	Cam.	7–14 d.	Bovista
				Brachyglottis r.
				Brassica n.
		Am. c., Cam., Clch. (?), Mag. c., Opi.	20–30 d.	Bromium
				Brucea ant.
				Brucinum
Calc.	Alum.,. amc., Ang. (some times) relieved pain and pyrosis of As. i., Chi., Chlm., Clem. (sometimes), Dph., Frg., Jg. c. (angina pectoris), Lc. x. (sometimes partly), Mlr. No. I., II., and III., Mns., Merc., Mez., Mu. x. (small doses), Ost., Rh. b., Rho., Rhs., Sll., Scro. (chest symptoms), Sga.	Aco., Alum., Ant. t. (sometimes), Cam., Cham., Chel., Clem., Cof.; Teste found by accident, Fe. m. the best antidote in his experience ; Ign., Mu. x., Nux, Pul., Rhs., Sga.	7–21 d.	Bryonia
		Lach., Sga.		Bufo

REMEDY	Complementary Remedies	Remedy Follows Well	Remedy is Followed Well by	Compatible Remedies
Cactus g.		Aco., Arn., Ars., Bel., Bry., Cham., Gel., Ip., K. br. (diaphragmitis), Lach., Nux, Rhs.		Dig. (tumultuous) action of heart, slow, irregular pulse, scanty urine, dropsy, E. pf., Lach., Nux, Sul. (pleurisy).
Cadmium bro.				
Cadmium sulph.		Ipc., Ars., Bel.	Alet. (nausea of pregnancy) Bel. (rolling of head with open eyes in cholera infantum), Cb. v., Lo. i. (in yellow fever Nt. x.	
Cainca		Ars.		
Cajuputum				
Caladium	Nt. x.		Aco., Caus., Pul., Sep.	Aco., Cth., Pul., Sep.
Calcerea arsen.		In case which have been heavily dosed with Quinine,	Con.,, Glo., Opi., Pul.	Con., Glo., Opi., Pul.
Calcarea bro.				
Calcarea carb.	Bel., Rhs.,	Cham., Chi., Con., Cup., Nt. x., Nux, Pul., Sul.)esp. if the pupils dilate)	Aga., Bel., Bis., Drs., Gph., Ipc., Lyc., Na. c., Nt. x., Nux, Pho., Plat., Pul., Rhs., Sars., Sep., Sil., Ther.	
Calcarea caus.				
Calcarea chlor.				
Calcarea fluor.			·	
Calcarea hypoph.				·
Calcarea iod.				

Incompatible Remedies	Remedy Antidotes	Remedy is Antidoted by	Duration of Action	R E M E D Y
	Aml. (cardiac constriction).	Aco., Cam., Chi., E. pf.		Cactus g.
				Cadmium bro.
				Cadmium sulph
		Clch. Rhs. (gastralgia), Ver.		Cainca
				Cajuputum
Ar. t. ; the Araceae	Cap., Merc.	Cap., Cb. v. (rash), Hyo. (night cough), Ign. (stitches in pit of stomach, and fever), Merc. (preputial symptoms), Zng. (asthma).	30–40 d.	Caladium
		Cb. v. (palpitation), Glo. (headache), Pul. (headache, tearing pains in face)		Calcarea arsen
				Calcarea bro.
Ba. c., Bry.; Kali b. (before Calc.), Nt. x. (after); Sul. (after)	Relieves icy coldness of Aga.; Ant. c., Bis., Chi. Ch. s., Cop., Dig., Mez. (headache), Nt. s. d., Nt. x., Ox. (?), Pho.	Bry., Cam., Chi., Hep., Iod., Ip., Nt. s. d., Nt. x., Nux, Sep., Sul.	60 d.	Calcarea carb.
				Calcarea caus.
				Calcarea chlor.
				Calcarea fluor.
				Calcarea hypoph.
				Calcarea iod.

REMEDY	Complementary Remedies	Remedy Follows Well	Remedy is Followed Well by	Compatible Remedies
Calcarea mur.				
Calcarea ov. t.				
Calcarea oxal.				
Calcarea phos.	Hep., Rut., Sul,., Zin.	Ars., Chi., Iod., Merc.	Rhs., Sul.	
Calcarea pi.				
Calcarea ren.				
Calcarea sil.				
Calcarea sulph.				
Calendula	Hep.	Ars.	Arn., Ars., Bry., Hep., Nt. x., Pho., Rhs.	Arn., Ars., Bry., Nt. x., Pho., Rhs.
Calotropis				
Caltha p.				
Camphora	Cth.		Ant. t., Ars., Bel., Coc. i., Nux, Rhs., Ver.	
Camphora bro.				
Canchalagua				
Cannabis ind.				

Incompatible Remedies	Remedy Antidotes	Remedy is Antidoted by	Duration of Action	REMEDY
				Calcarea mur.
				Calcarea ov. t.
				Calcarea oxal.
	Pul. (air passage)		60 d.	Calcarea phos.
				Calcarea pi.
				Calcarea ren.
				Calcarea sil
				Calcarea sulph.
Cam.		Arn.		Calendula
		Cam., Cof., caused vomiting when before there was only nausea, but antidoted many effects.		Calotropis
				Caltha p.
Caln., after Cof. (sometimes), < sufferings from K. n., < effects of Sac. l.	Am.c., Canth., Cb.v., Cup., Lau., Led., Lyc., Mag. m., Men., Mep. tempo-rarily),Mos. (unconsciousness and coldness) Mu. x. (small doses), Na. c., Na. m., Scil.; socalled worm medicines, tobacco, bitter almonds, and other fruits containing prussic acid; also the secondary affections remaining after poisoning with acids, salts, metals, poisonous mush rooms, &c.			Camphora
				Camphora bro.
				Canchalagua
				Cannabis ind.

REMEDY	Complementary Remedies	Remedy Follows Well	Remedy is Followed Well by	Compatible Remedies
Cannabis sat.			Bel., Hyo., Lyc., Nux, Opi., Pul., Rhs., Ver.	
Cantharis	Cam.		Bel., K. bi., Merc., Pho., Pul., Sep., Sul.	
Capsicum			Bel., Lyc., Pul., Sil.	
Carbo an.	Ca. p.		Ars., Bel., Bry. (Cb. v. ?), Nt. x., Pho., Pul., Sep., Sil., Sul., Ver.	
Carbo veg.	Chi., Drs., K. ca. (stitches in heart, (c.), Pho.		Aco., Ars., Chi., Drs., K. ca., Lyc., Nux, Ph. x., Pul., Sep., Sul.	
Carbolicum ac.				
Carboneum				
Carboneum hyd.				
Carboneum oxy.				
Carboneum sulph.				
Carduus ben.				
Carduus mar.				
Carisbad				
Carya alb.				

Incompatible Remedies	Remedy Antidotes	Remedy is Antidoted by	Duration of Action	R E M E D Y
Cam		Cam.	1–10 d.	**Cannabis sat.**
Cof.	Alcohol, Cam., Vinegar.	Aco; Aps. antidotes the cystitis of Cth., Cam. the strangury and retention of urine, K. n. the renal symptoms; Lau., Pul., Rhe., Symt.	30–40 d.	**Cantharis**
	Effects of Alcohol, Bis., Cof., Cf. t., Merc. high (?), Opi, Quinine.	Cam., Chi., Cin., Cld., Su. x., vapour of burning sulphur.	7 d.	**Capsicum**
Cb. v. (?)	Effects of Quinine Ziz.	Ars., Cam., Cof., Lach., Nux, Vinegar, Vinum	60 d.	**Carbo an.**
Cb. a. (?)	Athra., Cld. (rash), Ca. ar. (palpitation), Chi., Ch. s., Lach., Merc., Nt. s. d., effects of putrid meats or fish, rancid fats, salt or salt meats, relieved effects of Sla.	Ars., Caus., Cof., Fer., Nt. s. d.	60 d.	**Carbo veg.**
	Athra.	Chalk, Saccharated Lime. In burns milk gives immediate relief, also copious draughts of milk in poisoning cases.		**Carbolicum ac.**
				Carboneum
				Carboneum hyd.
				Carboneum oxy.
				Carboneum sulph
				Carduus ben.
				Carduus mar.
				Carlsbad
				Carya alb.

REMEDY	Complementary Remedies	Remedy Follows Well	Remedy is Followed Well by	Compatible Remedies
Cascara sag.				
Cascarilla				
Castanea V.				
Castor eq.				
Castoreum				
Caulophyllum		Gel.		
Causticum	Col., Pts., Mr. c. assists the action of Caus. and vice versa (in small pox).		Ant. t., Calc., Gui., K. i., Lyc., Nux, Pul., Rhs., Rut., Sep., Sil., Stn., Sul.	*Before:* Calc. K. i., (facial paralysis from an abscess), Lyc., Nux, Rhs., Rut., Sep., Sil., Sul. *Intercurrently :* Ars, Cup., Ig., Pod., Pul., Rhs., Sep., Stn. *After:* Calc., Coc. i., Col., Cup., Hyo., Ign., Pet., Pts., Rhs., Sep., Stn., Sul.
Ceanothus amer.			Ber., Con., My.c., Qer.	
Cedron				
Cenchris con.				
Centaurea tag.				
Cereus bon.				
Cereus ser.				
Cerium oxal.				
Cervus				
Cetraria islan.				
Chamomilla	Bel. in diseases of children (Cham. acts more on nerves of abdomen, Bel. more on cranial nerves), Mgn. c., Pul.	Mr. sol., Pul., Sul.	Aco., Ar., Bel., Bry., Cac., Calc., Coc. i., For., Merc., Nux, Pul., Rhs., Sep., Sil., Sul.	

Incompatible Remedies	Remedy Antidotes	Remedy is Antidoted by	Duration of Action	REMEDY
				Cascara sag.
				Cascarilla
				Castanea V.
		Hep. > the sore nipples; Thu. has removed the warts caused by Ct. eq.		Castor eq.
		Clch.		Castoreum
Cof.				Caulophyllum
Acids, Coc. i., Cof., Pho.	Asa., chi., Col., Ephr., Grt., Lyc., Nt. s. d., Pb. (leadipoisioning, abuse of Merc., and Sul. in scabies. Relieves paralysis of wrist of Hpm.	Ant. t. (sometimes), Asa., Cof., Col., Dul., gui. (rheumatic contractions), K. n. (renal symptoms), Nt. s. d., Nux.	50 d.	Causticum
		Na. m.		Ceanothus amer.
	Lach.	Bel., Lach.		Cedron
	Pul.	Am. c. (general symptoms), Cham. (internal haemorhage)		Cenchris con.
				Centaurea tag.
				Cereus bon.
				Cereus ser.
				Cerium oxal.
				Cervus
				Cetraria islan.
Nux, Zin.	Coffee and the narcotics, esp. Opium (useful in nervestorm when morphia is discontinued), the nightly toothache of Thu.	Aco., Alm., Bor., Cam., Coc. i., Cof., Col., Con., Ign., Nux, Pul., Val.	20–30 d.	Chamomilla

Remedy	Complementary Remedies	Remedy Follows Well	Remedy is Followed Well by	Compatible Remedies
Chaparro amar.				
Cheiranthus c.				
Chelidonium			Aco., Ars., Bry., Ipc., Led., Lyc., Nux, Sep., Spl., Sul.	Ars., Bry., Crl., (whooping-cough)
Chelone				
Chenopodium anthel.				
Chenopodium vul.				
Chimaphila mac.				
Chimaphila umb.				
China bol.				
China officin.	Fer.		Ac. x., Arn., Ars., Asa., Bel., Calc., Ca. p., Cb. v., Fer., Lach., Merc., Pho., Ph. x., Pul., Sul., Ver.	Ca. p., Fer.,
Chininum arsen.				
Chininum mur.				
Chininum sal.				
Chininum sulph.				
Chionanthus vir.				
Chloralum				

Incompatible Remedies	Remedy Antidotes	Remedy is Antidoted by	Duration of Action	R E M E D Y
				Chaparro amar.
				Cheiranthus c.
	Ang. (sometimes), Bry.	Acids, Aco., Cam., Cham., Cof., Coffee, Wine.	7–14 d.	Chelidonium
				Chelone
				Chenopodium anthel.
				Chenopodium vul.
				Chimaphila mac.
				Chimaphila umb.
				China bol.
After Dig., Kre. (when following Chi), after Sel.	Ant. t., Arn., Ars., Asa., Aur., Cac., Calc., Cap., Cham., cin., Cof., Cu. a., Fer., Gel., Gph., Ham., Hel., Hyo., Iod., Ipc., Merc., Mns., Pal. (diarrhoea), Ped., (sometimes), Sul. Is useful in bad effects of tea-drinking and after abuse of chamomile tea (uterine haemorrhages), Ver., Vis.	Aps., Aran., Arn., Ars., Asa., Bel., Bry., Calc., Cb. v., Caus., Cin., E. pf., Fer., Ipc., Lach., Led., Lyc., Men., Merc., Na. c., Na. m., Nux, Pul., Rhs., Sep., Sul., Ver.	7 d.	China officin.
				Chininum arsen.
				Chininum mur.
				Chininum sal.
	Ars. iod.,	Aran., Arn., Ars., Calc., Cb. v., Fer., Hep., Lach. and esp. Na. m., which antidotes overdosing with Quinine, Pul.		Chininum sulph.
				Chionanthus vir.
		Ammon., Atr., Dig. (heart), Electricity, Mos.		Chloralum

REMEDY	Complementary Remedies	Remedy Follows Well	Remedy is Followed Well by	Compatible Remedies
Chloroformum				
Chlorum		Pho.		
Cholesterinum				
Chromicum ac. Chromium oxida.				
Chrysophanicum ac.				
Cichorium				
Cicuta mac.				
Cicuta vir.		Ars. and Con. (Cancer of lip), Cup. (aphasia in chorea), Lach.	Bel., Hep., Opi., Pul., Rhs., Sep.	
Cimex				
Cimicifuga				
Cina		Ant. t., Drs.	Calc., Chi., Ign., Nux, Plat., Pul., Rhs., Sil., Stn.	
Cinchoninum s.				
Cineraria mar.				
Cinnabaris				
Cinnamomum				
Cistus can.	Bel., Cb., v., Magnesium. Pho.			
Citrus lim.		It increases the curative effects of Bel.		

Incompatible Remedies	Remedy Antidotes	Remedy is Antidoted by	Duration of Action	REMEDY
	Pho., Sty.	Aml., Brandy, Ice in rectum, Ipc.		**Chloroformum**
	Hy. x., Sulphuretted hydrogen.	Albumen, Bry., Sulphuretted hydrogen, Lyc. (impotence), Plumb. acet. (blood-spitting and pleurisy.		**Chlorum**
				Cholesterinum
		Dph. has cured the rheumaqtic pains, Mr. c. has counteracted the general effect in workmen, the rest-lessness and relief from motion suggest Rhs.,		**Chromicum ac.** **Chromium oxida.**
				Chrysophanicum ac.
				Cichorium
				Cicuta mac.
	Cup., Opium.	Arn., Cof., Cu. a., Opi., Tobacco for massive doses.		**Cicuta vir.**
				Cimex
		Aco., Bap.	8–12 d.	**Cimicifuga**
	Cap., Chi., Merc., Val.	Cam., Cap., Chi., Pip. n.	14–20 d.	**Cina**
				Cinchoninum s.
				Cineraria mar.
	Au. m.	Hep., Nt. x., Opi., Sul.		**Cinnabaris**
	Opium	Aco.		**Cinnamomum**
Coffee.		Cam., Rhs., Sep.		**Cistus can.**
	Aco., Euphorb., Stm., snake-bites and all animal poisons.	Aço., Asr., Datura, Euphorb., Hep., Sep.		**Citrus lim.**

REMEDY	Complementary Remedies	Remedy Follows Well	Remedy is Followed Well by	Compatible Remedies
Clematis erec.			Calc., Rhs., Sep., Sil., Sul.	Sil.
Cobaltum				
Coca				
Coccinella				
Cocculus		Aco. (endocarditis with fearfulness).	Ars. Bel., Hep., Ign., Lyc., Nux., Opi., Pul., Rhs,. Sul.	Cham. Ign., Nux.
Coccus cacti				
Codeinum				
Coffea cru.	Aco.		Aco., Aur., Bel., Lyc., Nux, Opi., Sul.	
Coffea tos.				
Coffeinum				
Colchicinum				
Colchicum		Lyc.	Cb. v. (ascites), Merc., Nux, Pul., Rhs., Sep.	
Collinsonia can.				
Colocynthinum				
Colocynthis	Merc. (dysentery with much tenesmus)		Bel., Bry., Caus., Cham., Merc., Nux, Pul., Spil, Stp.	Cham., Stp.

Incompatible Remedies	Remedy Antidotes	Remedy is Antidoted by	Duration of Action	R E M E D Y
	Bry., Merc., Rho., Rs. v. (sometimes), Tab. (sometimes)	Anac., Bry., (toothache, urinary symptoms), Cam., Cham., Ctn., Rn. b., Rhs.	14–20 d.	Clematis erec.
				Cobaltum
		Gel.		Coca
				Coccinella
Caus., Cof.	Alcohol, Ant. t., Aur., Cham., Clch., Cup., Ig., Nux, Pet., Ph., Spi., the fever of Thu, Yuc.	Cam., Cham., Cup., Ign., Nux, Stp.	30 d.	Cocculus
				Coccus cacti
				Codeinum
Ast. r.: inimical to Ag. n. (nervous headache); Cth., Caus., Cis., Coc. i., Ign.; aggravates symptoms of Lc. x.; Mil. (= congestion to head), Stm.	Amb., Am. m., Ana., Ang., Aur., Bel., Bor., Cb. v., Caus., Cham., Cic., Col,. Con., Cyc., Gam., Gel., Glo., Hy. x., Ign., Iod., K. ca., Lach., Lau., Lyc., Man., Mos., Nux, Par., Ph. x., Pho., Pul., Rhs., Sty., Tab., Val.	Ac. x., Aco., Asp., Cham., Ign., Merc., Nux, Sul., and esp. Tab.	1–7 do.	Coffea cru.
				Coffea tos.
				Coffeinum
				Colchicinum
Ac. x., disagrees when given after Clch.	Cai., Castor, Plat., Thu.	Bel., Cam., Coc. i., Led., Nux, Pul. (heart), Spi., honey and sugar. In poisoning give Amm. in sugar water	14–20 d.	Colchicum
		Nux.		Collinsonia can.
				Colocynthinum
	Caus., Cham., Gam., Magnes., Pod., Rhe.	Cam., Caus., Cham., Cof., Opi., Stp. Large doses are counteracted by Cam., infusion of galls, tepid milk Opi.	1–7 d.	Colocynthis

REMEDY	Complementary Remedies	Remedy Follows Well	Remedy is Followed Well by	Compatible Remedies
Colostrum				
Comocladia				
Conchiolinum				
Coniinum				
Coniinum bro.				
Conium mac.			Arn., Ars., Bel., Calc., Cic., Drs., Lyc., Nux, Pho., Pul., Rhs., Stm., Sul.	Arn., Ars., Bel., Calc., Lyc., Nux, Pho., Pul., Rhs., Stm.
Convallaria				
Convolvulus arv.				
Convolvulus duar.				
Copaiva				
Corallium rub.				
Coriaria rus.				
Cornus alter.				
Cornus cir				
Cornus flor.				
Corydalis				
Coto bark				
Cotyledon				
Crataegus oxy.				
Crocus			Nux, Pul., Sul.	Chi., Nux, Pul., Sul.
Crotalus cas.				
Crotalus hor.				

Incompatible Remedies	Remedy Antidotes	Remedy is Antidoted by	Duration of Action	REMEDY
				Colostrum
				Comocladia
				Conchiolinum
				Coniinum
				Coniinum bro.
Con. sometimes disagrees with patients who have been taking Pso.	Ant. t., (sometimes), Cham., Cu. a., Cup., Merc., Nr. s. d., Nt. x., Rum., Sbd., Sul.	Cof., Dul., Nt. x., Nt. s. d., (Wine)	30–50 d.	Conium mac.
				Convallaria
				Convolvulus arv.
				Convolvulus duar.
		Bel., Calc., Merc., Sul., Mr. c. in the male, and Mr. sol. in the female, according to Teste, neutralise the action of Cop. almost instantaneously.		
	Merc.	Calc.		Corallium rub.
				Coriaria rus.
				Cornus alter.
				Cornus cir
				Cornus flor.
				Corydalis
				Coto bark
				Cotyledon
				Crataegus oxy.
		Aco., Bel., Opi.	8 d.	Crocus
				Crotalus cas.
	It relieved eye symptoms of Mep.	Lach. Its effects are modified by Alcohol, Ammon., Cam., Cof., Opi., and radiant heat.		Crotalus hor.

REMEDY	Complementary Remedies	Remedy Follows Well	Remedy is Followed Well by	Compatible Remedies
Croton chl.				
Croton tig.			Rhs.	K. br.
Cubeba				Cop.
Cucurbita p.				
Culex mus.				
Cundurango				
Cuphea vis.				
Cupressus aus.				
Cupressus law.				
Cuprum acet.	Calc., Gel. (over-worked brain), Cicut. and Solanaceae (mental symptoms), Zin. (hydrocephalus and convulsions from suppressed exanthems).			
Cuprum arsen				
Cuprum met.	Calc.		Ars., Bel., Calc., Caus., Cic., Hyo., K. n., Pul., Stm., Ver.	
Cuprum sulph.				
Curare		Arn. (paralysis from injury). Bar. c. (in debility of the aged) Bel. (paralysis after epistaxis).		

Incompatible Remedies	Remedy Antidotes	Remedy is Antidoted by	Duration of Action	REMEDY
				Croton chl.
	Rhs.	Anac., Ant. t., Clem., Rhs., Rn. b.	30 d.	Croton tig.
				Cubeba
				Cucurbita p.
				Culex mus.
				Cundurango
				Cuphea vis.
				Cupressus aus.
				Cupressus law.
		Bel., Chi., Cicut., Dul., Hep., Ipc., Merc., Nux, In poisoning cases, by sugar or white of egg given freely.		Cuprum acet.
		See under Arsen		Cuprum arsen
	Coc. i., Dul.	*Dynamic:* Aur., Bel., Cham., Chi., Con,., Cic., Dul., Hep., Ipc., Merc., Nux, Pul,., Ver. Aggravations are > by smelling Cam. Hep., or Potash soap may be used after *poisoning* from food prepared in copper vessels,. Sugar, or white of egg mixed with milk, and given freely.		
		Eggs, milk, pure yellow prussiate of potash.		Cuprum sulph.
	The poison of rabies, and Strychnia	Bromine, Chlorine. In case of poisoning, artificial respiration must be resorted to. If the poinsoning is due to a punctured wound, rubbing in tobacco or salt will neutralise it.		Curare

REMEDY	Complementary Remedies	Remedy Follows Well	Remedy is Followed Well by	Compatible Remedies
Cyclamen			Pho., Pul., Rhs., Sep., Sul.	
Cypripedium				
Daphne ind.				
Datura arb.				
Datura fer.				
Datura met.				
Derris pin.				
Dictamnus				
Digitalinum (see under Digitalis)				
Digitalis			Bel., Bry., Cham., Chi., Lyc., Nux, Opi., Pho., Pul., Sep., Sul., Ver.	Bel., Bry., Cham., Chi., Lyc., Nux, Opi., Pho., Pul. Sep., Sul., Ver.
Digitoxinum				
Dioscorea				
Diphtherinum				
Dirca pal.				
Dolichos		Rhs. (in herpes).		
Doryphora				
Drosera	Nux.		Calc., Cin., Pul., Sul., Ver.	Calc., Gna., Pul., Ver.
Duboisinum				
Dulcamara	Ba. c.	Bry., Calc., Lyc., Rhs., Sep., Ver.	Bel., Cal., Lyc., Rhs., Sep.	

Incompatible Remedies	Remedy Antidotes	Remedy is Antidoted by	Duration of Action	REMEDY
		Cam., Cof., Pul.	14–20 d.	**Cyclamen**
	Rhs. poisoning			**Cypripedium**
	Chr., x., Merc.	Bry., Dig., Rhs.,, Sep., Sil., Zn.		**Daphne ind**
				Datura arb.
				Datura fer.
				Datura met.
				Derris pin.
				Dictamnus
				Digitalinum (*see under* **Digitalis**)
Chin. (increases the anxiety), Nt. s. d.	Chl. h. (heart), Dph., Gel., My. c. (jaundice), Wine.	Vegetable acids, Aps., Calc., Camphor, (Clch.), Ether, infusion of galls, Nt. x., Nux, Opi., Serpentaria, Vinegar.	40–50 d.	**Digitalis**
				Digitoxinum
				Dioscorea
				Diphtherinum
				Dirca pal.
		Aco., and "in cases of dentition with fever, Aco., should be given before Dol. to prevent convulsions" (Hering).		**Dolichos**
		The local effect by: Earth; other antidotes are: Vinegar and other vegetable acids, Stm.		**Doryophora**
		Cam.	20–30 d.	**Drosera**
				Duboisinum
Bel., Lach.	Ba. c., Cam., Con., Cup., Merc.	Cam., Cup., Ipc., K. ca., Merc.	30 d.	**Dulcamara**

REMEDY	Complementary Remedies	Remedy Follows Well	Remedy is Followed Well by	Compatible Remedies
Echinacea ang.				
Echinacea pur.				
Elaeis guin.				
Elaps				
Elaterium				
Electricitas				
Ephedra vul.				
Epigea rep.				
Epilibium pal.				
Epiphegus				
Equisetum				
Erechthites				
Ergotinum				
Erigeron				
Eriodictyon glu.				
Erodium				
Eryngium aq.				
Eryngium mar.				
Erythrinus				
Eserinum				
Etherum				
Ethylum nit.				

Incompatible Remedies	Remedy Antidotes	Remedy is Antidoted by	Duration of Action	R E M E D Y
	Rhus-poisoning			Echinacea ang.
				Echinacea pur.
				Elaeis guin.
		Alcohol, Ars., Radiated heat.		Elaps
				Elaterium
	(In attenuation) Chl. h., Mgt., Merc., Ph. h., Plumb	Mo. a., Pho. (the effect of storms). Effects on the back, recorded by Hahnemann as from the fumes of burning sulphur, were antidoted by electric shock.		Electricitas
				Ephedra vul.
				Epigea rep.
				Epilibium pal.
				Epiphegus
				Equisetum
				Erechthites
				Ergotinum
				Erigeron
				Eriodictyon glu.
				Erodium
				Eryngium aq.
				Eryngium mar.
				Erythrinus
				Eserinum
		Bel. for bronchitis as an after-result of Ether anaesthesia. Weakening effects removed by Hep., Hyo., Nux.		Etherum
				Ethylum nit.

Remedy	Complementary Remedies	Remedy Follows Well	Remedy is Followed Well by	Compatible Remedies
Eucalyptus		ars. in relapsing fevers. A cup of Coffee > the effects.		
Eugenia j.				
Euonyminum				
Euonymus atro.				
Euonymus eur.				
Eupatorium aro.				
Eupatorium perf.			Na. m., Sep.	Na. m., Sep., which also follow well.
Eupatorium pur.				
Euphorbia amyg.				
Euphorbio cor.				
Euphorbia cyp.				
Euphorbia het.				
Euphorbia hyper.				
Euphorbia ip.				
Euphorbia lath.				
Euphorbia pil.				
Euphorbium		Fer., Gph., Lach., Pul., Sep., Sul.	Fer., Lach, Pul., Sep., sul.	
Euphrasia			Aco., Calc., Con., Nux, Pho., Pul., Rhs., Sil., Sul.	Aco., Calc., Con., Nux, Pho., Pul., Rhs., Sil., Sul.
Eupionum				
Fagopyrum				
Fagus				
Fel. tauri				
Ferrum	Alm., Chi., Ham.		Aco., Arn., Bel., chi., Con., Lyc., Merc., Pho., Pul., Sul., Ver.	aco., Arn., Bel., Chi., Con., Lyc., Merc., Pho., Ver.

Incompatible Remedies	Remedy Antidotes	Remedy is Antidoted by	Duration of Action	REMEDY
	Sty. poisioning.			Eucalyptus
	Coffee, smoking tobacco			Eugenia j.
				Euonyminum
				Euonymus atro.
				Euonymus eur.
				Eupatorium aro.
	Cac., Cin.		1–7 d.	Eupatorium perf.
				Eupatorium pur.
				Euphorbia amyg.
				Euphorbio cor.
				Euphorbia cyp.
				Euphorbia het.
				Euphorbia hyper.
				Euphorbia ip.
				Euphorbia lath.
				Euphorbia pil.
	Ars., Cit., Grt., Nux.	Ac. x., Cam., Cit., large quantities of lemon-juice, Opi.	50 d.	Euphorbium
		Cam., Caus., Pul.		Euphrasia
		Gph. (effect on eye lids).		Euphrasia
				Fagopyrum
				Fagus
				Fel. tauri
Ac. x., Beer, Thea.	alcoholic drinks, Ars., Chi., Hy. x., Iod., Merc., Tea.	Arn., Ars., Beer., Bel., Chi., Hep., Ipc., Pul.	50 d.	Ferrum

REMEDY	Complementary Remedies	Remedy Follows Well	Remedy is Followed Well by	Compatible Remedies
Ferrum arsen				
Ferrum bro.				
Ferrum iod.				
Ferrum mag.				
Ferrum mur.				
Ferrum per.				
Ferrum pho.				Ant. t., (capillary bronchitis), Ca. fl. (haemorrhoids), Ca. p. (chlorosis, haemorrhoids), Ca. s. (hip-joint disease), K. m. (croup, pneumonia, palpitation, typhus), Kali p. (colic, threatened gangrene), Na. s. (diabetes)
Ferrum pho. hyd.				
Ferrum pic.				
Ferrum pyro.				
Ferrum sul.				
Ferrum tart.				
Ferula gl.				
Ficus rel.				
Filix mas.				
Fluoricum ac.	Sil.	ars. in ascites from gin-drinker's liver; Kali c. in hip-disease; Ph. x. in diabetes	Gph., Nt. x.	
Formica				
Fragaria v.				
Franciscea uni.				
Franzensbad				

Incompatible Remedies	Remedy Antidotes	Remedy is Antidoted by	Duration of Action	REMEDY
				Ferrum arsen
				Ferrum bro.
				Ferrum iod.
				Ferrum mag.
		Bry., Kre. (sometimes) (?)		Ferrum mur.
				Ferrum per.
Par.	According to Cooper, Fe. p. antidoted "violent dysuria, night and day," caused by Sto b.			Ferrum pho.
				Ferrum pho. hyd.
				Ferrum pic.
				Ferrum pyro.
				Ferrum sul.
				Ferrum tart.
				Ferula gl.
				Ficus rel.
				Filix mas.
	Sil.		30 d.	Fluoricum ac.
				Formica
				Fragaria v.
				Franciscea uni.
				Franzensbad

REMEDY	Complementary Remedies	Remedy Follows Well	Remedy is Followed Well by	Compatible Remedies
Fraxinus amer.				
Fucus ves.				
Gadus morr.				
Galega				
Galium				
Gallicum ac.				
Galvanismus				
Gambogia				
Gastein				
Gaultheria				
Gelsemium			Bap., Cac., Ipc.	Bap. (in typhoid, influenza); Ipc., (in dumb ague).
Genista				
Gentiana cru.				
Gentiana lut.				
Gentiana quin.				
Geranium mac.				
Gettysburg				
Geum ri.				
Ginseng				
Glonoinum				
Gnaphalium				

Incompatible Remedies	Remedy Antidotes	Remedy is Antidoted by	Duration of Action	REMEDY
				Fraxinus amer.
				Fucus ves.
				Gadus morr.
				Galega
				Galium
				Gallicum ac.
	Mgt.			Galvanismus
		Cam., Cof., Col., Kali. c., Opi.		Gambogia
				Gastein
				Gaultheria
Gel. antagonises Atr., Opi.	Coca Mag. p. Nx. m., Sol. Tab. (sometimes).	Atr., Chi., Cof., Dig., Na. m., Nx. m. In cases of poisoning, artificial respiration and faradisation of respiratory muscles. Foy found Nitroglycerine a perfect antidote in one case. Jephson antidoted his case with Strychnine.		Gelsemium
				Genista
				Gentiana cru.
				Gentiana lut.
				Gentiana quin.
				Geranium mac.
				Gettysburg
				Geum ri.
				Ginseng
	Ca. ar. (headache), Pal. (headache), Sol.	Aco., Cam., Cof., Nux.		Glonoinum
				Gnaphalium

REMEDY	Complementary Remedies	Remedy Follows Well	Remedy is Followed Well by	Compatible Remedies
Gossypium her.				
Granatum				
Graphites	Ars., Caus., Fer., Hep., Lyc.	Calc., Lyc., Pul., Sep., Sul.	Eub., Ntr. s., Sil.	
Gratiola				
Grindelia				
Guaco				
Guaiacum		Gui, is better than Caus., which it follows well when either gout or rheumatism causes distortion of limbs < every attempt of motion.	Calc. Merc.	After Caus. (in torticollis), after Merc., (rheumatism, gout, and syphilis), after Sul. (in cholers infantum).
Guarana				
Guarea				
Gymnema syl.				
Gymnocladus can.				
Haematoxylon				
Hall				
Hamamelis	Fer. in haemorrhages.			
Hecla				
Hedeoma				
Hedera he.				
Hedysarum lid.				
Helianthus				
Heliotropium				
Helix tosta				
Helleborus foe.				

Incompatible Remedies	Remedy Antidotes	Remedy is Antidoted by	Duration of Action	R E M E D Y
		Vb. p.		Gossypium her.
				Granatum
	Ars., effect on eyelid of Epn., Iod., Lyc., Rhs., Ther. (more chronic effects of).	Aco., Ars., Chi., Nux, Wine	40–50 d.	Graphites
	Iod.	Caus., Bel., Eub., Nux.		Gratiola
	Rhs.			Grindelia
		Kre. and Sul. (leucor-rhoea).		Guaco
	Caus., Merc., Na. hch., Rhs.	Nux.	40 d.	Guaiacum
				Guarana
				Guarea
				Gymnema syl.
				Gymnocladus can.
		Cam.		Haematoxylon
				Hall
		Arn., Cam., Chi., Pul., (toothache).	1–7 d.	Hamamelis
				Hecla
		Ver. (some of its effects).		Hedeoma
				Hedera he.
				Hedysarum lid.
				Helianthus
				Heliotropium
				Helix tosta
				Helleborus foe.

Remedy	Complementary Remedies	Remedy Follows Well	Remedy is Followed Well by	Compatible Remedies
Helleborus ni.			Bel., Bry., Chi., Lyc., Nux, Pho., Pul., sul., Zin.	Bel., Bry., Chi., Lyc., Nux, Pho., Pul., Sul., Zin.
Helleborus ori.				
Helleborus vir.				
Heloderma				
Helonias				
Hepar	Caln. in injuries.	Aco., Arn., Bel., Lach., Merc., Nt. x., Sil., Spo., Zin., (Boenninghausen's powders for croup were given in this order: (1) Aco. 200, (2) Hep.200, (3) Spo. 200).	Aco., Arn., Bel., Bry., Iod., Lach., Merc., Nt. x., Nux, Pul., Rhs., Sep., Sil., Spo., Sul., Zin.	
Heopatica				
Heracleum				
Hippomanes				
Hippozaeninum				
Hoang-nan				
Homarus				
Homeria				
Hura bra.				
Hura crep.				
Hydrangea arb.				
Hydrastininum mur.				

Incompatible Remedies	Remedy Antidotes	Remedy is Antidoted by	Duration of Action	REMEDY
		Cam., Chi.	20–30 d.	Helleborus ni.
Cof.				Helleborus ori.
				Helleborus vir.
				Heloderma
	The prolapse of Lil. and the mental depression of K. br.			Helonias
Spo. does not follow well, according to C. C. Smith; but see under "Follows Well."	Am. c., mant. c., Ars., Bel., Calc., Ch. s., Cnb., Cit., Cod-liver oil. It may be used after poisoning from food prepared in copper vessels. It removes the weakening effects of Ether. Cu. a., Cup., Fer., Iod., Iof., K. i., Lach., Metals, and esp. mercurial preparations, Nt. x., Osm. (pain in larynx,), Pb., Sil.			Hepar
				Heopatica
				Heracleum
		Caus. > the paralysis of wrist; Coffee.		Hippomanes
				Hippozaeninum
				Hoang-nan
				Homarus
				Homeria
		Cam., Opi.		Hura bra.
		Cam., Opi.		Hura crep.
				Hydrangea arb.
				Hydrastininum mur.

REMEDY	Complementary Remedies	Remedy Follows Well	Remedy is Followed Well by	Compatible Remedies
Hydrastinum mur.				
Hydrastis				
Hydrocotyle				
Hydrocyanicum ac.				
Hydrophobinum		Ag. n. (uterine disease); Tab. (headache)	Na. m.	
Hydrophyllum vir.				
Hyoscyaminum				
Hyoscyamus		Bel., Nux, Opi., Rhs.	Bel., Pho., Pul., Stm., Ver.	
Hypericum				
Iberis				
Ichthyolum				
Ictodes foe				
Ignatia	Na. m.		Ars., Bel., Calc., Chi., Lyc., Nux, Pul., Rhs., Sep., Sil., Sul.	Ars., Bel., Calc., Chi., Lyc., Nux, Pul., Rhs., Sep., Sul., Zin.
Ilex aqui.				
Illicium anis.		Aconite and Bryonia in haemoptysis.		
Indigo				
Indium				
Inula				

Incompatible Remedies	Remedy Antidotes	Remedy is Antidoted by	Duration of Action	REMEDY
				Hydrastinum mur.
	chlorate of potass, Merc., Ss. x. (constipation).	Sul. (head symptoms and sciatic pains).		**Hydrastis**
				Hydrocotyle
		Cam., Chlm., Cof., Fer., Ipc., Nux, Opi., Ver.		**Hydrocyanicum ac.**
		Agn., Bel., Ced., Fgs., Hyo., Lach., Stm.		**Hydrophobinum**
				Hydrophyllum vir.
				Hyoscyaminum
	Bel., Cld., (night cough), Eth., Merc., Plumb., Rum., Stm., Sty., (drowsiness).	Ac. x., Bel., Chi., Citric ac., Stm., Vinegar.	6–14 d.	**Hyoscyamus**
	Effects of mesmerism (Sul.)	Ars. (weakness or sickness on moving), Cham. (pains in face)		**Hypericum**
				Iberis
				Ichthyolum
				Ictodes foe
Cof. Nux (sometimes), Tab.	Arn., Brandy., Cld. (sometimes), Chamomile tea, Cham., Coc. i., Cof., Mgt., Mgt. n., Mgt. s., Phyt., Pul., Sel., Tab., Zin.	Ac. x., Arn., Cam., Cham., Coc. i., Cof., Nux, Pul. (chief antidote).	9 d.	**Ignatia**
				Ilex aqui.
				Illicium anis.
		Cam., Nux.		**Indigo**
				Indium
				Inula

Remedy	Complementary Remedies	Remedy Follows Well	Remedy is Followed Well by	Compatible Remedies
Iodium	Bad., Lyc.,	Ars., Hep. (croup), Merc.	Aco., Ag. n., Calc., K. bi., Lyc., Mr. sol., Pho., Pul.	
Iodoformum				
Ipecacuanha	Arn., Cup.		Ant. t., Arn., Ars., (cholera infantum, debility colds, croup, chills), Bel., Bry., Calc., Cd. s. (yellow fever) Cham., Chi., Cup., Ign., Nux, Pho., Pul., Rhe., Sep., Sul., Tab., Ver.	
Iridium				
Iris flor.				
Iris foe.				
Iris ger.				
Iris ten.				
Iris ver.				
Itu				
Jaborandi				
Jacaranda car.				

Incompatible Remedies	Remedy Antidotes	Remedy is Antidoted by	Duration of Action	REMEDY
	An. oc. (locally), Ars., Merc. (glands).	Starch or wheat flour mixed with water (to large doses). Antidotes to small doses : Ant. t., Aps., Ars., Bel., Cam., Ch. s., Cog., Fer., Gph., Grt., Hep., Opi., Pho., Spo., Sul., Thu.	30–40 d.	Iodium
		Hep., Sang. (skin)		Iodoformum
	Ago., alum., ant. t., aps. (Ipc. low antidotes medium doses and poisonings of Aps., also powdered Ipc., applied locally; Arn., ars., Calc., Chi., Chl., Chlf., Copper fumes, Cu. a., Cup., Dul., Fer., Hy. x., it relieved the cough of K.n., Lau., Ln. u. (?), Lo. i., Med. (dry cough), esp. useful for secondary effects of Mor., (Teste says it is the surest antidote to Mu. x.), Opi., Stil. (nausea from the fumes), Su. x., Tab., (primary effects : vomiting).	Arn., Ars., Chi., Nux, Tab.	7–10 d.	Ipecacuanha
				Iridium
				Iris flor.
				Iris foe.
				Iris ger.
				Iris ten.
	Merc., Nux, Ol. j. (sometimes), Phyt.	Nux		Iris ver.
				Itu
		Bel.		Jaborandi
				Jacaranda car.

REMEDY	Complementary Remedies	Remedy Follows Well	Remedy is Followed Well by	Compatible Remedies
Jacaranda gual.				
Jalapa				
Jasminum				
Jatropha				
Jatropha u.				
Jequirity				
Juglans cin.				
Juglans re.		Elp. (axillary affections black haemorrhages), Gnd. (pain over 1. eye), Sul. (head hot, cold extremities).		
Juncus				
Juniperus com.				
Juniperus vir.				
Kali acet				
Kall ars.				
Kali bi.		after Apis (scrofulous ophthalmia). After Cth. in dysentery, when, though scrapings continue, the discharge becomes jelly-like. After Iod. in croup.	Ant. t., (in catarrhal affections and skin diseases), Pul.	

Incompatible Remedies	Remedy Antidotes	Remedy is Antidoted by	Duration of Action	R E M E D Y
	Merc.	Merc.		Jacaranda gual.
				Jalapa
		Convulsive symptoms > by a bath.		Jasminum
		Placing hands in cold water.		Jatropha
				Jatropha u.
				Jequirity
	Ana.	Bry. (angina pectoris; Bry gtt. v. > immediately).		Juglans cin.
		Rhs.		Juglans re.
				Juncus
				Juniperus com.
				Juniperus vir.
				Kali acet
		In some cases of overdoses K. i., For other *antidotes* see Ars., which it greatly resembles, and with which it must be compared.		Kall ars.
	Arsenical vapour, effect of beer, Merc., Mr. i. f.; also it is the best general antodote to the effect of metallic poisoning among brass workers.	The same antidotes as for poisoning by Acids : Chalk, Eggs, Hydrated Peroxide of Iron, Magnesia, Milk, Almond or Olive Oil, Soap, Bicarbonates of Soda and Potash, any one of which should be administered almost immediately after the dose. Among the *dynamic antidotes* are Ars., Lach. (croup, diphtheria, & c.), Pul. (wandering pains.)	30 d.	Kali bi.

REMEDY	Complementary Remedies	Remedy Follows Well	Remedy is Followed Well by	Compatible Remedies
Kali br.		Aco. and Spo. in croup, Eng. in acne.		
Kali car.	K. ca. in complementary to : Cb. v., Na. m., Nt. x., Pho., Sep. Complementary to K. ca. are Cb. v., Nux.	Bry., K. sul., Lyc., Na. m., Pho., Stn.	Ars., Cb. v., Fl. x., Lyc., Nt. x., Pho., Pul., Sep., Sul.	
Kali chlori.				
Kali chloro.				
Kali cit.				
Kali cy.				
Kali fer.				
Kali iod.		Merc.	Nt. x.	
Kali mur.		Ca. fl., Ca. p., Fe. p.		
Kali nit.		Aco. in dysentery; Bel., Calc., Pul., Rhs., Sep.	Bel., Calc., Nux in dysentery, Pul., Rhs., Sep., Sul.	
Kali ox.				

Incompatible Remedies	Remedy Antidotes	Remedy is Antidoted by	Duration of Action	REMEDY
	Lead poisoning.	Vegetable acids, Cam., Hion (mental depression) Oils, Nux, Zin.		**Kali br.**
	Dul., Gam., Nt. s. d.	Cam., Cof., Nt. s. d.	40–50 d.	**Kali car.**
	Merc.	Hdr.		**Kali chlori.**
				Kali chloro.
				Kali cit.
		Nitrate of Cobalt (?)		**Kali cy.**
				Kali fer.
	It antidoted in some cases of over-dosing with K. as., Lead-poisoning, Merc., Mez.	Ag. n. > "fulness and indigestion after each dose" caused by K. i.; Aur., Hep., Nt. x., 12 or 30 often gives vast relief to syphilitics who have been saturated with K. i. under old-school treatment and are getting < under it. This includes cases of iritis. Actinomycosis affecting the anal region has been cured with Nt. x. 30, after massive doses of K. i. has been administered to patient under old-school doctors.		**Kali iod.**
	Merc.	Bel., Ca. s. Hdr., Pul.		**Kali mur.**
Smelling Cam. intensified the sufferings.	Cth. (sometimes), the renal symptoms of Caus., Nt. s. d.	Ipc. > the cough, smelling Nt. s. d.	30–40 d.	**Kali nit.**
				Kali ox.

REMEDY	Complementary Remedies	Remedy Follows Well	Remedy is Followed Well by	Compatible Remedies
Kali per.				
Kali phos.				Cyc. (disordered mental conditions), K.m. (puerperal fever), Mag.p. (bladder troubles),Zn.p. (brain paralysis with nephritic irritation, Na., m. and Nt x., (haemorrhages).
Kali pic.				
Kali sulphura.				
Kali sulphuri.			Ac. x., Ars., Calc., Hep., Pul., Rhs., Sep., Sil., Sul.	Ac. x. (itching and redness of the skin), Calc., Hep., Pul., Rhs., Sep., Sil., Sul,.
Kali tari.				
Kali tel.				
Kalmia lat.		Nux, Spi., Thyr.		
Kamala				
Kaolin				
Karaka				
Kerosolenum				
Kissingen				
Kousso				
Kreosotum			Ars. (in malignant disease), Bel., Calc., K. ca., Lyc., Nt. x., Nux, Rhs., Sep., Sul.	

Incompatible Remedies	Remedy Antidotes	Remedy is Antidoted by	Duration of Action	REMEDY
	Opium. (After ½ oz. laudanum taken, K, pm. in dilute solution (gr. ii. to the pint) was given repeatedly, and acted promptly.) Pho. (well diluted and given freely).			**Kali per.**
				Kali phos.
				Kali pic.
				Kali sulphura.
	Rhs. poisoning.			Kali sulphuri.
				Kali tari.
				Kali tel.
				Kalmia lat.
				Kamala
				Kaolin
				Karaka
				Kerosolenum
				Kissingen
				Kousso
After Cb. v., also after Chi.	Athra, Guac., Pb.	Aco. (vascular erethism). According to Teste Fer. is the best antidote, esp. for overaction of Kre. in lively, sanguine, and vigorous children. Nux (violent pulsations in every opart of the body).	15–20 d.	**Kreosotum**

REMEDY	Complementary Remedies	Remedy Follows Well	Remedy is Followed Well by	Compatible Remedies
Laburnum				
Lac can.				
Lac feli.				
Lac vac. coag.				
Lac vac. de.				
Lacerta				
Lachesis	Hep., Lyc., (the chief complement). Iod. and K. i., which are complementary to Lyc., are probably complementary to Lach.; Nt. x.		Aco., alm., Ars., Bel., Bro., Cac., Cb. v., Caus., Chi., Cic., Con., Eub., Hep., Hyo., K. bi., Lc. c., Lyc., Merc., Mr. i. f., Na. m., Nt. x., Nux, Pho., Pul., Rhs., Sil., Sul. Trn.	Aco., Ars., Bel., Bro., Cb. v., Chi., Hep., Hyo., K. bi., Lc. c., Lyc., Merc., Nt. x., Nux, Oln., Pho., Pul., Sil., Sul. (pneumonia), Trn., (Plat, followed well when Hep. and Lach. failed to evacuate pus from ovarian abscess).
Lachnanthes				
Lacticum ac.				Meat diet in diabetes.
Lactis vac. flos.				
Lactuca				
Lamium				
Lapathum				
Lapis alb.				
Lapasana com.				
Lathyrus				

Incompatible Remedies	Remedy Antidotes	Remedy is Antidoted by	Duration of Action	REMEDY
		Coffee and stimulants, hot and cold douches to chest.		Laburnum
				Lac can.
				Lac feli.
				Lac vac. coag.
				Lac vac. de.
				Lacerta
Aggravated by and incompatible with Ac. x. ; Am. c., Dul., Nt. x., inimical to Pso.; Sep. (?).	Athra., Aps., ars., Buf., Ch. s., Crt.h., K. bi. (croup, diphtheria, & c.), Mag. p. (cough), Rhs., Rum.	Alcohol inwardly, radiate heat outwardly, Salt (for effects of bite). *Antidotes to dilutions:* Alum., Ars., Bel., Calc., Cb. c., according to Teste the chief antidote is Ced.; Cham., Coc. i., Cof., Hep., Led., Merc., Nt. x., Nux, Ph,. x., Sep. (the visible tenesmus of rectum), Trn. (Henrig).		Lachesis
				Lachnanthes
Coffee < symptoms.	Art. t., Pod.	Bry. (> sharp pains upper third r,. side, but soreness remained).		Lacticum ac.
				Lactis vac. flos.
		Vegetable acids and Coffee. (In a proving of Lactucarium, Acetic Ether and Hock were more effectual than Coffee.)		Lactuca
				Lamium
				Lapathum
				Lapis alb.
				Lapasana com.
				Lathyrus

REMEDY	Complementary Remedies	Remedy Follows Well	Remedy is Followed Well by	Compatible Remedies
Latrodectus kat.				
Latrodectus mact.				
Laurocerasus			Bel., Cb. v., Pho., Pul., Ver.	Bel., Pho., Pul., Ver.
Ledum			Aco., Bel., Bry., Chel., Nux, Pul., Rhs., Sul.	Aco., Arn., Bel., Bry., Nux, Pul., Rhs., Sul.
Lemna min.		Calc., Merc., Pso.		
Leonurus card.				
Lepidium bon.				
Leptandra				
Levico				
Liatris spic.				
Lilium tigr.				
Limulus				
Linaria				
Linum cath.				
Linum usita.				
Lippia mex.				
Lippspringe				
Lithium benz.				
Lithium bro.				
Lithium carb.				
Lithium lac.				
Lithium mur.				
Lobelia card.				
Lobelia dort.				
Lobelia erin				

Incompatible Remedies	Remedy Antidotes	Remedy is Antidoted by	Duration of Action	REMEDY
				Latrodectus kat.
				Latrodectus mact.
	Ant. t., Cth., Nx. m.	Cam., Cof., Ipc., Nx. m., Opi.	4–8 d.	Laurocerasus
Chi. ("Cinchona bark given for the debility produced by Ledum is very injurious." — Hahnemann.)	Effects of alcohol, Aps., Chi., Vsp.	Cam., Rhs., (the best antidote, according to Teste).	30 d.	Ledum
				Lemna min.
		Ars.		Leonurus card.
				Lepidium bon.
	Pod.			Leptandra
				Levico
		Hlon. (anteversion), Nux (colic, Plat., Pul.		Liatris spic.
				Lilium tigr.
				Limulus
		Tea in milk.		Linaria
		Sul. (headache).		Linum cath.
		Asa. (?) Ipc. (?)		Linum usita.
				Lippia mex.
				Lippspringe
				Lithium benz.
				Lithium bro.
				Lithium carb.
				Lithium lac.
				Lithium mur.
				Lobelia card.
				Lobelia dort.
				Lobelia erin

Remedy	Complementary Remedies	Remedy Follows Well	Remedy is Followed Well by	Compatible Remedies
Lobelia infl.				
Lobelia pur.				
Lobelia syph.				
Lolium tem.				
Lonicera peri.				
Lonicera xylos.				
Luna				
Lupulus				
Lycopersicum				
Lycopodium	Chel., Iod., Ign., Ipc., (in capillary bronchitis, < r. side, sputa yellow and thick), K. i., Lach., Pul.	C a l c . , Lach, Sul.	Ana., Bel., Bry., Calc. (?), Clch., Drs., Gph., Hyo., K. ca., Lach., Led., Nux, Pho., Pul., Sep., Sil., Stm., Ther., Ver.	Bel., Bry., Calc., c. (predisposition to constipation hard stools evacuated with difficulty, or urging ineffective), Cb. v. (a dose of Cb. v. every eighth day facilitates action of Lyc.), Gph., Hyp., Lach., Led., Pho., Pul., Sep., Sil, Stm., Sul., Ver.
Lycopus				
Macrotinum				
Magnesia carb.	Cham.		Caus., Pho., Pul., Sep., Sul.	Caus., Pho., Pul., Sep., Sul.
Magnesia mur.			Bel., Lyc., Na. m., Nux, Pul., Sep.	Bel., Na. m., Pul., Sep., Sul.
Magnesia phos.				
Magnesia sulph.				
Magnetis po. am.				
Magnetis po. arc.				

Incompatible Remedies	Remedy Antidotes	Remedy is Antidoted by	Duration of Action	REMEDY
				Lobelia infl.
				Lobelia pur.
				Lobelia syph.
				Lolium tem.
				Lonicera peri.
				Lonicera xylos.
				Luna
				Lupulus
				Lycopersicum
Cof.; after Sul. except in cycle of Sul., Calc., Lyc., Sul., & c.	All., Alo. (relieves earache), Chi. (yellow face, liver and spleen swollen, flatulence, tension under short ribs < r. side, pressure in stomach, and constipation), Chlorine (effects of the fumes when they cause impotence), Merc., Mr. i. f., Tab. (sometimes).	Aco., Cam., Caus., Cham., Cof., Gph., Nux, Pul.	40–50 d.	Lycopodium
	Act. r. (?)			Lycopus
	Ost.			Macrotinum
		Ars., Cham., (neuralgia), Col., Mr. sol., Nux, Pul., Rhe. (abdominal troubles).	40–50 d.	Magnesia carb.
	Merc. (metrorrhagia).	Ars., Cam., Cham., Nux.	40–50 d.	Magnesia mur.
		Bel., Gel., Lach. (cough)		Magnesia phos.
				Magnesia sulph.
		Elc., Glv., Ign., Zin. (imposition of Zinc. plate).		Magnetis po. am.
				Magnetis po. arc.

REMEDY	Complementary Remedies	Remedy Follows Well	Remedy is Followed Well by	Compatible Remedies
Magnetis po. aust.				
Magnolia glau.				
Magnolia grand.				
Malandrinum				
Malaria offi.				
Mancinella				
Mandragora				
Manganum			Pul., Rhs., Sul.	Pul., Rhs., Sul.
Manganum mur.				
Manganum oxy. nat.				
Manganum sulph.				
Marum			Chi., Pul., Sil.	
Matthiola g.				
Medorrhinum				Sul. (esp. when stool drives out of bed.)

Incompatible Remedies	Remedy Antidotes	Remedy is Antidoted by	Duration of Action	REMEDY
	Mgt. n.	Ign., Mgt. n., Zin.		Magnetis po. aust.
				Magnolia glau.
				Magnolia grand.
	Vac., Var.			Malandrinum
		Bowen found the best antidotes to be: Bry., and Nux for the effects of No. I. (*see* Dr. Clarke's *Disc. of P.M.M.*, v. ii. p. 394); Ars. and Bry. for No. II.; Bry. and Rhs. for No. III. Chi and E. pf. gave negative results.		Malaria offi.
				Mancinella
		The effects were removed by free indulgence in cigars, coffee and wine. With regular dieting they lasted much longer, and were removed by Bel., Cam., and Nux.		Mandragora
		Cam., Cof., Mr. sol.	40 d.	Manganum
				Manganum mur.
				Manganum oxy. nat.
				Manganum sulph.
		Cam.	14–21 d.	Marum
	Cooper relates a case which seems to indicate that Mor. causes neuralgia, and that Mat. antidotes Mor.			Matthiola g.
		Ipc. (dry couth).		Medorrhinum

Remedy	Complementary Remedies	Remedy Follows Well	Remedy is Followed Well by	Compatible Remedies
Medusa				
Melastoma				
Melliotus			‒	
Mellitagrinum				
Menispermum				
Mentha pi.				
Mentha pu.				
Menyanthes		Cup., Lach., Lyc., Pul., Rhs., Ver.	Cap., Lyc., Pul., Rhs.,	
Mephitis		Drs. (in cough of consumptives)		
Mercurialis per.				
Mercurius	Bad.	Aco., Bel., Hep., Lach., Sul.	Ars., Asa., Bel., Calc., Cb. v., Chi., Gui., Hep., Iod., Lyc., Mu. x., Nt. x., Pho., Pul., Rhs., Sep., Sul., Thu.	

Incompatible Remedies	Remedy Antidotes	Remedy is Antidoted by	Duration of Action	REMEDY
				Medusa
				Melastoma
				Melliotus
				Mellitagrinum
		Bry., Chi.		**Menispermum**
				Mentha pi.
				Mentha pu.
	Effects of China and Quinine.	Cam.	14–20 d.	**Menyanthes**
		Cam., but only temporarily. Crotal. > eye symptoms.		**Mephitis**
		Aco., Bel.		**Mercurialis per.**
It is < by Ac. x., Sil. (Merc. and Sil. should never be g i v e n i m m e d i - a t e l y before or after each other).	Ailments from arsenic or cop- per vapours, stings of insects, bad effects of sugar. Ant. c., ant. t., Arg., Asa., Aur., Ba. c., Bel., Cld. (sometimes), Can. s. (small doses), Chi., Cof., Cop. (in the female), Cu.s., Cup., Dul., Ja. g., Mag. c., Man., Mez., Mr. c., Nt. x., Opi., Osm. (laryngeal catarrh), Plnt. (toothache), Rhs., Sar., Sul., Vi. t.	Arn., Ars., As a (bone affec- tions—Asa. is distinguialsed by extreme sensitiveness of diseased parts, extreme sore- ness of bones round eye); Aur (suicidal mania, caries of bones esp. of patella and nose), Bel., Bry., Cld., Cap. (abuse of Merc.) Cb. v., Caus. (sometimes), Chi (chronic ptylism), Cin., Clem., Con., Cup., Dph., Dul. (Ptylism < by every damp change), Elc., Fer., Gui., Hep. (mental symp- toms—anxiety, distress, sui- cidal and even homicidal mood—bone pains, sore mouth, ulcers and gastric symptoms), Hdr., Hyo., Iod., (glands), Iris, Ja. g., K. bi., K. chl., K. i. (syphilis and mercurialism combined, bones, periosteum, glands, ozoena, thin watery dis- charge, upper lip sore and raw, repeated catarrhs after Merc., every little exposure to damp or wet air = coryza, eyes hot watery, swollen, ceuralgic pains in one or	Antidote d by *(contd..)* b o t h cheeks , nose stuffed a n d swolle n and a t s a m e t i m e p r o - f u s e , watery , scald- i n g coryza , sore throat every fresh expo- sure), K. m. (scor- butus, feter),	**Mercurius** Antidoted by *(contd..)* Lyc., Mag., m. (metrorrhagia), Mez. (nervous system, neural- gia in eyes, face, anywhere), Mu. x., Nux (tremors), Opi., Pod., (vapours) Pul., Spi., Stp., (depressed sys- tem, wasted sal- low, dank rings round eyes, spongy gms, ulcers on tongue), Stil., Sul., Ter., Thu.;, "all symptoms agreeing, Merc. high" (Guernsey).

REMEDY	Complementary Remedies	Remedy Follows Well	Remedy is Followed Well by	Compatible Remedies
Mercurius ac.				
Mercurius bin.		Bel.		
Mercurius bin. *cum* k. iod.				
Mercurius cor.		Aco., Ag. n. (which follows Pul.).		
Mercurius cyan.				
Mercurius dul.				
Mercurius nit.				
Mercurius pr.alb				
Mercurius pr. rub.				
Mercurius prot.		Lach. (scarlatina)		
Mercurius sulpho.				
Mercurius sulphur				
Methylene-blue				
Mezereum			Calc., Caus., Ign., Lyc., Merc., Nux, Pho., Pul.	Calc., Caus., Ign., Lyc., Merc., Nux, Pho., Pul.
Millefolium				
Mimosa				
Mitchella				
Momordica				
Morphinum				

Incompatible Remedies	Remedy Antidotes	Remedy is Antidoted by	Duration of Action	REMEDY
				Mercurius ac.
		Hep.		Mercurius bin.
				Mercurius bin. cum k. iod.
	Chr.o.(sometimes), Trb. (diarrhoea)	(*Poisonous doses*) White of egg. *Dynamic antidotes :* Lo. i. (Teste), Mr. sol., Sep., Sil. (Hering). Also antidotes to the Mercuries generally (*see* Merc.).		Mercurius cor.
				Mercurius cyan.
		Hep.		Mercurius dul.
				Mercurius nit.
				Mercurius pr.alb
				Mercurius pr. rub.
		Hep., Lys., (palpitation).		Mercurius prot.
				Mercurius sulpho.
				Mercurius sulphur
				Methylene-blue
	Alcohol, Merc., Nt. x., Pho., Phy.	Acids, Aco., Bry., Calc. (headache), Cam., K. i., Merc.., Nux.	80–60 d.	Mezereum
Coff (= congestion to the head)	Ar.m.		1–3 d.	Millefolium
				Mimosa
				Mitchella
				Momordica
Vinegar (it increases the painful symptoms, vertigo, &c.).	Elc. (Mo. as., *see* Electricitas).	Aco. and Ipc. useful for secondary effects, Atr., Avn., Bel., Strong Coffee (poisoning), Oxg., Oxygen inhalations. [Keaney (H.P.), xv. 195) cured with one dose of Sul. c.m. (Swan) a man who had taken 2 grs. of morphine daily for fifteen years].		Morphinum

REMEDY	Complementary Remedies	Remedy Follows Well	Remedy is Followed Well by	Compatible Remedies
Moschus				
Mucuna ur.				
Murex				
Muriaticum ac.		Bry., Merc., Rhs.	Calc., K. ca., Nux, Pul., Sep., Sil., Sul.	
Musa				
Mygale				
Myosotis				
Myrica cer.				
Myristica seb.				
Myrtis com.				
Nabalus				
Naja				
Napthalinum				
Narcissus				
Narcotinum				
Natrum ars.				
Natrum caco.				
Natrum carb.	Sep. (Kali salts)		Calc., Nt. x., Nux, Pul., Sep., Sul.	Calc., Nux, Pul., Sep., Sul.
Natrum hypo.	Sep.			
Natrum iod.				
Natrum lac.				

Incompatible Remedies	Remedy Antidotes	Remedy is Antidoted by	Duration of Action	REMEDY
	Chl. h., Ther. (headaches).	Cam. (unconsciousness and coldness), Cof.		Moschus
				Mucuna ur.
				Murex
	Bry., Merc., Opi. (it "cures the muscular weakness following the excessive use of Opium" — Hering), Sel.	Carbonates of alkalies and earths (poisoning cases), small doses : Bry., Cam. (Teste says the surest antidote is Ipc.).		Muriaticum ac.
				Musa
				Mygale
				Myosotis
		Dig. (jaundice).		Myrica cer.
				Myristica seb.
				Myrtis com.
				Nabalus
		Ammonia, Stimulants (effects of bite), Tab. (potencies)		Naja
				Napthalinum
				Narcissus
				Narcotinum
				Natrum ars.
				Natrum caco.
	As. mt., Chi., Nt. s. d.	Cam., Nt. s.d.	30 d.	Natrum carb.
		Gui., Pul. (rheumatic and myalgic symptoms; also, probably, the antidotes to Na. m.).		Natrum hypo.
				Natrum iod.
				Natrum lac.

REMEDY	Complementary Remedies	Remedy Follows Well	Remedy is Followed Well by	Compatible Remedies
Natrum mur.	Aps., Cap., Ign., Sep., Na. m. is the *Chronic* of : Aps., Cap., Ign., (its vegetable analogue)	Ca. p., Fe. p., K. m., K. p., K. s., Na. s.	Bry., Calc., Hep., K. ca., Pul., Rhs., Sep., Sul., Thu.	
Natrum nitri.				
Natrum nitro.				
Natrum phos.				
Natrum sal.				
Natrum sel.				
Nitrum sil.				
Natrum sulphuri	Ars., Thu.			Bel., Fe. p. (poly-uria), Na. m. (skin disease), Thu. (sycosis and hydrogenoid con-stitution)
Natrum sum-phuro.				
Nectrianinum				
Niccolum				
Niccolum sul.				
Nicotinum				
Nitri sp. dul.				

Incompatible Remedies	Remedy Antidotes	Remedy is Antidoted by	Duration of Action	REMEDY
It increases the action of Pod. (?).	Ac. x. (for gastric, pulmonary, and febrile symptoms), Agn. (headache), Aps., (bee-stings), Ag. n. (abuse of, as in cautery), Cean, Cin., Nt. s. d., Quinine (when diseases continue intermittent, and patients suffer from headache, constiopation, disturbed sleep). Na. m. should not be given *during* the paroxysm of fever.	Ars. (bad effects of sea-bathing), Cam.,, Smelling Nt. s. d.; Nux will > headache if persistant, or prostration if prolonged after Na. m.; Pho., (esp. abuse of salt in flood), Sep.		Natrum mur.
				Natrum nitri.
		Coffee		Natrum nitro.
		Aps. (urticaria) Sep. (esp. eruption and swelling about joints).		Natrum phos.
				Natrum sal.
				Natrum sel.
				Nitrum sil.
			30–40 d.	Natrum sulphuri
				Natrum sumphuro.
				Nectrianinum
				Niccolum
				Niccolum sul.
		See under Tab.		Nicotinum
Dig. Rn. b.	Cam., Cb. v., Caus., Con., K. ca. (smelling), K. n., Na. c., Na. m. (crude or in potencies), Plat, Phyt. (smelling), Sep.	Calc., Cb. v., Caus., Con., K. ca., K. n., Na. c., Na. m., Opi., Sep.		Nitri sp. dul.

REMEDY	Complementary Remedies	Remedy Follows Well	Remedy is Followed Well by	Compatible Remedies
Nitricum ac.	Ars. Cld.	Aur. (abuse of Merc.), Calc., Ch. a. (bubo), Hep. (throat, &c), K. ca. (phthisis, &c), Mez. (secondary syphilis), Na. c., Pul., Sul., Thu.	Arn. (collapse in dysentery), Calc., Cb. v., K. ca., Kre. (diphtheritic dysentery), Merc. Pho., Pul., Sec. (gangrene of mucous membrane), Sep., Sil., Sul. (scrofulous ophthalmia), Thu.	
Nitrogenum oxy.				
Nitroso-mur ac.				
Nuphur lut.				
Nux mos.			Ant. t., Lyc., Pul., Rhs., Stm.	Ant. t., Lyc., Nux, Pul., Rhs., Stm.
Nux vom.	(Calc.), K. ca., Sep., Sul.	Ars., Ipc., Mag. m., Pho., Sep., Sul.	Act. s., Ars., Bel., Bry., Cac., Calc., Cb. v., Clch., Coc. i., Hyo., Lyc., Pho., Pul., Rhs., Sep., Sul.	

Incompatible Remedies	Remedy Antidotes	Remedy is Antidoted by	Duration of Action	REMEDY
Lach *After* : C a l c . — Hahnemann.	Calc., Cnb., Con., Dig., K. i. (?), Lach., Merc., Rs. v.	Calc., Con., Hep., Merc., Mez., Pet., Sul.		Nitricum ac.
		Bel. (?)		Nitrogenum oxy.
				Nitroso-mur ac.
				Nuphur lut.
	Alcohol, bad yeasty beer, Ars., Gel., Lau., Lead colic, Rho., Turpentine.	Cam., Gel., Lau., Nux, Opi., Val., Zin.		Nux mos.
Ac. x. disagrees whcn given after Nux. Nux disagrees when followed by Ac. x., Acids, Ast. r., Ign. (sometimes), Zin.	Narcotic, drastic, and vegetable remedies. Bad effects of anomalies in foods, *e.g.* Ginger, Nutmeg., Pepper and so called "hot" medicines, Aesc. (pile symptoms). Ail., Alcohol, Alo,. (relieves earache), Aln. (nausea and vomiting), Amb., Am. m., Ars., As. h., Bis., Bry., Calc., Cb. a., Caus., Cep. (coryza recurring in August), Cham, Chil, Coc. i., Cof., Clch., Coll., Cu. a., Cup., Ether, Glo., Gph., Grt., Gui., Hy. x., Ind., Ipc., Iris., K. br., Kre. (sometimes), Lach., Lil., Lyc., Mag. c., Mag. cit., Mag. m., Mlr. (effects of No. 1), Merc., Mez (neuralgia), Nux will relieve headache if persistent, or prostation if prolonged.	Aco., Amb., Ars., Bel., Cam., Cham., Coc. i., Cof., Eub., Ign., Iris., Opi., Pal., Plat., Pul., Stm., Thus., Wine. A n t i d o t e s (*contd.*) after Na.m.; Ol a., Opi., Ost. (l u m b a g o), Pet., Pho., Plumb., Pod., Pul., Rhe., Sin. n., Stm., Tab. (sometimes), Tel. (epigastric oppression), Thu. (urination).		Nux vom.

REMEDY	Complementary Remedies	Remedy Follows Well	Remedy is Followed Well by	Compatible Remedies
Nyctanthes				
Nymophaea oror.				
Ocimum can.			Dio.	
Cenanthe croc.				
Cenothera				
Oleander			Con., Lyc., Na. m., Pul., Rhs., Sep., Spi.	Con., Lyc., Na. m., Pul., Rhs., Sep., Spi.
Oleum an.				
Olem j. asel.				
Oniscus				
Ononis				
Onosmodium				
Oophorinum				
Opium			Aco. Ant. t., Bel., Bry., Hyo., Nux, Nx. m.	
Opuntia				
Orchitinum				

Incompatible Remedies	Remedy Antidotes	Remedy is Antidoted by	Duration of Action	REMEDY
				Nyctanthes
				Nymophaea oror.
				Ocimum can.
				Cenanthe croc.
				Cenothera
		Cam. (acute effects), Sul. (chronic effects.)	20–30 d.	Oleander
				Oleum an.
		Iris. (chill with sick stomach and diarrhoea).		Olem j. asel.
				Oniscus
				Ononis
				Onosmodium
				Oophorinum
	Amg. (convulsions), Ant. t. (Opium in large doses is the best antidote to Ant. t.), Atr., Bel., Bro., Cam., Cic., Cnb., Col. (large doses), Cro., Dig., Eub., Gam., Hur. Hur.c., Hy. x., Iod., Lach., Lau., Merc., Nt. s. d., Nx.m., Nux, Ol. a., Pb., Phyt. (large doses), Stm., Sty.	Strong Coffee K. pm. solution (about 1 gr. to the pint of water; the patient is made to swallow half-a-point every five minutes, and then caused to vomit; later a somewhat stronger solution may be given and retained); oxygen inhalations; (patient must be kept walking about; if allowed to sleep, it may be impossible to wake him again); Ag. n., Bel., Cam., Cham., (nerves irritability), Ipc., Nux, Sars., Sul. (marasmus), Vanil., Vinum.	7 d.	Opium
				Opuntia
				Orchitinum

REMEDY	Complementary Remedies	Remedy Follows Well	Remedy is Followed Well by	Compatible Remedies
Oreodaphne				
Origanum				
Ornithogalum				
Osmium				
Ostrya				
Ovi. gal. pel.				
Oxalicum ac.				
Oxydendron				
Oxygenium				
Oxytropis lamb.				
Paeonia				
Palladium	Plat.			
Pancreatinum				
Paraffinum				
Pareira				
Parietaria				
Paris			Calc., Led., Lyc., Nux, Pho., Pul., Rhs., Sep., Sul.	Calc., Led., Lyc., Nux, Pho., Rhs., Sep., Sul.
Parthenium				
Passiflora				
Pastinaca				
Paullinia pin.				
Pecten				
Pediculus				

Incompatible Remedies	Remedy Antidotes	Remedy is Antidoted by	Duration of Action	REMEDY
				Oreodaphne
				Origanum
				Ornithogalum
		Bel. and Merc. (laryngal catarrh), Hep. and Spo. (pain in larynx), Sulphuretted Hydrogen, Ph. x., Sil. (swollen gums).		Osmium
		Bry., Mac., Nux (lumbago).		Ostrya
				Ovi. gal. pel.
		Carbonates of Lime and Magnesia		Oxalicum ac.
				Oxydendron
	Morphia and Strychnine poisoning.			Oxygenium
				Oxytropis lamb.
		Alo., Rat.		Paeonia
	Nux.	Bel. and Glo. (headache), Chi. (diarrhoea).		Palladium
				Pancreatinum
				Paraffinum
				Pareira
				Parietaria
Fe. ph.	Aco.	Cam., cof.	2-4 d.	Paris
	Quinine			Parthenium
	Sty. (?)			Passiflora
				Pastinaca
				Paullinia pin.
				Pecten
		Chi. (anasarca)		Pediculus

REMEDY	Complementary Remedies	Remedy Follows Well	Remedy is Followed Well by	Compatible Remedies
Pelargonium ren.				
Penthorum sed.				
Pepsinum				
Persica				
Pestinum				
Petiveria				
Petroleum	Before Sep.		Bry., Calc., Lyc., Nt.x., Nux, Pul., Sep., Sil., Sul.	Bry., Calc., Lyc., Nt.x., Nux, Pul., Sep., Sil., Sul.
Petroselinum				
Phallus imp.				
Phaseolus				
Phellandrium				
Phenacetinum				
Phlorizinum				
Phosphoricum ac.			Ars., Bel., Ca. p., Caus., Chi., Fer., Fe. p., K. ph., Lyc., Na. p. Nux, Pul., Sep., Sul., Ver.	Chi., before or after, in colliquative sweats, diarrhoea, and debility. After Nux in fainting after a meal, after Rhs. in typhoid.
Phosphorus	Ars., Cep. (all three have alliaceous odours), Cb. v., Ipc.		Ars., Bel., Bry., Calc., Cb. v., Chi., K. ca., Lyc., Nux, Pul., Rhs., Sep., Sil., Sul.	Ars., Bapt., Bel., Bry., Calc., Cb. v., Chi., K. ca., Lyc., Nux, Pul, Rhs., Sep., Sil., Sul.
Phosphorus hydro.				
Phosphorus mur.				
Physalia				
Physostigma				

Incompatible Remedies	Remedy Antidotes	Remedy is Antidoted by	Duration of Action	REMEDY
				Pelargonium ren.
				Penthorum sed.
				Pepsinum
				Persica
				Pestinum
				Petiveria
	Lead poisoning (one of the best remedies), Nt. x.	Aco., Coc. i., Nux, Pho.	40–50 d.	Petroleum
				Petroselinum
				Phallus imp.
				Phaseolus
		Rhe. (diarrhoea).		Phellandrium
				Phenacetinum
				Phlorizinum
		Cam., Cof., Stp.	40 d.	Phosphoricum ac.
Aps., Caus.	Cam., Iod., Na. m. (excessive use of salt), Pet., Rs. v., Rum., it relieved the effects of Sla., Tab. (sometimes), Ter.	Ars., Calc., Cam., Chlf., Cof., K. pm. well diluted and given freely (Dr. Antal), Mez., Nux, Sep., Ter., Wine.	40 d.	Phosphorus
		Electricity.		Phosphorus hydro.
				Phosphorus mur.
				Physalia
	Atr.	Injection of Atr. antagonises its effects. Arn., Coffee; Emetics are of the first importance. Lil. curedastigmatism of Phst., Sinapisms.		Physostigma

REMEDY	Complementary Remedies	Remedy Follows Well	Remedy is Followed Well by	Compatible Remedies
Phytolacca				
Pichi				
Picricum ac.				
Picrotoxinum				
Pilocarpinum		Merc. (in sweating of rheumatic fever).		
Piminta				
Pimpinella				
Pinus lamb.				
Pinus syl.				
Piper meth.				
Piper nig.				
Piperazinum				
Piscidia				
Pix liquida				
Plantago				
Platinum	Pal. (both affect r. ovary, but Pal. has > from pressure.		Ana., Arg., Bel., Lyc., Pul., Rhs., Sep., Ver.	Bel., Ign., Lyc., Pul., Rhs., Sep., Ver.
Pllatinum mur.				
Platinum mur. nat.				
Plectranthus				
Plumbago				

Incompatible Remedies	Remedy Antidotes	Remedy is Antidoted by	Duration of Action	REMEDY
	Bap.	Bel., Coffee (vomiting); Ign., Iris., Merc., Mez., Milk, Nt. s. d., Opi. (large doses), Salt, Sul. (eyes).		Phytolacca
				Pichi
				Picricum ac.
				Picrotoxinum
		Atr., Am. c. (salvolatile), Brandy.		Pilocarpinum
				Piminta
				Pimpinella
				Pinus lamb.
				Pinus syl.
		Pul. and Rhs. (partially).		Piper meth.
	Cin.			Piper nig.
				Piperazinum
				Piscidia
				Pix liquida
	Aps., Rhs., Tab.	Merc. (toothache).		Plantago
	Lead, Sil. (?), Nux	Bel., Nt. s. d., Pul., (Teste, who classes Plat. with Thu., Bro., and Castor, says Colch. is the best antidote to all four.		Platinum
				Pllatinum mur.
				Platinum mur. nat.
				Plectranthus
				Plumbago

REMEDY	Complementary Remedies	Remedy Follows Well	Remedy is Followed Well by	Compatible Remedies
Plumbum			Ars., Bel.., Lyc., Merc., Pho., Pul., Sil., Sul.	Ars., Bel., Lyc., Merc., Pho., Pul., Sil., Sul.
Plumbum chro.				
Plumbum iod.				
Podophyllum	(Sul.)			After Ipc., and Nux in vomiting, after Calc. and Sul. in liver diseases.
Polygonum				
Polyporus pin.				
Populus can.				
Populus trem.		Cannab, Cth. (Pop.t. succeeded after these had only partially helped).		
Primula obcon.				
Primula ver.				
Primula vulg.				
Prinos vert.				
Prunus pad.				
Prunus spl.				
Prunus virg.				

Incompatible Remedies	Remedy Antidotes	Remedy is Antidoted by	Duration of Action	REMEDY
	Ast. r., bad effects of long sbuse of vinegar.	Ac. x. (colic) Alcohol is a preventive, Alm., Aln., Ant. c., Bel., Caus., (lead poisoning), Coc. i., Hep., Kre., Na n. (?), Nx. m. (lead colic), Nux, Opi, Pet., Plat., Ppz., Sulphuric acid diluted is one of the best sntidotes to the chronic effects of lead, Zin. (Teste, who classes Pb. with Merc. and Ars., says Aeth. is the best antidote in his experience; he names also Elc., Hyo., Ple., Strm.).	20–30 d.	Plumbum
				Plumbum chro.
				Plumbum iod.
Salt, which ibncreases its action.	Merc. it relieved the diarrhoea of Lo. s., but not the acute abdom- inal pains, Src.	Col., Lc. x., Lpt., Nux.	30 d.	Podophyllum
				Polygonum
				Polyporus pin.
		Rhs.		Populus can.
				Populus trem.
				Primula obcon.
				Primula ver.
				Primula vulg.
				Prinos vert.
				Prunus pad.
				Prunus spl.
				Prunus virg.

REMEDY	Complementary Remedies	Remedy Follows Well	Remedy is Followed Well by	Compatible Remedies
Psorinum	After Arn. (blow on ovary), Bac. (Bac. is the *acute* of Pso.), after Lc. x. (vomiting of pregnancy), Sul., Sul. after Pso, in mammary cancer.	Arn., Lc. x., Sul.	Alm., Bor., Cb. v.., Chi., Hep., Sul.	Cb. v., Chi., Sul. (if Sul. is indicated but fails to act give Pso.).
Ptelea				
Pulmo vulp.				
Pulsatilla	Ag. n. (if Ag. n. flags give Pul., Ag. n. follows Pul. in o p h t h a l m i a), Cham., Cep., Lyc., Sil., Stn. (Stn. has menses too early and too profuse), Su. x.		Ana., Ant. t., Ars., Asa., Bel., Bry., Calc., Eub., Gph., Ign., K. bi., Lyc., Nt. x., Nux, Pho., Rhs., Sep., Sul.	Ars., Bel., Bry., Ign., K. bi., Lyc., Nux, Pho., Rhs., Sep., sul.
Pulsatilla nutt.				
Pyrethrum par.				
Pyrogenium				
Pyrus amer.				
Quassia				

Incompatible Remedies	Remedy Antidotes	Remedy is Antidoted by	Duration of Action	REMEDY
Con. (some-times), Lach., Sep. (?).		Coffee.	30–40 d.	**Psorinum**
				Ptelea
				Pulmo vulp.
	Amb., Ant. t., Athra., Arg., Ar. t., Asa., Aur., Bel., Bry., Ca. ar. (sometimes), Cth., Cham., Chi., Ch. s., Cof., Clch., Cyc., Ephr., Fer. (in chlorotic girls who have been dam-aged by Iron, Pul. has an excellent effect), Gel., Ham. (thooth-ache), Ign.. (chief antodote), K. bi,. (wan-dering pains), K. m., Lil., Lyc., vapours of Mercury and Copper, Mag. c., Na. hch. (rheu-matic and myalgic symptoms), Pip. m. (partially), Plat., Rn., b., Rn. s., Rhe., Sbd., Sbl. (sometimes), Sbi., Sel., Spi., Stn., Stm., Sul., Su. x., Tab. (some-times), Thu., Toadstool poisoning, Val., Vi. t., Whisky, Ziz. (migraine).	Acids, Ant. t., Cen., Cham., (Cham and Pul. antidotes each other and follow each other well. If either one has over-acted the otherwill probably neutralise the ill effect and carry on the good); Cof., Ign., Nux, Stn., (Teste adds Sul., and says when the improper use of Pul. has affected the air passages Ca. p. has proved the best antidote).	40 d.	**Pulsatilla**
		Ant. c.		**Pulsatilla nutt.**
				Pyrethrum par.
				Pyrogenium
		Cam.		**Pyrus amer.**
				Quassia

REMEDY	Complementary Remedies	Remedy Follows Well	Remedy is Followed Well by	Compatible Remedies
Quebracho				
quercus				
Ranunculus ac.				
Ranunculus bulb.			Bry., Ign., K. ca., Nux, Rhs., Sep.	
Ranunculus fic.				
Ranunculus flam.				
Ranunculus gla.				
Ranunculus rep.				
Ranunculus scel.		Ars. in pemphigus.	Bel. Lach., in diphtheria with denuded tongue, Pho., Pul., Rhs., Sil.	
Raphanus		Lyc.		
Ratanhia		Bov., Sep. (in uterine affections, Teste), Sul.		
Rhamnus cath.				
Rhamnus frang.				
Rheum	After Mag. c. when milk disagrees and child has sour odour.		Bel., Pul., Rhs., Sul.	Ipc.
Rhodium oxy. nit.				
Rhododendron			Arn., Ars., Calc., Con., Lyc., Merc., Nux, Pul., Sep., Sil., Sul.	

Incompatible Remedies	Remedy Antidotes	Remedy is Antidoted by	Duration of Action	REMEDY
				Quebracho
	Alcohol.			quercus
				Ranunculus ac.
Ac. x. disagrees when given after Rn. b., Rn. b. disagrees when followed by Ac. x. Alcohol, Nt. s. d., Stp., Sul., Vinegar, Wine.	Rs. v. (Rheumatic pains < on taking cold).	Anac. Bry., Cam., Clem., Ctn., Pul., Rhs.		Ranunculus bulb.
				Ranunculus fic.
				Ranunculus flam.
		> by Coffee		Ranunculus gla.
		> by ether in milk		Ranunculus rep.
		Cam., Pul., Coffee and Wine antidote only partially. The ulcers were somewhat > by Peruvian Balsam		Ranunculus scel.
		copious draughts of cold water. (Milk and water < the pains in abdomen).		Raphanus —
	Paeo			Ratanhia
				Rhamnus cath.
				Rhamnus frang.
	Cth., Mag. c. ("Rhe. may be given after abuse of Magnesia, with or without Rhubarb, if stools are sour"), Phel. (diarrhoea).	Cam., Cham., Col., Merc., Nux, Pul.	2–3 d.	Rheum
				Rhodium oxy. nit.
		Bry., Cam., Clem., Nx. m., Rhs.,	35–40 d.	Rhododendron

REMEDY	Complementary Remedies	Remedy Follows Well	Remedy is Followed Well by	Compatible Remedies
Rhus arom.				
Rhus diver.				
Rhus glab.				
Rhus rad. Rhus tox.	Bry., Calc.		Arn., Ars., Bel., Bry., Cac., Calc., Ca. p., Cham., Cons., Drs., Gph., Hyo., Lach., Merc., Mu. x., Nux, Pho., Pul., Sep., Sul.	Arn., Ars., Bry., Calc., Ca. p., Cham., Con., Lach., Ph. x., Pul., Sul.
Rhus ven.	Rhs.			
Ricinus				
Robinia				
Rosa can.				
Rosa damasc.				
Rosmarinus				
Rubia tinct.				
Rumex acet.				
Rumex crisp.			Calc.	
Russula				

Incompatible Remedies	Remedy Antidotes	Remedy is Antidoted by	Duration of Action	R E M E D Y
				Rhus arom.
				Rhus diver.
				Rhus glab.
Aps., before or after esp. in skin affections.	Aga., Ail., An. oc., Ant. t., Athra., (Ars.), Bry., Cai., Chi., Cis., Dph., Jg. r., Mlr. (effects of No. III), Pip. m. (partially), Pop. c., Rn. b., Rho., Sap., Sep., Sin. n., Sul., Vi. t.	Ana. (if there are gastric symptoms or symptoms going from r. to l.), Am. c., Bel., Bry., Cam., Clem., Cof., Ctn., Cup., (poisoning), Gph., Gnd., Gui. (poisoning), K. sc., Lach., Led. (Teste), Merc., Plnt., Rn., b., Sang., Sep., Sul., Vbn.	1–7 d.	**Rhus rad.** **Rhus tox.**
		Bry., Clem., (itching on hands and genitals, anus, lips mouth and nose), Nt. x. (sprained) pain in r. hip), Pho., Ranun (rheumatic pains < on taking cold). Blue clay applied externally > itching and burning entirely (Hering). Coffee had no effect on the symptoms.		**Rhus ven.**
				Ricinus
				Robinia
				Rosa can.
				Rosa damasc.
				Rosmarinus
				Rubia tinct.
				Rumex acet.
		Bel. Cam., Con., Hyo., Lach., Pho.		**Rumex crisp.**
				Russula

REMEDY	Complementary Remedies	Remedy Follows Well	Remedy is Followed Well by	Compatible Remedies
Ruta	Ca. p. in joint affecdtions.	Arn., Symt.	Calc., Caus., Lyc., Ph. x., Pul., Sep., Sul., Su. x.	After arn. in joinmt affections, after Symt. in bone injuries. Calc., Caus., Lycs., Ph. x., Pul., Sul.,. Su. x., (diseases of bone).
Sabadilla	Sep.	Bry. (pleurisy).	Ars., Bel., Merc., Nux, Pul.	
Sabal ser.				
Sabina	Thu.		Ars., Bel., Pul., Rhs., Spo., Sul.	Ars., Bel., Rhs., Spo.
Saccharum lac.				
Saccharum off.				
Salicinum				
Salicylicum ac.				
Salix mol.				
Salix nig.				
Salix pur.				
Salol				
Salvia				
Sambucus can.				
Sambucus nig.		Ars., Opi., (effects of fright)	Ars., Bel., Con., Nux, Pho., Rhs., Sep.	Bel., Con., Nux, Pho., Rhs., Sep.
Sanguinaria				Bel. (scarlatina)
Sanguinarinum				
Sanguinarinum nit.				
Sanguinarinum tart.				
Sanguisuga				
Sanicula				

Incompatible Remedies	Remedy Antidotes	Remedy is Antidoted by	Duration of Action	REMEDY
	Merc.	Cam.	30 d.	**Ruta**
	Bel. (salivation)	Cam., Con., Pul.		**Sabadilla**
		Sil. (Sbl. grows on the sandy shore), Pul. (delayed menses, Pul. also grows on sandy soils).		**Sabal ser.**
		Cam., Pul.	20–30 d.	**Sabina**
				Saccharum lac.
		Ac. x., (?).		**Saccharum off.**
				Salicinum
	Athra.			**Salicylicum ac.**
				Salix mol.
				Salix nig.
				Salix pur.
		Bry.		**Salol**
				Salva
				Sambucus can.
	Ars. (> aliments from abuse of Ars.)	Ars., Cam.	3–4 hours.	**Sambucus nig.**
	Bap. Iof. (skin), Opium, Rhs.			**Sanguinaria**
				Sanguinarinum
				Sanguinarinum nit.
				Sanguinarinum tart.
				Sanguisuga
				Sanicula

REMEDY	Complementary Remedies	Remedy Follows Well	Remedy is Followed Well by	Compatible Remedies
Santalum				
Santonimum				
Saponinum				
Sarracenia				
Sarsaparilla	Cep., Merc., Sep.		Bel., Cep., Hep., Mere., Pho., Rhs., Sep., Sul.	Cep., Hep., Pho., Rhs., Sep., Sul.
Scammonium				
Schinus				
Scilla mar.		Bry.	Ars., Ign., Nux, Rhs., Sil.	*After :* Bry.
Scirrhinum				
Scolopendra				
Scorpio				
Scrophularia			Dig. (in enlarged g l a n d s . — R.T.C.)	
Scutellaria				
Secale corn.				Aco., Ars., Bel., Chi, (Teste classes Sec. with Chi. in his Ferrum group), Merc., Pul.
Selenium			Calc., Merc., Nux, Sep.	*After:* Cld., Na. c., Ph. x., (in sexual weakness), Stp. Itch checked by Merc. or Sul. often requires Sel.
Sempervivum tect.				
Senecio aur.				
Senecio jac.				
Senega			Calc., Lyc., Pho., Sul.	
Senna				

Incompatible Remedies	Remedy Antidotes	Remedy is Antidoted by	Duration of Action	REMEDY
				Santalum
				Santonimum
		(Ars.), Phs.		Saponinum
	Var.	Pod.		Sarracenia
Ac. x., (it disagrees when given after Sars.)	Merc. Opi.	Bel., Merc., Sep.	35 d.	Sarsaparilla
				Scammonium
				Schinus
All., Cep.		Cam.		Scilla mar.
				Scirrhinum
				Scolopendra
				Scorpio
		Bry. (chest symptoms).		Scrophularia
				Scutellaria
Aco., Ars., Bel., Chi., Merc., Pul.		Cam., Opi.	20–30 d.	Secale corn.
Chi., Wine.		Ign., (Mu. x. in a case of mine.—J.H.C.), Pul.	40 d.	Selenium
				Sempervivum tect.
				Senecio aur.
				Senecio jac.
	Bry., Buf.	Arn., Bel., Bry., Cam.	30 d.	Senega
	Stm. (cerebral symptoms).			Senna

REMEDY	Complementary Remedies	Remedy Follows Well	Remedy is Followed Well by	Compatible Remedies
Sepia	Na. c., Na. m. (the cuttlefish is a *salt water* animal), and other *Natrum* salts, Nux, Sbd., Sul.		Bel., Calc., Cb. v., Con., Eub., Gph., Lyc., Nt.x., Nux, Pho., Pul., Rhs., Sars., Sil., Sul.	
Septicaeminum				
Silica	Fl. x., Pul. (Sil is the "chronic" of Pul.), Snc., Thu.	Bel., Bry., Calc., Ca. p. (in rickets when Ca. p. fails), Cin., Gph., Hep., Ign., Nt. x., Pho.	Ars., Asa., Bel., Calc., Clem., Gl.x., Gph., Hep., Lach., Lyc., Nux, Pho., Pul., Rhs., Sep. (if improvement ceases under Sil., a dose or two of Sul. will set up reaction, and Sil. will then complete the cure).	
Silica mar.				
Silphium				
Sinapis alb.				
Sinapis nig.				
Sium				
S k o o k u m Chuck				
Slag				
Sol				

Incompatible Remedies	Remedy Antidotes	Remedy is Antidoted by	Duration of Action	REMEDY
Bry. Lach. (but in one case in which *Lach.* in very high potency has caused intensely distressing rectal tenesmus with alternate inversion and eversion of the anus, *Sep.*, high, proved to be the antidote).	Ac. x. (gastric, pulmonary and febrile symptoms), Ant. t., Calc., Chi., Cis., Cit., Dph., Lach. (s o m e t i m e s), Merc., Mr. c. (dynamic), Na. m., Na. p. (exp. eruption and swelling about joints), Nt. s. d., Pho., Sars., Sil., Tab. (sometimes).	Vegetable acids, Aco., Ant. c., Ant. t., Smelling Nt. s. d., Rhs., Sul.	40–50 d.	Sepia
				Septicaeminum
Merc.	Artha., Dph, Hep., Mr. c., Osm. (swollen gums), Sbl., Sul., Vac.	Cam., F. x., Hep.	40–60 d.	Silica
				Silica mar.
				Silphium
				Sinapis alb.
		Smelling Bread (immediate effects of taking excess of condiment), Nux, Rhs. When blistering has been produced by a mustard poultice, Soap is the remedy.		Sinapis nig.
				Sium
		Tab.		S k o o k u m Chuck
		> By Cb. v., Pho., Ph. x.		Slag
		Aco., Bel.., Gel., Glo., and other sunstroke remedies.		Sol

REMEDY	Complementary Remedies	Remedy Follows Well	Remedy is Followed Well by	Compatible Remedies
Solaninum				
Solanum arr.				
Solanum car.				
Solanum mam.				
Solanum nig.				
Solanum oler.				
Solanum pseu cap.				
Solanum tu.				
Solanum tu. ae.				
Solidago				
Sphingurus				
Spigelia			Aco., Arn., Ars., Bel., Calc., Cimic., Dig., Iris., K. ca., Nux, Pul., Rhs., Sep., Sul., Zin.	Aco (endocarditis) Arn. (carbuncle) Ars., Dig., Iris (prosopalgia), K. ca., Zin. (heart).
Spigelia mar.				
Spiraea ulm.				
Spiranthes				
Spongia tost.			Aco., Hep., (Boenninghausen's croup powders consisted of a sequence of Aco., Hep., Spo., given in that order. Spo. is dry, Hep. rattling Spo. < before midnight, Hep. < after).	Bro., Bry., Cb. v., Con., Hep., K. br., Nux, Pho., Pul.
Squill, *see* Scilla mar.				
Stachys bet.				
Stannum	Pul.	Caus., Cin.	Bac., Calc., Hfb., Nux, Pho., Pul., Rhs., Sel., Sul.	

Incompatible Remedies	Remedy Antidotes	Remedy is Antidoted by	Duration of Action	R E M E D Y
				Solaninum
				Solanum arr.
				Solanum car.
				Solanum mam.
	Aur.			Solanum nig.
				Solanum oler.
				Solanum pseu cap.
				Solanum tu.
				Solanum tu. ae.
				Solidago
				Sphingurus
	Aur., Clch., (heart), Merc., Tab., (sometimes).	Aur. (restlessness in limbs); Cam., Coc. i., Pul.		Spigelia
				Spigelia mar.
				Spiraea ulm.
				Spiranthes
	Iod., Osm. (pain in larynx).	Aco., Cam.	20–30 d.	Spongia tost.
				Squill, *see* Scilla mar.
				Stachys bet.
		Pul..	35 d.	Stannum

REMEDY	Complementary Remedies	Remedy Follows Well	Remedy is Followed Well by	Compatible Remedies
Stannum iod.				
Staphisagria	Caus., Col.		Calc., Caus., Col., Ign., Lyc., Nux, Pul., Rhs.,Sul.	Caus. (Caus., Col., Stp. follow well in this order).
Stellaria med.				
Sticta pul.				
Stillingia syl.				
Stramonium		Bel;., Cup.	Aco., Bel. Bry., Cup., Hyo., Nux.	
Strontium br.				
Strontium carb.			Bel., Caus., K. ca., Pul., Rhs., Sep., Sul.	
Strontium nit.				
Strophanthus				
Strychninum				

Incompatible Remedies	Remedy Antidotes	Remedy is Antidoted by	Duration of Action	REMEDY
				Stannum iod.
Rn. b., before and after.	Amb., coc. i., Col., Merc., Ph. x., Tax. (sometimes), Thu., Trb. (thoothache), ver. (most cases—Teste).	Cam.	20–30 d.	Staphisagria
				Stellaria med.
				Sticta pul.
				Stillingia syl.
Cof.	Cor., Hyo., Merc., Nux, Pb.	Lemon-juice, Senna for cerebral symptoms, Tobacco injection, Bel., Cam. (particularly. — Teste), Nux, Opi., Pul.		Stramonium
				Strontium br.
		Cam.		Strontium carb.
				Strontium nit.
				Strophanthus
	Bz. n., large doses of Can. s., Gel. (poisoning. — Jephson	Aco., Cam., Chlf. and Tobacco have been advised. Aml. (convulsions), Ars. Black draught (Senna and Epson Salts) relieved the constipation better than any other aperient. Cof. (poisoning), Hyo. (drowsiness, respiratory affection). See also under Nux. Opi (large doses), Pas. (suggested by Hale). Osterwald found inhalation of Oxygen an effective antidote in animals. Ve. v., Sul. 30 in globules dry on the tongue brought about a rapid and almost	antidoted by (Contd.)

complete relief of all the rectal symptoms of Robinson's male prover. | Strychninum |

REMEDY	Complementary Remedies	Remedy Follows Well	Remedy is Followed Well by	Compatible Remedies
Succinum				
Sulfonal				
Sulphur	Aco., Nux, Pul. (Sul. is the "chronic" of these three. If a patient is sleepless, Sul. may be given at night; if the patient sleeps well, it is best given in the morning, as it may disturb sleep if given at night; Nux may be given at night and Sul. in the morning when their complementary action is desired). Alo. (Sul. is generally the remedy when Alo. has been abused as a purgative). Sul,. follows and Complements Ant. t. and Ipc. in lung affections, esp.l., and atelectasis. Ars., Bad.; Pso. complements Sul., Pso. loves heat, Sul. hates it. sul. complements Rhs. in paralysis. An interpolated dose of Sul. helps Sil.	Merc.	Aco., Alm., Ars., Bel., Bry., Calc., Cb. v., Drs., Eub., Gph., Gui., Merc., Nt. x., Nux, Pho., Pul., Sars., Sep.	Calc., Ca. p., Lyc., Pul., Sars., Sep. (Sul., Calc., Lyc., and Sul., Sars., Sep. frequently follow in this order. It is generally said that Calc. should not be used *before* Sul).
Sulphur hydro.				
Sulphur iod.				
Sulphur tereb.				
Sulphuricum ac.	Pul.	In injuries: Arn., Con., Rut.	Arn., Calc., Con., Lyc., Plat., Sep., Sul.	
Sulphurosum ac.				

Incompatible Remedies	Remedy Antidotes	Remedy is Antidoted by	Duration of Action	REMEDY
				Succinum
		Symptoms > by cold douches.		Sulfonal
Sulphur springs are compatible with Au.m. Hahnemann said Sul. should not be given after Calc.	Aco., Aln., alo., Calc., Chi., Cnb., Cof., Con., Cop., Guac. (sometimes), Hdr. (sometimes), Iod., Ln.c. (headache), Merc., Nt. x., Oln. (chronic effects), Opi. (marasmus), Phyt. (eyes), Pul. (?), Rhs., Sep.; sul. 30 in globules dry on the tongue brought about a rapid and almost complete relief of all the rectal symptoms of Robinson's male prover of Sty.; Thu., Vac., ailments from abuse of metals generally.	Aco., Cam., Cham., Chi., Merc., Pul., Rhs., Sep., Sil., Thu.	40–60 d.	Sulphur
	(Chlm.) Osm.	Chlm.		Sulphur hydro.
				Sulphur iod.
				Sulphur tereb.
	Cap., Lead poisoning. "Sulphuric acid, diluted, taken as a lemonade, is one of the best antidotes to the chronic effects of lead."	Ipc., Pul.	30–40 d. or 40–60 d.	Sulphuricum ac.
		Hdr. (constipation).		Sulphurosum ac.

Remedy	Complementary Remedies	Remedy Follows Well	Remedy is Followed Well by	Compatible Remedies
Sumbul.				
Symphoricarpus rac.				
Symphytum		Arn. (for pricking pains, and after the bruising of the soft parts is healed).		
Syphilinum				
Syzygium				
Tabacum			Cb. v., Hfb.	
Tamus				
Tanacetum				
Tanghinia				
Tannin				

Incompatible Remedies	Remedy Antidotes	Remedy is Antidoted by	Duration of Action	REMEDY
				Sumbul.
				Symphoricarpus rac.
	Cth. (Green's Herbal).			Symphytum
				Syphilinum
				Syzygium
Ign.	Ac. x., ars., Cic., Cof., Ipc., Naj. (potencies), Sko., Stm.	Ac. x., Ars. (effects of chewing tobacco), Cam., Clem. (toothache), Cof., Gel. (occipital headache and vertigo), Ign., Ipc. (primary effects : vomitting), Klm., Lyc. (impotence), Nux (bad taste in mouth in morning, amblyopia), Pho. (palpitation, tobacco heart, amblyopia, sexual weakness), Plnt. has sometimes caused aversion to tobacco. Pul. (hiccough), Sep. (neuralgia in face and dysopepsia, chronic nervousness), Sour Apples, Spi. (heart affections), Tab. 200, or 1,000 for the craving when discontinuing its use, Ver,. Vinegar, Wine (spasms, cold sweat from excessive smoking).		Tabacum
				Tamus
				Tanacetum
				Tanghinia
				Tannin

REMEDY	Complementary Remedies	Remedy Follows Well	Remedy is Followed Well by	Compatible Remedies
Taraxacum			Ars., asa., Bel., Chi., Lyc.,Rhs., Stp., Sul.	Ars. (night sweats)
Tarentula				
Tarentula cub.				
Tartaricum ac.				
Taxus bac.				
Tellurium				
Teplitz				
Terebinthina			Mr. c.	
Tetradymite				
Teucrium mar.				Chi., Pul., Sil.
Teucrium scor.				
Thallium				
Thea				
Theridion			Sul., Calc., Lyc. (scrofula).	
Thevetia				

Incompatible Remedies	Remedy Antidotes	Remedy is Antidoted by	Duration of Action	REMEDY
		Cam		**Taraxacum**
	Lach. (Hering).	*Partial antidotres:* Bov., Cb. v., Chel., Cup., Gel., Mg. c., Mos., Pul.		**Tarentula**
				Tarentula cub.
				Tartaricum ac.
		Stp. (prostration with oppression after an embrace).		**Taxus bac.**
		Nux (epigastric opression).		**Tellurium**
				Teplitz
	Merc. Pho.	Pho.		**Terebinthina**
				Tetradymite
		Cam.	14–21 d.	**Teucrium mar.**
				Teucrium scor.
				Thallium
Fer.		Beer, Fer., Thu. Hering says Coffee-drinkers should drink wine, tea-drinkers should drink beer. Beer caused in one tea-dinker relasation of bowels, which was > by port wine. But beer relieved in other nausea, irregularity of pulse, weakness, sleeplessness, nervousness and want of confidence.		**Thea**
		Aco., (sensitiveness to noises), Mos. (nausea), Gph. (more chronic effects).		**Theridion**
				Thevetia

REMEDY	Complementary Remedies	Remedy Follows Well	Remedy is Followed Well by	Compatible Remedies
Thiosinaminum				
Thlaspi bur. pas.				
Thuja	ars., Med., Na. s. in sycosis, Sbi., Sil.	Med., Merc., Nt. x.	Merc., Sul. (these follow best — H.N.G.); also Asa., Calc., Ign., K. ca., Lyc., Pul., Sbi., Sil., Sul., Vacc.	Nt. x., Sbi.
Thyroidinum				
Thyroiodinum				
Tilia				
Titanium				
Tongo				
Toxicophis				
Trachinus				
Tradescantia				
Trifolium pra.				
Trifolium re.				
Trillium	Ca. p. (menstrual and haemorrhagic affections).			
Trimethylaminum				
Triosteum				
Triticum re.				
Trombidium				
Tropaeolum				
Tuberculinum				Calc., Ca. i., Ca. p., Hdr. "it actually seems to fatten up tuberculous patients" (Burnett; confirmed by Nebel), Pho., Pul., Sep., Thu.

Incompatible Remedies	Remedy Antidotes	Remedy is Antidoted by	Duration of Action	REMEDY
				Thiosinaminum
				Thlaspi bur. pas.
	Cep. (offensicve breath and diarroea after eating onions), Iod., Merc., Nux, Sul., Tea., Vac., Var. (Ailments from abuse of metals generally)	Cam., Cham. (nightly toothache), Coc. i. (fever); Teste found Clch. the best antidote in his experience; Merc., Nux (sometimes), Pul., Stp., Sul.	60 d.	Thuja
				Thyroidinum
		Ars.		Thyroiodinum
				Tilia
				Titanium
		Vinegar		Tongo
				Toxicophis
				Trachinus
				Tradescantia
				Trifolium pra.
				Trifolium re.
				Trillium
				Trimethylaminum
				Triosteum
				Triticum re.
		Mr. c. (diarrhoea), Stp. (toothache).		Trombidium
				Tropaeolum
				Tuberculinum

REMEDY	Complementary Remedies	Remedy Follows Well	Remedy is Followed Well by	Compatible Remedies
Turnera aph.				
Tussilago far.				
Tussilago fra.				
Tussilago pet.				
Ulmus ful.				
Upas				
Uranium nit.				
Urea				
Uricum ac.				
Urinum				
Urtica urens				
Usnea barb				
Ustilago				
Uva-ursi				
Vaccininum				
Valeriana			Pho. Pul.	
Vanadium				
Variolinum				
Veratrinum				
Veratrum alb.	Arn.	Am. c., Arn., Ars., Bov. (dysmenorrhoea with vomiting and purging), Cam. (cholera), Cb. v., Chi., Cup., Ipc., Lyc. and Nux in painful constipation of infants.	Aco., Arn., Ars., Bel., Cb. v., Cham., Chi., Cup., Drs., Ipc., Pul., Rhs., Sep., Sul.	

Incompatible Remedies	Remedy Antidotes	Remedy is Antidoted by	Duration of Action	REMEDY
				Turnera aph.
				Tussilago far.
				Tussilago fra.
				Tussilago pet.
				Ulmus ful.
				Upas
				Uranium nit.
				Urea
				Uricum ac.
				Urinum
	Apis (bee-stings).	Dock leaves (Rumex obtus.) rubbed on the stung part lessen the pain; also nettle's own juice, and the juice from the common snail.		Urtica urens
				Usnea barb
				Ustilago
				Uva-ursi
	Var.	Aps., Ant. t., Mld., Sil., Thu.		Vaccininum
	Asa. Merc. Nx. m., abuse of Chamomile tea.	Bel., Cam., Cin., Cof., Merc., Pul.	8–10 d.	Valeriana
				Vanadium
		Ant. t., Mld., Src., Thu., Vac.		Variolinum
		Coffee mixed with a little lemon-Juice.		Veratrinum
	Ars., Cai., Cep. (colic with despondency), Chi., Cup. (colic), Hdm. (some of its effects), Hy. x., Opi., Tab., Vb. o. (diarrhoea).	Aco. (anxious, distracted state with coldness of body, or burning in brain — Hahn.), Ars. Cam. (preserve pain in head with coldness of body and unconsciousness after — Hahn.), Chi. (other chronic affections from abuse of Ver.— e.g., daily forenoon fever. — Hahn,)	Antidoted by (Contd.) Cof., Stp. (most cases — Teste). Poisoning doses; Strong Coffee.	Veratrum alb.

REMEDY	Complementary Remedies	Remedy Follows Well	Remedy is Followed Well by	Compatible Remedies
Veratrum n.				
Veratrum v.				
Verbascum			Bel., chi., Lyc., Pul., Rhs., Sep., Stm.	
Verbena hast.				
Vesicaria				Cac., Thl.
Vespa				
Viburnum op				
Viburnum pru.				
Viburnum ti.				
Vichy				
Vinca mi.				
Viola od.			Bel., cin., Crl., Nux, Pul.	Cina in helmin-thi-asis, Crl. in whooping-cough
Viola tri.			Pul., Rhs., Sep., Stp.	Pul., Rhs., Sep., Stp.
Vipera				
Viscum alb.				
Voeslau				
Wiesbaden				
Wildbad				
Wyethia				
Xanthoxylum				
Yohimbinum				
Yucca filam.				
Zea				
Zincum	Ca. p. in hy-drocephalus.	Aps., Bel.	Hep., Ign., Pul., Sep., Sul. (best — H.N.G.).	
Zincum ac.				

Incompatible Remedies	Remedy Antidotes	Remedy is Antidoted by	Duration of Action	REMEDY
				Veratrum n.
	Sty.	Hot Coffee.		Veratrum v.
		Cam	8–10 d.	Verbascum
	Rhs. poisoning			Verbena hast.
				Vesicaria
Ag. n.		Aps., Cam., Led., Salt-water, vinegar		Vespa
		Aco. (epididymitis), Ver. diarrhoea).		Viburnum op
	Gos.			Viburnum pru.
				Viburnum ti.
				Vichy
				Vinca mi.
	Used externally, stings and snake-bites.	Cam.	2–4 d.	Viola od.
		Cam., Merc., Pul., Rhs.	8–14 d.	Viola tri.
				Vipera
				Viscum alb.
				Voeslau
				Wiesbaden
				Wildbad
				Wyethia
				Xanthoxylum
				Yohimbinum
				Yucca filam.
				Zea
Cham., Nux., Wine.	Ba. c.	Cam., Hep., Ign., (Lobel.—Teste).	30–40 d.	Zincum
				Zincum ac.

REMEDY	Complementary Remedies	Remedy Follows Well	Remedy is Followed Well by	Compatible Remedies
Zincum br.				
Zincum cy.				
zincum iod.				
Zincum mur.				
Zincum phos.				
Zincum sulph				
Zincum val.				
Zingiber				
Zizia				

Incompatible Remedies	Remedy Antidotes	Remedy is Antidoted by	Duration of Action	REMEDY
				Zincum br.
				Zincum cy.
				zincum iod.
				Zincum mur.
				Zincum phos.
				Zincum sulph
				Zincum val.
	Cld. (asthma)	Nux.		Zingiber
		Cb. a.		Zizia

□□

Part V

REPERTORY OF
NATURAL RELATIONSHIPS

REPERTORY OF
NATURAL RELATIONSHIPS

NOTE

THE Homoeopathic Materia Medica consists potentially, we may say, of anything and everything that may be found in the universe. Man himself epitomises the universe, and nothing in the universe can therefore be said to be unrelated to him. It is his business to find out the indications for the uses of the substances at his command, and the methods in which they are to be prepared and applied. Some of them he has discovered, and the substances thus rescued from the unknown constitute the Homoeopathic Materia Medica as it is at present developed.

The following lists will show remedies belonging to the different kingdoms of nature arranged in the order of their natural kinship Readers will be able to discover how far natural relationship and clinical relationship correspond so far as the Homoeopathic Materia Medica at rpesent extends The lists will enable readers to find how almost any given remedy in the Materia Medica is related to any other remedy in nature The lists comprise—(1) Metals or Elements; (2) The Vegetable Kingdom; (3) The Animal Kingdom; (4) Sarcodes; (5) Nosodes.

1. Metals or Elements

An alphabetical list of the elements represented is given, each with its symbol and atomic weight. Prefixed to each name is a number. This number shows its position in the succeeding list, which gives the elements *in the order of their atomic weights*. In addition to this distinguishing number in the second list is affixed the letter "G" and a Roman numeral. This refers to a third list—a list of the Mendeleeffian Groups; and the numeral shows in which of these groups any given element is to be found.

2. Vegetable Kingdom

There are two lists given in this section—a list of natural orders in alphabetical order, and a list of natural orders in systematic or evolutionary order. In the first, or alphabetical list, under the name of each order, all the remedies of the order are given, also alphabetically. The alphabetical list is distinguished by numbers which correspond with the numbers of the systematic list, so that the place of any remedy in each list can be once be found.

Suppose, for example, that it were desired to find out all the relations of Belladonna in the Materia Medica. On consulting the *Dictionary* it would be found that Belladonna belongs to the *Solanacece* Looking up *Solanacece* in the alphabetical list, we find 20 other remedies belonging to the same order. Affixed to the name of the order we find the number "68". Turning to the systematic list, we find *Solanacece* bracketed with *Convolvulacece* (67), *Boraginacece* (66), and *Hydrophyllacece* (65) and followed by *Scrophulariacece* (69), &c Under each of these orders, in the alphabetical list, all their members will be found. Thus the relation of Belladonna to any or all of them may be traced.

3. Animal Kingdom

Of the animal kingdom a similar arrangement has been adopted—an alphabethical list distinguished by numbers corresponding to numbers in the succeeding systematic list In arranging the latter I have been governed mainly by Francis P Pascoe's "Zoological Classification." In the *Dictionary,* and the authorities on which it has relied, no very definite distinction between "Orders" and "Families" has been observed in describing the place or the various animals; but I do not think this will occasion any difficulty in tracing any animal remedy and its natural relations.

4. Sarcodes

I have found the term "Sarcodes" useful for designating the remedies prepared from healthy animal tissues and organs. They are "flesh" remedies, and   is Greek for "flesh " These are remedies of very great importance, and I have given a list of them, together with a supplementary list of remedies *derived* from *altered* tissues and secretions, as Urea and Uric acid from Urine, Thyro-iodin from Thyroid glands, &c.

5. Nosodes

Nosodes are remedies derived from morbid tissues and secretions containing the specific virus of diseases. A list of these remedies, the importance of which is becoming daily more recognized, concludes this section.

ELEMENTS

Alphabetical Lists

10	Aluminium	Al	27·10	9	Magnesium	Mg	24·36
36	(Antimonium)	Sb	120·20	20	(Manganum)	Mn	55·00
32	Argentum	Ag	107·93	45	Mercurius	Hg	200·00
26	Arsenicum	As	75·00	8	(Natrum)	Na	23·05
44	Aurum	Au	197·20	22	Niccolum	Ni	58·70
39	(Barium)	Ba	137·40	5	(Nitrogenium)	N	14·04
48	Bismuthum	Bi	208·50	41	Osmium	Os	191·00
3	(Boron)	B	11·00	6	Oxygenium	O	16·00
28	Bromium	Br	79·96	31	Palladium	Pd	106·50
33	(Cadmium)	Cd	112·40	12	Phosphorus	P	31·00
16	(Calcium)	Ca	40·10	43	Platinum	Pt	194·80
4	(Carbon)	C	12·00	47	Plumbum	Pb	206·90
40	(Cerium)	Ce	140·00	30	(Rhodium)	Rh	103·00
14	Chlorum	Cl	35·45	27	Selenium	Se	79·20
19	(Chromium)	Cr	52·10	11	(Silicon)	Si	28·4
23	Cobaltum	Co	59·00	35	Stannum	Sn	119·00
24	Cuprum	Cu	63·60	29	(Strontium)	Sr	87·60
21	Ferrum	Fe	55·90	13	Sulphur	S	32·06
7	(Fluorinum)	F	19·00	38	Tellurium	Te	127·60
1	(Hydrogenium)	H	1·008	46	Thallium	Tl	204·10
34	Indium	In	114·00	17	Titanium	Ti	48·10
37	Iodium	I	126·85	49	(Uranium)	U	238·50
42	Iridium	Ir	193·00	18	Vanadium	V	51·20
15	(Kali)	K	39·15	25	Zincum	Zn	65·40
2	(Lithium)	Li	7·03				

List in Order of Atomic Weights

1	G I	Hydrogenium	1·008	14	G VII	Chlorum	35·45
2	G I	Lithium	7·03	15	G I	Kali	39·15
3	G III	Boron	11·00	16	G II	Calcium	40·10
4	G IV	Carbon	12·00	17	G IV	Titanium	48·10
5	G V	Nitrogenium	14·04	18	G V	Vanadium	51·20
6	G VI	Oxygenium	16·00	19	G VI	Chromium	52·10
7	G VII	Fluorinum	19·00	20	G VII	Manganum	55·00
8	G I	Natrum	23·05	21	G VIII	Ferrum	55·90
9	G II	Magnesium	24·36	22	G VIII	Niccolum	58·70
10	G III	Aluminium	27·10	23	G VIII	Cobaltum	59·00
11	G IV	Silicon	28·40	24	G I	Cuprum	63·60
12	G V	Phosphorus	31·00	25	G II	Zincum	65·40
13	G VI	Sulphur	32·06	26	G V	Arsenicum	75·00

* The numerals prefixed to the names in this list show the place of each element in the list following, arranged in order of the atomic weights. The brackets signify that the element named is represented in the Materia Medica only by its salts.

† The letter "G. I," &c., refers to the list following, and show the group of elements to which the particular element belongs.

27	G VI	Selenium	79·20	39	G II	Barium	137·40
28	G VII	Bromium	79·96	40	G IV	Cerium	140·00
29	G II	Strontium	87·60	41	G VIII	Osmium	191·00
30	G VIII	Rhodium	103·00	42	G VIII	Iridium	193·00
31	G VIII	Palladium	106·50	43	G VIII	Platinum	194·80
32	G I	Argentum	107·93	44	G I	Aurum	197·20
33	G II	Cadmium	112·40	45	G II	Mercurius	200·30
34	G III	Indium	114·00	46	G III	Thallium	204·10
35	G IV	Stannum	119·00	47	G IV	Plumbum	206·90
36	G V	Antimonium	120·20	48	G V	Bismuthum	208·50
37	G VII	Iodium	126·85	49	G VI	Uranium	238·50
38	G VI	Tellurium	127·60				

Groups According to Mendeleeff

Group I

a { Lithium
Natrum
Kali

b { Hydrogenium
Cuprum
Argentum
Aurum

Group II

a { Magnesium
Calcium
Strontium
Barium

b { Zincum
Cadmium
Mercurius

Group III

a { Scandium
Yttrium

b { Boron
Aluminium
Indium
Thallium

Group IV

a { Titanium
Cerium

b { Carbon
Silicon
Stannum
Plumbum

Group V

a { Vanadium
Niobium

b { Nitrogenium
Phosphorus
Arsenicum
Antimonium
Bismuthum

Group VI

a { Chromium
Molybdenum
Tungsten
Uranium

b { Oxygenium
Sulphur
Selenium
Tellurium

Group VII

a Manganum

b { Fluorinum
Chlorum
Bromium
Iodium

Group VIII

Ferrum
Rubidium
Osmium
Cobaltum
Rhodium
Iridium
Niccolum
Palladium
Platinum

NATURAL BOTANICAL ORDERS

II Vegetable Kingdom*

1 ALPHABETICAL LIST OF NATURAL BOTANICAL ORDERS REPRESENTED IN THE MATERIA MEDICA*

Abietineae, *see* **Coniferae (114)**

Algae (119)
Fucus vesiculosus

Amaryllidaceae (101)
Agave Americana
Narcissus

Anacardiaceae (32)
Anacardium ocidentale
Anacardium orientale
Comocladia
Rhus aromatica
Rhus diversiloba
Rhus glabra
Rhus radicans

Rhus toxicodendron
Rhus venenata
Schinus

Andromedeae, *see*
Ericaceae, (56)
Anonaceae   (3)
Asimina triloba

Antirrhineae, *see*
Scrophulariaceae (70)

Apocynaceae (62)
Alstonia constricta.
Apocynum androsaemifolium
Apocynum cannabinum
Oleander
Quebracho

* The number affixed to each natural order shows the place of the order in the systematic arrangement given in the succeeding section

Strophanthus
Tanghinia
Thevetia
Vinca minor

Aquifoliaceae (*or***
Ilicaceae), (27)**
Ilex aquifolium
Prinos verticillatus

Araceae (110)
Arum dracontium
Arum dracunculus
Arum italicum
Arum maculatum
Arum triphyllum
Caladium

Arbuteae, *see* **Ericaceae
(56)**

Araliaceae (49)
Aralia racemosa
Ginseng
Hedera helix

Aristolochiaceae (79)
Aristolochia milhomens
Aristolochia serpentaria
Asarum europaeum

Asclepiadaceae (63)
Asclepias syriaca
Asclepias tuberosa

Calotropis
Cundurango
Gymnema sylvestre

Berberidaceae (05)
Berberis aquifolium
Berberis vulgaris
Caulophyllum
Podophyllum

Bignoniaceae (72)
Jacaranda Caroba
Jacaranda Gualandai

Boraginaceae (67)
Heliotropium
Myosotis
Onosmodium
Symphytum

Cactaceae (47)
Anhalonium lewinii
Cactus grandiflorus
Cereus bonplandii
Cereus serpentinus
Opuntia

Caesalpinieae, *see*
Leguminosae (34)

Camelliaceae, *see*
Ternstroemiaceae (17)

Campanulaceae (*including*

Lobeliaceae) (55)
Lobelia cardinalis
Lobelia dortmanna
Lobelia erinus
Lobelia inflata
Lobelia purpurascens
Lobelia syphilitica

Cannabinaceae (89)
Cannabis indica
Cannabis sativa
Lupulus

Caprifoliaceae (51), *sub-order* **Lonicereae**
Lonicera periclymenum
Lonicera xylosteum
Symphoricarpus racemosus
Triosteum

————, *sub-order* **Sambuceae**
Sambucus canadensis
Sambucus nigra
Viburnum opulus
Viburnum prunifolium
Viburnum tinus

Caryophyllaceae (14)
Agrostemma githago
Stellaria media

Celastraceae (28)
Euonymus atropurpurea
Euonymus europaea

Chenopodiaceae (76)
Chenopodium anthelminticum
Chenopodium vulvaria

Cichoriaceae, *see*
Composite (54)

Cinchonaceae, *see*
Rubiaceae (52)

Cistaceae (11)
Cistus Canadensis

Clematideae, *see*
Ranunculaceae (01)

Commelynaceae (108)
Tradescantia

Compositae (54)
Ambrosia artemisiaefolia
Calendula
Echinacea angustifolia
Echinacea purpurea
Erechthites
Grindelia
Guaco
Silphium
Wyethia

————, *sub-order* **Cichoriaceae**
Cichorium
Lactuca
Lapsana communis

Liatris spicata
Nabalus
Taraxacum

————, *sub-order* **Corymbiferae**
Abrotanum
Absinthium
Anthemis nobilis

Compositae (54), *sub-order*
corymbiferae *(continued)*
Arnica
Artemisia vulgaris
Bellis perennis
Brachglottis repens
Chamomilla
Cina
Cineraria maritima
Erigeron
Eupatorium aromaticum
Eupatorium perfoliatum
Eupatorium purpureum
Gnaphalium
Helianthus annuus
Inula
Millefolium
Parthenium hysterophorus
Pyrethrum parthenium
Senecio aureus
Senecio jacobaea
Solidago
Tanacetum
Tussilago farfara
Tussilago fragrans

Tussilago petasites

————, *sub-order*
Cynarocephalae
Arctium lappa
Carduus benedictus
Carduus marianus
Centaurea tagana

Coniferae (*or* **Pinaceae)**
(114), *Sub-order*
Cupressineae
Cupressus australis
Cupressus lawsoniana
Juniperus communis
Juniperus virginiana
Sabina
Thuja

————, *sub-order* **Taxeae**
Taxus baccata

————, *sub-order* **Abietineae**
Abies canadensis
Abies nigra
Pinus lambertiana
Pinus sylvestris
Terebinthina

Convolvulaceae (68)
Convolvulus arvensis
Convolvulus duratinus
Jalapa
Scammonium

Coriariaceae, (33)
Coriaria ruscifolia

Cornaceae (50)
Cornus alternifolia
Cornus circinata
Cornus florida

Corylaceae, *see*
Cupuliferae (94)

Corymbiferae, *see*
Compositae (54)

Crassulaceae (37)
Cotyledon
Penthorum sedoides
Sempervivum tectorum

Cruciferae (10)
Armoracea sativa
Brassica napus
Cheiranthus cheiri
Iberis
Lepidium bonariense
Matthiola graeca
Raphanus
Sinapis alba
Sinapis nigra
Thlaspi bursa pastoris
Vesicaria

Cucurbitaceae (46)
Bryonia

Colocynthis
Cucurbita pepo
Elaterium
Momordica

Cupressineae, *see*
Coniferae (114)

Cupuliferae (*or*
Corylaceae) (94)
Alnus
Castanea Vesca
Fagus
Ostrya
Quercus

Cynarocephalae, *see*
Compositae (54)

Dioscoreaceae (102)
Dioscrorea
Tamus

Droseraceae (38)
Drosera

Drupaceae, *see* **Rosaceae
(35)**

Equisetaceae (106)
Equisetum

Ericaceae (56)
Gaultheria

————, *tribe* **Arbuteae**

Arbutus andrachne

Uva ursi

————, *tribe* **Andromedeae**

Oxydendron

————, *tribe* **Rhodoreae**

Epigea repens

Kalmia latifolia

Ledum

Rhododendron

————, *tribe* **Pyroleae**

Chimaphila maculata

Chimaphila umbellata

Erythroxylaceae, *see*
Linaceae (20)

Eupatoriaceae, *included in*
Compositae (54)

Euphorbiaceae (86)

Acalypha indica

Cascarilla

Croton tiglium

Euphorbia amygdaloides

Euphorbia corollata

Euphorbia cyparissias

Euphorbia hetrodoxa

Euphorbia hypericifolia

Euphorbia ipecacuanhae

Euphorbia lathyris

Euphorbia peplus

Euphorbia pilulifera

Hura brasiliensis

Hura crepitans

Jatropha

Jatropha urens

Kamala

Mancinella

Mercurialis perennis

Ricinus

Stillingia sylvatica

Filices (117)

Filix mas

Fumariaceae (09)

Corydalis

Fungi (120)

Agaricus emeticus

Agaricus muscarius

Agaricus phalloides

Boletus laricis

Boletus luridus

Bovista

Phallus impudicus

Polyporus pinicola

Russala

Secale cornutum (Claviceps purpurea)

Ustilago (*on* Zea Mays)

Galiaceae, *see* **Rubiacae (52)**

Gentianaceae (65)
Canchalagua
Gentiana cruciata
Gentiana lutea
Gentiana quinqueflora
Menyanthes

Geraniaceae (22)
Erodium
Geranium maculatum
Pelargonium reniforme

Gnetaceae (115)
Ephedra Vulgaris

Graminaceae (113)
Anantherum
Arundo mauritanica
Avena sativa
Lolium temulentum
Triticum repens

————, *tribe* **Phalarideae**
Anthoxanthum
Zea

Guttiferae (*or* Clusiaceae) (16)
Gambogia

Haemodoraceae (99)
Aletris Farinosa
Lachnanthes

Hamamelidaceae (39)
Hamamelis

Helloboreae, *see* Ranunculaceae (01)

Hydrangeaceae, *see* Saxifragaceae (36)

Hydrophyllaceae (66)
Eriodictyon glutinosum
Hydrophyllum virginianum

Hypericaceae (15)
Hypericum

Ilicaceae, *see* Aquifoliaceae (27)

Iridaceae (100)
Crocus
Homeria
Iris florentina
Iris fcetidissima
Iris germanica
Iris tenax
Iris versicolor

Jasminaceae (61)
Jasminum
Nyctanthes

Juglandaceae (95)
Carya alba

Juglans cinerea
Juglans regia

Juncaceae (107)

Juncus

Labiatae (74)

Collinsonia canadensis
Hedeoma
Lamium
Leonurus cardiaca
Lycopus
Mentha pulegium
Ocimum canum
Origanum
Plectranthus
Rosmarinus
Salvia
Scutellaria
Stachys betonica
Teucrium marum
Teucrium scorodonia

Lauraceae (82)

Benzoin
Camphora
Cinnamomum
Coto bark
Oreodaphne

Leguminosae (34)

Derris Pinnata

Leguminosae (34), *sub-*

order **Papilionaceae**

Astragalus menziesii
Balsamum peruvianum
Baptisia confusa acetica
Baptisia tinctoria
Dolichos
Galega
Genista
Hedysarum ildefonisanum
Indigo
Jequirity
Kino
Laburnum
Lathyrus
Melilotus
Mucuna urens
Ononis
Oxytropis lamberti
Phaseolus
Physostigma
Robinia
Trifolium pratense
Trifolium repens

————, *sub-order* **Caesalpinieae**

Copaiva
Gymnocladus Canadensis
Haematoxylon
Senna
Tongo

————, *sub-order* **Mimoseae**

Mimosa

Lemnaceae (or Pistiaceae) (112)
Lemna minor

Lichenes (121)
Cetracia islandica
Sticta pulmonaria
Usnea barbata

Liliaceae (103)
Agraphis nutans
Allium cepa
Allium sativum
Aloe
Asparagus
Convallaria
Lilium tigrinum
Ornithogalum
Scilla maritima
See also **Melanthaceae (00)**, **Smilaceae (00)**, and **Trilliaceae (00)**

Linaceae (including Erythroxylaceae) (105)
Linum cathrticum
Linum usitatissimum
Coca

Lobeliaceae, see
Campanulaceae (55)

Loganiaceae (64)
Brucea antidysenterica

Curare
Gelsemium
Hoang-nan
Ignatia
Nux vomica
Spigelia anthelmia
Spigelia marilandica
Upas

Lonicereae, see
Caprifoliaceae (51)

Loranthaceae (84)
Viscum Album

Lycopodiaceae (118)
Lycopodium

Lythraceae (42)
Cuphea Viscosissma

Magnoliaceae (02)
Illicium anisatum
Magnolia glauca
Magnolia grandiflora

Malvaceae (18)
Gossypium herbaceum

Melanthaceae (105)
Colchicum
Helonias
Sabadilla
Veratrum album

Veratrum nigrum
Veratrum viride
Yucca filamentosa

Melastomaceae (41)
Melastoma

Meliaceae (26)
Azadirachta indica
Guarea

Menispermaceae (04)
Cocculus
Menispermum
Pareira

Mimoseae, *see*
Leguminosae (34)

Moraceae (88)
Ficus religiosa

Musaceae (98)
Musa

Myricaceae (92)
Myrica cerifera

Myristicaceae (81)
Myristica sebifera
Nux moschata

Myrsinaceae (59)

Karaka

Myrtaceae (40)
Angophora
Cajuputum
Eucalyptus
Eugenia jambos
Granatum
Myrtus communis
Syzygium

Nymphaeaceae (06)
Nuphar luteum
Nymphaea odorata

Oleaceae (60)
Chionanthus virginica
Fraxinus americana

Onagraceae (43)
Epilobium palustre
Oenothera

Orchidaceae (96)
Cypripedium
Spiranthes

Orobanchaceae (71)
Epiphegus

Orontiaceae (111)
Ictodes Foetida

Paeoneae, *see*

Ranunculaceae (01)

Palmaceae (109)
Areca
Elaeis guineensis
Musa, see **Musaceae**
Sabal serrulata

Papaveraceae (08)
Chelidonium
Opium
Sanguinaria

Papilionaceae, *see*
Leguminosae (34)

Passifloraceae (45)
Passiflora

Phalarideae, *see*
Graminaceae (113)

Phytolaccaceae (77)
Petiveria
Phytolacca

Pinaceae, *see* **Coniferae
(114)**

Piperaceae (80)
Cubeba
Piper methysticum
Piper nigrum

Pistiaceae, *see*
Lemnaceae

Plantaginaceae (75)
Plantago

Platanaceae (91)
Platanus

Plumbaginaceae (57)
Plumbago

Polygalaceae (13)
Senega

Polygonaceae (78)
Fagopyrum
Lapathum
Polygonum
Ratanhia
Rheum
Rumex acetosa
Rumex crispus

Pomeae, *see* **Rosaceae
(35)**

Primulaceae (58)
Anagallis arvensis
Cyclamen
Primula obconica
Primula veris
Primula vulgaris

Pseudo-solaneae, *see*
Scrophulariaceae (70)

Pyroleae, *see* **Ericaceae**

Ranunculaceae, *tribe*
Clematideae (01)
Clematis erecta

Ranunculaceae, *tribe*
Anemoneae
Adonis
Hepatica
Hydrastis
Pulsatilla
Pulsatilla nuttalliana

————, *tribe* **Ranunculeae**
Ranunculus acris
Ranunculus bulbosus
Ranunculus ficaria
Ranunculus flammula
Ranunculus glacialis
Ranunculus repens
Ranunculus sceleratus

————, *tribe* **Helleboreae**
Aconitum cammarum
Aconitum ferox
Aconitum lycoctonum
Aconitum napellus
Actaea racemosa
Actaea spicata
Aquilegia vulgaris

Caltha palustris
Helleborus fcetidus
Helleborus niger
Helleborus orentalis
Helleborus viridis
Staphisagria

————, *tribe* **Paeoneae**
Paeonia

Ranunculeae, *see*
Ranunculaceae (01)

Rhamnaceae (29)
Cascara sagrada
Ceanothus americanus
Rhamnus catharticus
Rhamnus frangula

Rhinantheae *see*
Scrophulariaceae (70)

Rhodoreae, *see*
Ericaceae (56)

Rosaceae (35), *sub-order*
Drupaceae
Amygdalae amarae aqua
Laurocerasus
Persica
Prunus padus
Prunus spinosa
Prunus virginiana

———, *sub-order* **Pomeae**
Crataegus oxyacantha
Pyrus americana

———, *sub-order* **Rosea**
Fragaria vesca
Geum rivale
Kouss
Rosa canina
Rosa damascena
Spiraea ulmaria

Roseae, *see* **Rosaceae (35)**

Rubiaceae (52)
Cainca
Coffea cruda
Coffea tosta
Mitchella

———, *sub-order* **Cinchonaceae**
China boliviana
China officinalis
Ipecacuanha

———, *sub-order* **Galiaceae** (*or* **Stellatae**)
Galium
Rubia tinctorum

Rutaceae (24)
Angustura vera
Aurantium

Barosma
Citrus limonum
Dictamnus
Jaborandi
Ruta

———, *sub-order*
Xanthoxylaceae
Ptelea
Xanthoxylum

Salicaceae (93)
Populus candicans
Populus tremuloides
Salix mollissima
Salix nigra
Salix purpurea

Sambuceae, *see*
Caprifoliaceae (51)

Santalaceae (85)
Santalum

Sapindaceae (31)
Aesculus glabra
Aesculus hippocastanum
Guarana
Paullinia pinnata

Sarraceniaceae (07)
Sarracenia

Saxifragaceae (*including*

Hydrangeaceae) (36)
Hydrangea arborescens

Scrophulariaceae (70),
sub-order **Pseudo-solaneae**
Franciscea uniflora

————, *sub-order* **Antirrhineae**
Digitalis
Gratiola
Leptandra
Linaria
Scrophularia
Verbascum

————, *sub-order* **Rhinantheae**
Chelone
Euphrasia

Simarubaceae (25)
Ailanthus glandulosa
Cedron
Chaparro amargoso
Quassia

Smilaceae (104)
Sarsaparilla

Solanaceae (69)
Belladonna
Capsicum
Datura arborea
Datura ferox

Datura metel
Duboisinum
Dulcamara
Hyoscyamus
Lycopersicum
Mandragora
Pichi
Solanum arrebenta
Solanum carolinense
Solanum mammosum
Solanum nigrum
Solanum oleraceum
Solanum pseudo-capsicum
Solanum tuberosum
Solanum tuberosum aegrotans
Stramonium
Tabacum

Taxeae, *see* **Coniferae (114)**

Ternstroemiaceae (*or*** Camelliaceae) (117)**
Thea

Thymelaceae (83)
Daphne indica
Dirca palustris
Mezereum

Tiliaceae (19)
Tilia

Trilliaceae (106)
Paris
Trillium

Tropaeolaceae (23)
Tropaeolum

Turneraceae (44)
Turnera aphrodisiaca

Ulmaceae (*of the* Urticales) (90)
Ulmus Fulva

Umbelliferae (48)
Aethusa
Ammoniacum
Apium graveolens
Asafoetida
Athamanta
Cicuta maculata
Cicuta virosa
Conium maculatum
Eryngium aquaticum
Eryngium maritimum
Ferula glauca
Heracleum
Hydrocotyle asiatica
Imperatoria
Oenanthe crocata
Pastinaca
Petroselinum
Phellandrium
Pimpinella

Sium
Sumbul
Zizia

Urticaceae (87)
Parietaria
Urtica urens

Valerianaceae (53)
Valeriana

Verbenaceae (73)
Agnus castus
Lippia mexicana
Verbena hastata

Violaceae (12)
(An order most members of which contain Emetin)
Viola odorata
Viola tricolor

Vitaceae (30)
Ampelopsis

Xanthoxylaceae, *see* Rutaceae (24)

Zingiberaceae (97)
Zingiber

Zygophyllaceae (21)
Guaiacum

NATURAL BOTANICAL ORDERS

II Vegetable Kingdom

2 LIST OF NATURAL BOTANICAL ORDERS REPRESENTED IN THE MATERIA MEDICA IN SYSTEMATIC ARRANGEMENT

Division 1—**PHANEROGAMIA.**
Sub-division 1—**Angiospermia.**
Class 1—DICOTYLEDONES.
Sub-class 1—Polypetalae.

Series 1—*Thalamiflorce.*

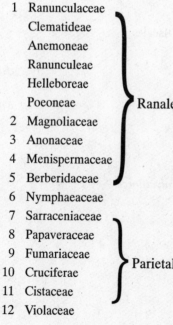

1 Ranunculaceae
  Clematideae
  Anemoneae
  Ranunculeae
  Helleboreae
  Poeoneae } Ranales
2 Magnoliaceae
3 Anonaceae
4 Menispermaceae
5 Berberidaceae
6 Nymphaeaceae
7 Sarraceniaceae
8 Papaveraceae
9 Fumariaceae } Parietales
10 Cruciferae
11 Cistaceae
12 Violaceae

13 Polygalaceae Polygalineae
14 Caryophyllaceae Caryophyllineae
15 Hypericaceae
16 Guttiferae (or Clusiaceae)   } Guttiferales
17 Ternstroemiaceae (or Camelliaceae)
18 Malvaceae
19 Tiliaceae   } Malvales

Series 2—Disciflorce.

20 Linaceae (including Erythroxylaceae)
21 Zygophyllaceae
22 Geraniaceae
23 Tropceolaceae
24 Rutaceae   } Geraniales
     Xanthoxylaceae
25 Simarubaceae
26 Meliaceae
27 Aquifoliaceae (or Ilicaceae) Olacales
28 Celastraceae
29 Rhamnaceae   } Celastrales
30 Vitaceae
31 Sapindaceae
32 Anacardiaceae   } Sapindales
33 Coriariaceae

Series 3—Calyciflorce

34 Laguminosae
     Papilionaceae
     Caesalpinieae
     Mimoseae   } Rosales
35 Rosaceae
     Drupaceae
     Pomeae

Roseae

36 Saxifragaceae (including Hydrangeaceae)

37 Crassulaceae   } Rosales

38 Droseraceae

39 Hamamelidaceae

40 Myrtaceae

41 Melastomaceae

42 Lythraceae   } Myrtales

43 Onagraceae

44 Turneraceae

45 Passifloraceae   } Passiflorales

46 Cucurbitaceae

47 Cactaceae.   Ficoidales

48 Umbelliferae

49 Araliaceae   } Umbellales

50 Cornaceae

SUB-CLASS 2—GAMOPETALAE (OR COROLLIFLORAE)
Series 1—Inferce (or Epigynce)

51 Caprifoliaceae

Lonicereae

Sambuceae

52 Rubiaceae   } Rubiales

Cinchonaceae

Galiaceae (or Stellatae)

53 Valerianaceae

54 Compositae

Cichoriaceae   } Asterales

Corymbiferae

Cynarocephalae

55 Campanulaceae (including Lobeliaceae) Campanales

Series 2—Superce (or Heteromerce)

56 Ericaceae } Ericales

Arbuteae
Andromedeae
Rhodoreae
Pyroleae
} Ericales

57　Plumbaginaceae
58　Primulaceae 　} Primulales
59　Myrsinaceae

Series 3—Dicarpice (or *Bicarpellatce*)

60　Oleaceae
61　Jasminaceae
62　Apocynaceae
63　Asclepiadaceae　} Gentianales
64　Loganiaceae
65　Gentianaceae

66　Hydrophyllaceae
67　Boraginaceae
68　convolvulaceae　} Ploemoniales
69　Solanaceae

70　Scrophulariaceae
　　Pseudo-solaneae
　　Antirrhineae
　　Rhinantheae　} Personales
71　Orobanchaceae
72　Bignoniaceae

73　Verbenaceae
74　Labiatae 　} Labiales
75　Plantaginaceae

SUB-CLASS 3—MONOCHLAMYDEAE (or INCOMPLETAE)
Series 1—Curvembryece

76　Chenopodiaceae } Chenopodiales

77 Phytolaccaceae
78 Polygonaceae } Chenopodiales

79 Aristolochiaceae Asarales
80 Piperaceae Piperales

81 Myristicaceae
82 Lauraceae } Laurales

83 Thymelaceae Daphnales

84 Loranthaceae
85 Santalaceae } Santalales

86 Euphorbiaceae Euphorbiales

87 Urticaceae
88 Moraceae
89 Cannabinaceae } Urticales
90 Ulmaceae

91 Platanaceae
92 Myricaceae } Platanales
93 Salicaceae

94 Cupuliferae (*or* Corylaceae)
95 Juglandaceae } Quernales

Class 2—MONOCOTYLEDONES.

96 Orchidaceae Orchidales

97 Zingiberaceae
98 Musaceae } Amomales

99 Haemodoraceae
100 Iridaceae } Narcissales
101 Amaryllidaceae

102 Dioscoreaceae Dioscorales

Division 2

103 Liliaceae
104 Smilaceae } Liliales
105 Melanthaceae

106 Trilliaceae ⎫
107 Juncaceae ⎬ Liliales
108 Commelynaceae Commelynales
109 Palmaceae Palmales
110 Araceae ⎫
111 Orontiaceae ⎬ Arales
112 Lemnaceae
113 Graminaceae
        Phalarideae

Sub-division 2—**Gymnospermia**

114 Coniferae (or Pinaceae)
        Cupressineae
        Taxeae
        Abietineae
115 Gnetaceae

Division 2—**CRYPTOGAMIA**

116 Equisetaceae
117 Filices
118 Lycopodiaceae
119 Algae
120 Fungi
121 Lichenes

NATURAL ZOOLOGICAL ORDERS

III Animal Kingdom
1 ALPHABETICAL LIST OF NATURAL ORDERS*

Acaridea (*Class* Arachnida)
Trombidium

Araneidea (*Class* Arachnida)
Aranea diadema
Aranea scinencia
Latrodectus Katipo
Latrodectus mactans
Mygale
Tarentula cubensis
Tarentula (hispanica)
Theridion

Asteroidea (*or* Radiata)
Asterias rubens

Bufonidae (*Class* Batrachia *or* Amphibia)
Bufo

Carnivora
Mephitis

Cephalopoda
(Sepia)

Chilopoda (*Class* Myriapoda)
Scolopendra

Coleoptera (*Class* Insecta)
Cantharis
Coccinella septempunctata
Doryphora decemlineata

Crotalidae
Bothrops lanceolatus

* The number refer to the place of the order in the Systematic List of Orders of the Animal Kingdom following.

Crotalus cascavella
Crotalus horridus

Decapoda (*Class*
Crustacea, *of the*
Articulata)
Astacus fluviatilis
Homarus

Diptera (*Class* **Insecta)**
Culex musca

Elapidae
Elaps
Naja

Erythrineae (*Class*
Pisces)
Erythrinus

Fibrospongiae (*Class*
Spongiae)
· Badiaga (Spongilla fluviatilis)
Spongia

Gadidae (*Class* **Pisces)**
(Gadus morrhua)
(Oleum jecoris aselli)

Gasteropoda
(Helix tosta)
Murex

Gorgoniaceae

Corallium rubrum

Helodermidae
Heloderma

Hemiptera (*Class* **Insecta)**
Aphis chenopodii glauci
Cimex
Coccus cacti
Pediculus

Hirudinea
Sanguisuga

Hymenoptera (*Class*
Insecta)
Apis
Formica
Vespa

Insecta, *see under the Orders*
of the Class

Isopoda (*Class* **Crustacea,**
of the **Articulata)**
Oniscus

Lacertilia
Amphisbaena
Lacerta

Lamellibranchiata
(Calcarea ostrearum)
Pecten

Lepidoptera (*Class*** Insecta)**
Bombyx processionea

Mammalia (*Class***),** *see* **Carnivora, Rodentia,** *and* **Ruminantia**

Merostomata (*or*** Poecilopoda,** *of the* **Crustacea)**
Limulus

Ophidia, *see* **Crotalidae, Elapidae,** *and* **Viperidae**

Orthoptera (*Class*** Insecta)**
Blatta americana
Blatta orientalis

Physophorae
Physalia

Radiata (*more recently named*** Asteroidea)**
Asterias rubens

Rodentia
(Castoreum)
(Sphingurus)

Ruminantia
(Cervus)

(Fel tauri)
(Moschus)

Scorpiodea (*Class*** Arachnida)**
Scorpia

Spongiae (*Class***),** *see* **Fibrospongiae**

Trachinidae
Trachinus

Viperidae
Cenchris contortrix
Lachesis
Toxicophis
Vipera

NATURAL ZOOLOGICAL ORDERS

III Vegetable Kingdom (*Continued*)
NATURAL ZOOLOGICAL ORDERS IN SYSTEMATIC ARRANGEMENT

Sub-Kingdom 1—Protozoa.
(Not represented).

Sub-Kingdom 2—Coelenterata

Class—SPONGIAE	*Class*—HYDROZOA	*Class*—ACTINOZOA
1 Fibrospongiae	2 Physophorae	3 Gorgoniaceae

Sub-Kingdom 3—Echinodermata
4 Asteroidea (*or* Radiata)

Sub-Kingdom 4—Vermes
Class—ANNELIDA
5 Hirudinea

Sub-kingdom 5—**Articulata,** *section* **Arthropoda**

Class—INSECTA
6 Coleoptera
7 Diptera
8 Hemiptera
9 Hymenoptera
10 Lepidoptera
11 Orthoptera

Class—MYRIAPODA
12 Chilopoda

Class—CRUSTACEA
13 Isopoda
14 Merostomata (*or*
 Poecilopoda)
15 Decapoda

Class—ARACHNIDA
16 Acaridea
17 Araneidea
18 Scorpiodia

Sub-kingdom 6—**Mollusca**

19 Cephalopoda   20 Gasteropoda   21 Lamellibranchiata

Sub-Kingdom 7—**Vertebrata**

i PISCES
  22 Erythrineae
  23 Gadidae
  24 Trachinidae

ii BATRACHIA (or AMPHIBIA)
  25 Bufonidae

iii REPTILIA
a Ophidia
  26 Crotalidae

27 Elapidae
28 Viperidae
b Sauria
  29 Lacertilia
  30 Helodermidae

iv MAMMALIA
  31 Carnivora
  32 Rodentia
  33 Ruminantia

IV. SARCODES

Adrenalinum
Aranearum tela
Calcarea carbonica (ostrearum)
Calcarea ovi testae
Carbo animalis
Castor equi
Cervus
Colostrum
Conchiolinum
Fel tauri
Gadrus morrhua
Helix tosta
Hippomanes
Lac caninum
Lac felinum
Lac vaccinum
Oleum jecoris aselli
Oophorinum
Orchitinum
Ovi gallinae pellicula
Ovi gallinae testa, see Calcarea
ovi testae
Pulmo vulpis
Sphingurus
Thyroidinum
Urinum

SARCODE-DERIVATIVES †

Cholesterinum
Lac vaccinum coagulatum
Lac vaccinum defloratum
Lacticum acidum
Lactis vaccini flos
Pancreatinum
Pepsinum
Pyrogenium (or Sepsinum)
Saccharum lactis
Thyroiodinum
Urea
Uricum acidum

* This list contains remedies made from preparations of healthy animal tissues and secretions Preparations of poisonous animals (Homarus, Sanguisuga Erythrinum, &c) are not included under this head.
† Preparations *derived from* healthy animal tissues and secretions are included under this head.